Spine Oncology

Guest Editors

RAKESH DONTHINENI, MD, MBA

ONDER OFLUOGLU, MD

ORTHOPEDIC CLINICS OF NORTH AMERICA

www.orthopedic.theclinics.com

January 2009 • Volume 40 • Number 1

SAUNDERS an imprint of ELSEVIER, Inc.

W.B. SAUNDERS COMPANY
A Division of Elsevier Inc.

1600 John F. Kennedy Blvd. ● Suite 1800 ● Philadelphia, PA 19103-2899.

http://www.orthopedic.theclinics.com

ORTHOPEDIC CLINICS OF NORTH AMERICA Volume 40, Number 1
January 2009 ISSN 0030-5898, ISBN-10: 1-4377-0514-6, ISBN-13: 978-1-4377-0514-0

Editor: Debora Dellapena

Orthopedic Clinics of North America (ISSN 0030-5898) is published quarterly (For Post Office use only: Volume 40 issue 1 of 4) by Elsevier Inc., 360 Park Avenue South, New York, NY 10010-1710. Months of publication are January, April, July, and October. Business and Editorial Offices: 1600 John F. Kennedy Blvd., Suite 1800, Philadelphia, PA 19103-2899. Customer Service Office: 6277 Sea Harbor Drive, Orlando, FL 33887-4800. Periodicals postage paid at New York, NY and additional mailing offices. Subscription prices are $244.00 per year for (US individuals), $424.00 per year for (US institutions), $288.00 per year (Canadian individuals), $508.00 per year (Canadian institutions), $355.00 per year (international individuals), $508.00 per year (international institutions), $122.00 per year (US students), $177.00 per year (Canadian and international students). Foreign air speed delivery is included in all *Clinics* subscription prices. All prices are subject to change without notice. **POSTMASTER:** Send address changes to *Orthopedic Clinics of North America*, Elsevier Periodicals Customer Service, 11830 Westline Industrial Drive, St. Louis, MO 63146. Customer Service (orders, claims, online, change of address): Elsevier Periodicals Customer Service, 11830 Westline Industrial Drive, St. Louis, MO 63146. Tel: 1-800-654-2452 (U.S. and Canada); 314-453-7041 (outside U.S. and Canada). Fax: 314-453-5170. E-mail: journalscustomerservice-usa@elsevier.com (for print support); journalsonlinesupport-usa@elsevier.com (for online support).

Reprints. For copies of 100 or more, of articles in this publication, please contact the Commercial Reprints Department, Elsevier Inc., 360 Park Avenue South, New York, NY 10010-1710. Tel.: 212-633-3812; Fax: 212-462-1935; Email: reprints@elsevier.com.

Orthopedic Clinics of North America is covered in MEDLINE/PubMed (Index Medicus), Cinahl, Excerpta Medica, and Cumulative Index to Nursing and Allied Health Literature.

Printed and bound by CPI Group (UK) Ltd, Croydon, CR0 4YY
Transferred to Digital Print 2011

Contributors

GUEST EDITORS

RAKESH DONTHINENI, MD, MBA
Associate Clinical Professor, Department of Orthopaedics, University of California Davis, Sacramento; Spine and Orthopaedic Oncology, Oakland; Alta Bates Summit Medical Center, Berkeley, California

ONDER OFLUOGLU, MD
Vice Chairman, Department of Orthopedics, Lutfi Kırdar Research Hospital, Istanbul, Turkey

AUTHORS

YASUMITSU AJIRO, MD
Assistant Professor, Department of Orthopaedic Surgery, Nihon University School of Medicine, Tokyo, Japan

TODD ALAMIN, MD
Assistant Professor, Stanford University, Department of Orthopaedic Surgery, Spinal Surgery Section, Stanford University School of Medicine, Stanford, California

L. AMENDOLA, MD
Rizzoli Institute; Department of Orthopaedics and Traumatology — Spine Surgery Maggiore 'C.A. Pizzardi', Bologna, Italy

LAURENT BALABAUD, MD
Institut Mutualiste Montsouris, Paris, France

STEFANO BANDIERA, MD
Department of Orthopaedics and Traumatology — Spine Surgery Maggiore Hospital 'C.A. Pizzardi', Bologna, Italy

S. BENNIS, MD
Institut Mutualiste Montsouris, Paris, France

STEFANO BORIANI, MD
Department of Orthopaedics and Traumatology — Spine Surgery Maggiore Hospital 'C.A. Pizzardi'; Professor, Rizzoli Institute of Orthopaedics and Traumatology, Bologna, Italy

ISTVAN BORS, MD
National Center for Spinal Disorders, Buda Health Center, Budapest, Hungary

MICHELE CAPPUCCIO, MD
Department of Orthopaedics and Traumatology — Spine Surgery Maggiore Hospital 'C.A. Pizzardi', Bologna, Italy

SATORU DEMURA, MD
Assistant Professor, Department of Orthopedic Surgery, School of Medicine, Kanazawa University, Takaramachi, Kanazawa, Japan

RAKESH DONTHINENI, MD, MBA
Associate Clinical Professor, Department of Orthopaedics, University of California Davis, Sacramento; Spine and Orthopaedic Oncology, Oakland; Alta Bates Summit Medical Center, Berkeley, California

ALESSANDRO GASBARRINI, MD
Department of Orthopaedics and Traumatology — Spine Surgery Maggiore Hospital 'C.A. Pizzardi', Bologna; Professor, Catholic University of Orthopaedics and Traumatology, Rome, Italy

ZIYA L. GOKASLAN, MD
Professor of Neurosurgery, Oncology,
Orthopaedic Surgery; Vice Chairman,
Department of Neurosurgery, Johns Hopkins
University, Baltimore, Maryland

S. HANSEN, MD
Institut Mutualiste Montsouris, Paris, France

JÜRGEN HARMS, MD
Professor; Chairman of the Department
of Orthopaedics and Spine Surgery,
Klinikum Karlsbad-Langensteinbach,
Karlsbad-Langensteinbach, Germany

NORIO KAWAHARA, MD
Associate Professor, Department of
Orthopedic Surgery, School of Medicine,
Kanazawa University, Kanazawa, Japan

ARON LAZARY, MD
National Center for Spinal Disorders, Buda
Health Center; 1st Department of Internal
Medicine, Semmelweis University, Budapest,
Hungary

ROBERT MAYLE, MD
Stanford University Department of
Orthopaedic Surgery, Stanford University
School of Medicine, Edwards Building,
Stanford, California

CHRISTIAN MAZEL, MD
Professor and Chairman, Institut Mutualiste
Montsouris, Paris, France

ROBERT P. MELCHER, MD
Oberarzt, Department of Orthopaedics
and Spine Surgery, Klinikum
Karlsbad-Langensteinbach,
Karlsbad-Langensteinbach, Germany

HIDEKI MURAKAMI, MD
Assistant Professor, Department of Orthopedic
Surgery, School of Medicine, Kanazawa
University, Kanazawa, Japan

TRANG NGUYEN, BS
Department of Neurosurgery, Johns Hopkins
University, Baltimore, Maryland

ONDER OFLUOGLU, MD
Vice Chairman, Department of Orthopedics,
Lutfi Kırdar Research Hospital, Istanbul,
Turkey

MASASHI OSHIMA, MD
Assistant Professor, Department of
Orthopaedic Surgery, Nihon University School
of Medicine, Tokyo, Japan

GERALD ROSEN, MD
Director, Cancer Center, St Vincent's Hospital,
New York, New York

DANIEL M. SCIUBBA, MD
Chief Resident in Neurological Surgery,
Department of Neurosurgery, Johns Hopkins
University, Baltimore, Maryland

NARAYAN SUNDARESAN, MD
Clinical Professor of Neurosurgery, Mount
Sinai Medical School, New York, New York

PATRICK S. SWIFT, MD
Medical Director, Radiation Oncology, Alta
Bates Comprehensive Cancer Center,
Berkeley, California

YASUAKI TOKUHASHI, MD
Associate Professor, Department of
Orthopaedic Surgery, Nihon University School
of Medicine, Tokyo, Japan

KATSURO TOMITA, MD
Professor and Chairman, Department of
Orthopedic Surgery, Graduate School of
Medical Science, Kanazawa University,
Kanazawa, Japan

PETER PAUL VARGA, MD
National Center for Spinal Disorders, Buda
Health Center, Budapest, Hungary

Contents

> Persistent axial pain with or without neurologic changes should prompt workup for a possible tumor of the spine. Metastatic disease is more predominant than primary tumors, but still needs adequate evaluation before any management. The various steps of evaluation, diagnosis, and staging are reviewed.

> In the treatment of primary tumors, complete local eradication is the main goal, as an oncologically appropriate surgical treatment can substantially improve the prognosis and even be considered a life-saving procedure. In deciding the best treatment for primary bone tumors of the spine, the choice of surgery, radiation therapy, chemotherapy, selective arterial embolization, or other medical treatments alone or in combination is based on diagnosis, staging, and a deep understanding of the biology and the behavior of each tumor. This article is a guide to diagnosing and treating such rare tumors.

> Primary malignant tumors of the spine account for less than 5% of primary bone tumors. Data from the SEER program suggest that the most common bone sarcomas are osteosarcoma, chondrosarcoma, Ewing's sarcoma, chordoma, and malignant fibrous histiocytoma/fibrosarcoma. During the last two decades, tremendous progress has been made in clinical aspects, surgical approaches, and reconstruction with instrumentation at all levels of the spine. Stabilization procedures, including vertebroplasty and kyphoplasty, have further allowed palliation of pain and symptom relief from compression fractures. Improved radiation techniques have offered the potential for improved local control. This article reviews the changes in surgical philosophy in the management of malignant spinal tumors during the past two decades.

> Metastatic spine tumors cause the loss of the supporting function of the spine through vertebral destruction or invade and compress the spinal cord or cauda

equine. As a result, metastatic spine tumor causes severe pain, paralysis, or impairment of activities of daily living (ADL). Also, because the finding of metastatic foci in the spine suggests a generalized disorder, life expectancy and treatment options have many limitations. For this reason, treatment is primarily symptomatic, and the major goals in selecting therapeutic modalities are to relieve pain, prevent paralysis, and improve ADL. This article discusses the selection of treatment for metastatic spine tumors and, in particular, the indications for surgical treatment.

The authors' group has developed a new surgical technique of spondylectomy (vertebrectomy) called "total en bloc spondylectomy" (TES). This technique is different from spondylectomy in that it involves en bloc removal of the lesion, that is, removal of the whole vertebra, body and lamina, as one compartment. The surgical technique of TES has been remarkably improved based on adequate knowledge and consideration of the surgical anatomy, physiology, and biomechanics of the spine and spinal cord. Review of the developmental process of this operation leads to recognition of the tips, pitfalls, and solutions.

We initially review the general biomechanical principles that should be considered in surgical reconstruction of spinal tumors. This will be further clarified by more detailed descriptions for individual spinal regions in the subsequent part of the article. In the case of patients with spinal metastases, especially in patients with a median survival time less than a few months, a thorough review of the risks and benefits regarding surgical intervention must be discussed with the patient. However, once the decision for surgery has been made, a biomechanically sound reconstruction should be performed to help restore or maintain the patient's mobility.

Since the first pioneering work in the area of tumors of the spine, medical professionals have sought to determine the proper role of spine surgery in the management of spinal tumors. Experience has proven that spine surgery is effective in the treatment of spinal cord compression for decreasing pain and improving quality of life with low rates of surgical complications. We use several staging systems to assess the patient's prognosis, to determine the best type of tumoral resection in preoperative surgical planning, and to provide guidance as to the best therapeutic option for the patient. In the surgical treatment of spine tumors, one of two opposing strategies must be chosen: (1) palliative surgery with cord decompression and spine stabilization or (2) curative surgery with en bloc radical resection of the tumor and stabilization. In this article, we describe indications and surgical techniques related to cervical spinal tumors: fixation and laminectomy of the upper and lower cervical spines, corporectomy, and partial and total vertebrectomy. For tumors of the cervicothoracic region, the most frequent level of spine metastasis and thoracic spine tumors, we describe the fixation and laminectomy technique, en bloc tumor resection, and partial and total vertebrectomy. The last part of the article addresses outcomes following spinal surgery, including outcomes related to en bloc Pancoast Tobias tumor resection, malignant dumbbell schwanomas, and metastasis.

Lumbar Tumor Resections and Management   93

Todd Alamin and Robert Mayle

More than one-third of patients with cancer have vertebral metastases found at autopsy. Primary and metastatic tumors to the spinal column can lead to pain, instability, and neurologic deficit. Symptomatic lesions are most prevalent in the thoracic spine (70%), followed by the lumbar spine (20%) and cervical spine (10%). Lesions in larger vertebral bodies tend to be asymptomatic given the increased ratio between the diameter of the spinal canal and the traversing nerve roots.

Sacral Tumors and Management   105

Peter Paul Varga, Istvan Bors, and Aron Lazary

The evaluation and complex treatments of sacral tumors require a multidisciplinary approach. Because of the complex anatomy conditions and biomechanics of the lumbo-pelvic junction, surgical treatment of sacral neoplasms is one of the most challenging fields in spine. Here, diagnostic process and surgical and nonsurgical treatment options for sacral tumors are summarized based on the literature and on the authors' own experiences.

Complications of En Bloc Resections in the Spine   125

Stefano Bandiera, Stefano Boriani, Rakesh Donthineni, L. Amendola, Michele Cappuccio, and Alessandro Gasbarrini

Morbidity of surgical procedures for spine tumors is expected to be worse than for other conditions. This is particularly true for en bloc resections, a technically demanding procedure. En bloc resections can help improve the prognosis of aggressive benign and malignant tumors in the spine, but the related morbidity is high and sometimes fatal. Reoperations have higher risks because of dissection through scar/fibrosis from previous surgeries and possibly from radiation. Careful planning for treatment is mandatory, and if the surgeon is unsure, referral to a specialty center is necessary.

Radiation for Spinal Metastatic Tumors   133

Patrick S. Swift

Radiotherapeutic management of vertebral metastases varies based on the extent of disease within the spine and systemically, the histology of the tumor, and the life expectancy of the patient. The goals of pain reduction, structural stability of the axial skeleton, and maintenance of local control for the remainder of the patient's life guide the decision to proceed with a short simple course of standard therapy or a more complex approach with stereotactic regimens. The complex and rigorous processes involved in stereotactic radiotherapy for the spine require close cooperation among the radiation oncologist, neurosurgeon, orthopedic surgeon, and medical oncologist, but the clinical results show that the result is an enhanced quality of life for the patient.

> As survival time increases for many cancers, it is likely that the incidence and prevalence of spinal metastases will increase also. Given that most patients first present with solitary lesions in the spine, proper initial diagnosis and management are of paramount importance in minimizing pain, improving neurologic function, and potentially lengthening survival. Although pain control and standard radiation are still used, spinal stereotactic radiosurgery, vertebroplasty and kyphoplasty, and spinal cord decompression and fusion are now consistently used in aggressive management and offer exciting preliminary results.

> In most patients who have spinal metastases, treatment is mainly palliative. The conventional surgical methods carry higher risks of complications and postoperative morbidity. Minimally invasive spinal interventions seem to be reasonable alternatives to treat spinal metastatic disease. These procedures can result in less soft tissue trauma, lower blood loss, shorter hospitalization time and are better tolerated by the patients. In this review, the techniques and results of minimally invasive management in spinal metastasis, including percutaneous image-guided interventions (vertebroplasty, kyphoplasty, and radiofrequency ablation) and minimally invasive surgical techniques (endoscopic and minimal access operations), are presented.

> Over the past three decades, progress has been dramatic in the management of spine tumors. For example, advanced imaging technologies made available at manageable costs have lowered the threshold for scanning. CT, MRI, and PET imaging modalities have greatly enhanced the ability of the surgeon to accurately delineate the extension of the lesion within the bone, the soft tissue, and the spinal canal. Such enhancements have led to great leaps forward in preoperative planning and postoperative evaluation, including improved reconstruction options are resulting in improved outcomes. This article introduces the theme of this volume.

Orthopedic Clinics of North America

THE CLINICS ARE NOW AVAILABLE ONLINE!

Access your subscription at:
www.theclinics.com

Preface

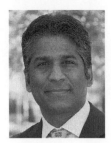 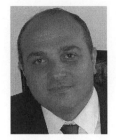

Rakesh Donthineni, MD, MBA   Onder Ofluoglu, MD
Guest Editors

The management of spine tumors has progressed dramatically over the last few decades. The emerging diagnostic technologies, novel adjuvant agents, and improved surgical techniques have helped the survival and quality of life for these patients. A wide array of reconstructive options of the vertebral body, along with the preoperative planning assisted by the modern imaging modalities, have boosted the confidence of surgeons to tackle more challenging cases. Daedalean efforts are needed to not only contain the tumor but also to eradicate it. As the experts in spine oncology from around the world are gaining and sharing their knowledge of the management of these difficult diseases, it is helping formulate better studies to validate our present methods, as well as develop new ones.

A collection of esteemed specialists from around the world have contributed their thoughts in this issue of *Orthopedic Clinics of North America* focused on spine oncology. We are indebted to them for not only bringing forward the latest ideas and expertise, but in the process allowing the vast others to extract the relevant information pertaining to their patients' diseases.

We are grateful to Deb Dellapena and Elsevier for this creative opportunity; and our families, friends, and colleagues for their patience, understanding, and support.

Rakesh Donthineni, MD, MBA
Spine and Orthopaedic Oncology
5700 Telegraph Avenue
Suite 100
Oakland, CA 94609, USA

Department of Orthopaedics
University of California Davis
Suite 3800, Y Street
Sacramento, CA 95817, USA

Onder Ofluoglu, MD
Department of Orthopedics
Lutfi Kırdar Research Hospital
Şemsi Denizer Cd. E-5
Karayolu Cevizli Mevkii 34890
Kartal/Istanbul, Turkey

E-mail addresses:
rdmd.inc@gmail.com (R. Donthineni)
oofluoglu@gmail.com (O. Ofluoglu)

doi:10.1016/j.ocl.2008.10.003

Diagnosis and Staging of Spine Tumors

Rakesh Donthineni, MD, MBA[a,b,*]

KEYWORDS
- Spine • Tumor • Diagnosis • Benign
- Malignant • Metastasis

As the expected incidence of cancers in the United States approaches 1.5 million cases for 2008, and with more than 0.5 million deaths, it ranks second only to cardiovascular disease in significance. Nearly three quarters of all cancers are diagnosed in persons 55 years and older. The incidence per year of breast and prostate cancers are approximately 180,000 each, and slightly more for lung cancer. With the improvement in diagnosis and treatment methods, there is an increasing trend in long-term survival by about 30%.[1] As patients with cancers have longer survival, there is an expected increase in the prevalence of metastatic disease.

With a higher incidence and prevalence of cancers of other organs of the body, there are more symptomatic or asymptomatic cases of metastatic disease to the spine than primary tumors.[2] Autopsy studies demonstrated between 30% and 90% of spinal metastases in patients with a history of other malignancy. The common primaries were lung, breast, lymphoma, and myeloma. Nearly 17% of patients with other primaries may present with spinal cord compression as a result of metastases.[3–5] Metastases to the spine have a predilection toward the thoracic spine, followed by the lumbar and cervical.[6]

More than 2000 bone and joint cancers and about 10,000 soft tissue cancers are diagnosed per year.[1] The incidence of benign tumors of the spine is a little more than 1% of all primary skeletal tumors, and nearly 5% for malignant tumors.[7] Within the benign tumors, giant cell tumors, osteoid osteomas, osteoblastomas, and hemangiomas are more likely. Although the incidence of hemangioma of the spine is about 10% in the general population, only a small percentage develop symptoms.[8,9] Apart from the hematopoietic tumors, including myeloma and lymphoma, the primary malignant tumors of the spine include chordoma, chondrosarcoma, osteosarcoma, and others.

PRESENTATION

Patients with spinal tumors most often present with axial pain, and some with radicular pain (if the tumor is extends to and compresses the nerves). A lesser percentage present with cauda equina syndrome and most of these are a result of metastatic disease and rapidly growing tumors. The cervical lesions tend to progress slowly in terms of neurologic symptoms, whereas the thoracolumbar lesions are more aggressive and are more clinically affected. About 60% will present with central or nerve root symptoms, and more than a third will present with a motor deficit. Sphincter function alterations in isolation are less frequent (less than 3%).[10]

Patients with cord compression not only have symptoms of sensory or motor disturbances, but most of them (>90%) have pain. There is often a delay from the time of the presentation of symptoms to the alterations in signs, and therefore, a delay in evaluation by the primary care doctor to the point of full diagnosis and management by a specialist. Plain radiographs may help in diagnosis in a fifth of the patients, whereas an MRI is much more useful in identifying the level of compression.[11] As part of the patient evaluation and follow-up, the extent of the neurologic dysfunction should be carefully mapped.[12]

Financial disclosure: no funding of any sort was obtained to conduct this review.
a Spine and Orthopaedic Oncology, 5700 Telegraph Avenue, Suite 100, Oakland, CA 94609, USA
b Department of Orthopaedics, University of California Davis, Suite 3800, Y Street, Sacramento, CA 95817, USA
* Spine and Orthopaedic Oncology, 5700 Telegraph Avenue, Suite 100, Oakland, CA 94609.
E-mail address: rdmd.inc@gmail.com

Orthop Clin N Am 40 (2009) 1–7
doi:10.1016/j.ocl.2008.10.001

The cause of the axial pain in patients with spinal tumors is because of the destructive effect of the tumor, the cortical breakdown, and also from extension into the canal with compression of the cord. Weakening of the vertebrae will likely lead to fractures, micro or macro, causing pain. The posterior longitudinal ligament is the weakest barrier for tumor growth, and the tumor often extends at points of perforating vessels. Spread to adjacent vertebrae is likely at the edge of the level involved beneath the longitudinal ligament, and via paravertebral muscles.[13,14]

The extension of metastatic tumors to the axial spine is mainly through the vascular mechanism, either by seeding via the arterial system or a closer spread via the valveless extradural venous system (Batson's venous plexus). A more direct extension is seen in the pulmonary apical tumors. Although the mechanical spread of the tumors seems logical, the tendency of the tumors to settle in some environments more than others, as related to the molecular and surface protein behavior, should not be ignored.[15–18]

In patients with a history of a previous adenocarcinoma or other malignancies, a new focus of tumor in the skeletal system often correlates with the historical primary, but needs to be corroborated. Without such a history, an unidentified focus should prompt the search for the primary. A thorough history, examination, the basic laboratory studies, plain radiographs, and other appropriate imaging of the affected site, whole body technetium-99m-phospate bone scan, and CT scan of the chest, abdomen, and pelvis often identifies most of the primary sites. Biopsy of the lesion adds significant information, but if done alone has a lesser yield than the combine effort. There may still be a small percentage where the primary may not be identifiable.[4,19–22]

Once identified, whether a primary or secondary tumor, the next step should be the appropriate planning for management. Although imaging studies, such as MRI and CT, have greatly assisted in diagnosing based on radiographs, only a few tumors can be diagnosed without a histologic evaluation. Osteoid osteoma is one such tumor that can be diagnosed on the plain radiographs and CT, and one can proceed with the treatment, whether it be a surgical excision or a percutaneous ablation (radiofrequency ablation). With regard to metastatic disease, the indications for surgical intervention are intractable pain, worsening neurologic deficit, a pathologic fracture, and instability.

LABORATORY AND IMAGING STUDIES

Apart from the basic workup of a patient with the spine tumor, most of the blood and serum studies do not contribute much to the diagnosis in primary tumors of the musculoskeletal system. Elevated erythrocyte sedimentation rate can be found in round cell tumors, benign or malignant, and also in infections. Serum and urinary protein electrophoresis are helpful in identifying myeloma. Low hematocrit may suggest a marrow infiltrative process, although it could also signify an advanced stage malignancy.

As part of the workup, imaging studies follow suit. Plain radiographs should be included, as they are easily accessible and allow approximate localization of the disease process (if visible on the radiographs), but also assist in evaluating the curvature of the spine and any changes in its structural appearance secondary to changes in the biomechanics.

Lytic tumors are not easily identified on plain radiographs until close to 50% of bone destruction occurs. Increasing destruction (cross-sectional area) and a poor bone mineral density in combination contribute to a higher likelihood for compressive fractures. In the thoracic vertebrae, although a larger defect may portend to a compression fracture, the intact costovertebral joints play a significant support to the overall structure, and as such, any involvement of these joints rapidly leads to a vertebral collapse.[23–26]

Once the involved level is identified, CT and MRI are the studies of choice to give much more data on the distribution of the tumor within the vertebrae, its extension, and effects on the local anatomy. MRI with intravenous contrast (Gadolinium) will assist in identifying the areas of most activity, and may direct the placement of the biopsy needle to achieve a high yield. Whole-body technetium-99m bone scan will help identify other sites of involvement, and hence help stage the disease, or even identify another location that may be an easier site for obtaining a piece of tissue for diagnostic purposes (**Fig. 1**).

Angiography may be used, but more as a treatment in benign highly vascular tumors (eg, ABC, GCT) or in preparation for the surgical treatment of a vascular tumor (eg, renal and thyroid metastases, and multiple myeloma) and thereby decreasing the blood loss intraoperatively.[27–30]

BIOPSY

A biopsy is mandatory if the isolated spinal lesion is unknown, even in the face of a distant history of a primary malignancy, as occasionally a new primary may be encountered. If the patient has a known history of metastatic disease with multiple lesions, the new troublesome spinal lesion may be

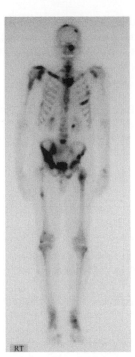

Fig. 1. Whole body bone scan demonstrating the extensive metastatic disease.

treated without the need for further histologic proof before dealing with the offending lesion.

Before planning the biopsy, the imaging studies need to be evaluated to ascertain the exact location of the tumor within the spinal column, and also to identify the most viable area on the MRI (with intravenous contrast), henceforth yielding the best tissue for diagnosis. The process of obtaining the tissue may be with a fine needle, core, incisional, or excisional. Needle and core biopsies are conducted percutaneously, with the difference being in the diameter of the bore. Incisional biopsy is conducted when an open approach to the tumor is conducted and a small piece of the tumor is obtained for analysis, leaving the rest in situ. In excisional biopsy, the whole tumor is removed with an intralesional, marginal, or wide margin.

Percutaneous biopsies, with fine needle aspiration or core biopsy, for musculoskeletal lesions have a favorable outcome in about 75% of the cases.[31] Fine needle aspiration may be adequate in metastatic tumors or in recurrences, whereas in cases of primary tumors, adequacy of tissue helps in the accuracy of diagnosis. Also, sufficient tissue is needed for not only for the standard stains in histology, but also possibly for immunostains and other studies, including cytogenetics. Increasing the diameter of the needle will obtain more

tissue and is helpful in sclerotic lesions, but the associated rates of complications increase.[32]

Albeit the varying results, image-guided transpedicular biopsy of the vertebral lesion is still the favored technique, the choice of imaging either fluoroscopy or CT (**Figs. 2** and **3**).[33] Percutaneous CT guided (via the pedicle or otherwise) is often the standard approach by the interventional radiologists, as they have access to the appropriate imaging machines, and the overall accuracy has been reported to be about 89%, with lytic lesions having a better yield (93%) versus the sclerotic/blastic lesions (76%). The sclerotic lesion accuracy is less than that for lytic or mixed lytic-sclerotic lesions or compression fractures, and also the false negative biopsies are higher in the sclerotic lesions. The accuracy is also lower if the lesion is visible on the MRI but not clear on CT imaging at the time of the biopsy.[34] MRI-guided biopsies are available and can helpful in locating the biopsy needle in the viable part of the tumor to give a higher diagnostic yield.[35]

Open incisional or excisional biopsies must be properly planned and approached with an incision small enough to allow a future resection, in cases of recurrence or when dealing with a primary malignancy. Contamination of neighboring structures should be limited as much as possible, and the path of approach should be away from any vital neurovascular structures, as any contamination would require resection of these structures to prevent or decrease recurrences. Meticulous hemostasis is a must, as the seeping blood may

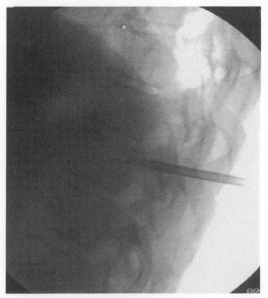

Fig. 2. Fluoroscopy-guided transpedicular approach for a vertebral body biopsy.

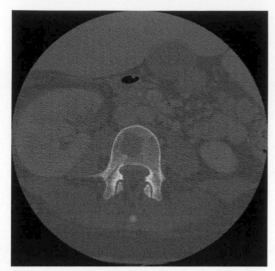

Fig. 3. CT scan demonstrating the lytic tumor, and the biopsy track through the pedicle.

act as a low-barrier pathway for tumor invasion. Any cortical windows created to obtain tumor specimen need to be covered with either bone wax or cement (PMMA) to contain hemorrhage and tumor spillage.

During the surgical preparation and draping, if a frozen section pathologic analysis is being considered, before the final treatment at the same surgical setting, a new set of instruments and drapes are mandatory to prevent accidental tumor seeding. This also applies when harvesting bone autograft from another site.[36]

Excisional biopsy may be performed for osteoid osteoma. In tumors such as osteoblastoma, aneurysmal bone cyst, and unknown metastatic adenocarcinoma, an intraoperative frozen section analysis is necessary before the definitive treatment of excision or cord decompression.

STAGING

As the imaging modalities and reconstruction options improved, the confidence to resect complicated large tumors also followed suit.[37,38] Whether it be primary (benign or malignant) or metastatic tumors, if the goal is to eradicate the tumor, then detailed imaging studies are necessary. Also, as part of understanding the extent of the tumors (primary malignant or metastatic), staging the disease helps prepare how to approach the local spinal tumor. After obtaining the history and physical examination and appropriate imaging studies of the local disease and a biopsy-proven diagnosis, the next step of the staging is to evaluate other sites of involvement. Apart from giant cell tumors

and occasionally chondroblastomas, benign skeletal tumors do not metastasize. Primary malignant tumors of the skeletal system often metastasize to lungs, and also to bones. A chest CT and a whole body bone scan will help identify these other locations.

The Musculoskeletal Tumor Society's staging system (adapted from Enneking and colleagues)[39] is used extensively for tumors of the pelvis and extremities. The staging is based on either benign (1 = latent, inactive; 2 = active, but slow growing; 3 = active and aggressive growth) or malignant tumors (I, II, and III). Low-grade primary malignant tumors are graded "I" and high are graded "II." The tumor's location within the compartment is denoted as "A" or extracompartmental as "B." Those with spread beyond the local site (skip metastases or distant metastases) are denoted "III." Although there was a notable difference between the outcomes of stages I, II, and III, the location of the tumor within a compartment or its extension outside does not affect the long-term outcome significantly.[40]

Systematic evaluation of spine tumors was developed by Tomita and colleagues[41] and also by Weinstein-Boriani-Biagini.[42,43]

The WBB (Weinstein-Boriani-Biagini) staging system is based on viewing the affected vertebra in an axial view and dividing it into 12 equal radial segments ("clock-face"). The five outer to inner concentric layers are labeled A to E, with "A" as the extraosseous layer, and sequentially layering in to "E" as the dural involvement (**Fig. 4**). In the cervical vertebrae, "F" indicates involvement of the vertebral foramen (**Fig. 5**).

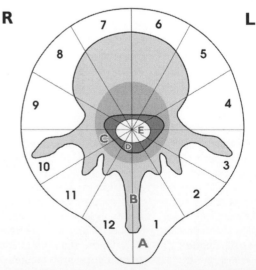

Fig. 4. WBB diagram of the thoracolumbar vertebra. (*Courtesy of* S. Boriani, MD, New York, NY.)

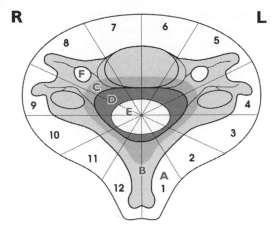

R   L

Fig. 5. WBB diagram of the cervical vertebra. (*Courtesy of* S. Boriani, MD, New York, NY.)

Tomita's scoring system describes the location of the tumor within the body (Type 1–3), extension outside the vertebra (Type 4–6), and involvement of other vertebrae (Type 7) (**Fig. 6**). Within the types 1 to 3, the extent of the tumor is either located within the body, extending to the pedicle, or to the lamina respectively. In Types 4 to 6, there is extension into the spinal canal alone, canal and lateral extraosseous extension, and to adjacent levels respectively. The categories help assist in planning the type of resection, either vertebrectomy (partial or total) and palliative surgery because of extensive involvement and spread.

The use of these systems mandates adequate imaging studies (MRI and CT), allows adequate planning of the surgery, and assists in interinstitutional comparison of data for long-term outcomes.

With regard to metastatic disease, various algorithms have been developed to help in planning the management. These systems help in evaluating the patient's general condition, the primary malignancy, systemic and the extent of local involvement, and other variables. Newer systems are being developed to improve management.[6,44–46]

As part of systemic staging, following tumor removal, the margin of the resection should be evaluated. There has been much confusion with the terminology for the type of surgery and the final margin. A more standardized approach should be recognized, both for universal use and understanding, but also for the comparison of multi-institutional data for long-term outcome studies.

TERMINOLOGY
Intralesional Excision

Intralesion excision is defined as piecemeal removal of the tumor. This is further subcategorized based on the capsule. The "capsule" is the reactive zone at the periphery of the tumor.

1. Intracapsular, if tumor removal is incomplete, as gross or histologic remnants inside the tumor capsule can be expected.
2. Extracapsular, if tumor removal includes all of the tumor mass and a surrounding layer of healthy tissue, but microscopic tumor may be left behind as a result of intralesional excision.

En Bloc Resection

En bloc resection is defined as in toto removal of the tumor mass, including a cuff of healthy tissue encasing the tumor (margin). The pathologist's evaluation of the margin allows further subclassification of en bloc resections:

1. Intralesional, if the tumor is violated intentionally (trying to save some of the vital structures

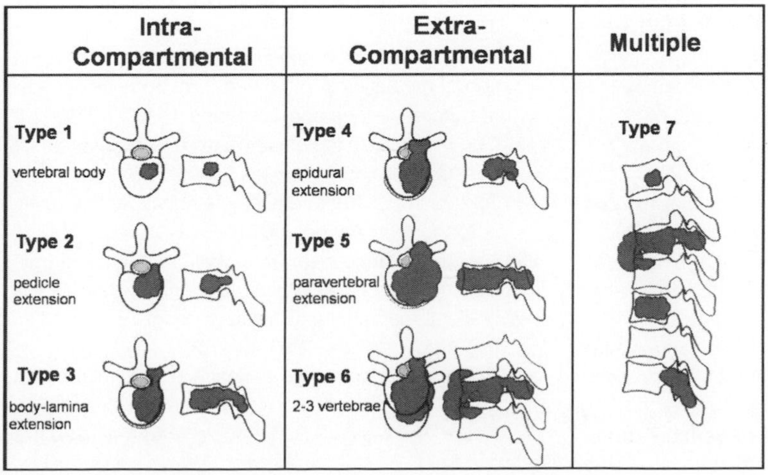

Intra-Compartmental	Extra-Compartmental	Multiple
Type 1 vertebral body	**Type 4** epidural extension	**Type 7**
Type 2 pedicle extension	**Type 5** paravertebral extension	
Type 3 body-lamina extension	**Type 6** 2-3 vertebrae	

Fig. 6. Tomita's classification of vertebral tumor involvement. (*Courtesy of* Katsuro Tomita, MD, Norio Kawahara, MD, and Hideki Murakami, MD, Kanazawa, Japan.)

adhered or encased by the tumor) or unintentionally.

2. Marginal, if the dissection is through the reactive outer area of the tumor (pseudocapsule), potentially leaving microscopic tumor behind.

3. Wide, if a layer of peripheral healthy tissue, a dense fibrous cover (eg, fascia), or an anatomic barrier not yet infiltrated (eg, pleura), fully cover the tumor and the pathologist reading shows a negative margin.

Radical resection, as described by Enneking and colleagues,[39] suggests en bloc removal of the tumor including the whole compartment and is very rarely if at all used in the spine. An attempt at the radical resection of an affected vertebra would require the removal of the whole vertebra, and ergo, transection of the spinal cord or nerves. Also, if the tumor extends into the spinal canal, a radical resection would require the removal of the whole spinal canal and associated structures, a theoretic but ethically unreasonable concept. As such, the use of "radical resection" has to be carefully used to avoid unnecessary confusion.

SUMMARY

The incidences of cancers are increasing, and as patients live longer, the risk of systemic and spinal metastases increases. Proper evaluation of the patient with history, examination, and imaging studies should help identify the cause of the symptoms, and after a histologic diagnosis, the next step is to strategize the management options. Detailed planning and staging will help not only in the surgical resection and reconstruction, but also achieve better outcomes for these patients.

ACKNOWLEDGMENTS

Figs. 4 and **5** were used with the kind permission of Dr. Stefano Boriani and **Fig. 6** from Drs. Katsuro Tomita, Norio Kawahara, and Hideki Murakami.

REFERENCES

1. American Cancer Society. Cancer Facts & Figures 2008. Atlanta: American Cancer Society; 2008.

2. Schuster JM, Grady MS. Medical management and adjuvant therapies in spinal metastatic disease. Neurosurg Focus 2001;11:e3.

3. Wong DA, Fornasier VL, MacNab I. Spinal metastases: the obvious, the occult, and the imposters. Spine 1990;15:1–4.

4. Ortiz Gómez JA. The incidence of vertebral body metastases. Int Orthop 1995;19:309–11.

5. Loblaw DA, Laperriere NJ, Mackillop WJ. A population-based study of malignant spinal cord compression in Ontario. Clin Oncol 2003;15:211–7.

6. Gasbarrini A, Cappuccio M, Mirabile L, et al. Spinal metastases: treatment evaluation algorithm. Eur Rev Med Pharmacol Sci 2004;8:265–74.

7. Unni K. Introduction and scope. In: Unni K, editor. Dahlin's bone tumors—general aspects and data on 11,087 cases. Philadelphia: Lippincott-Raven; 1996. p. 1–9.

8. Dagi TF, Schmidek HH. Vascular tumors of the spine. In: Sundaresan N, Schmidek HH, Schiller AL, editors. Tumors of the spine: diagnosis and clinical management. Philadelphia: W.B. Saunders Co; 1990. p. 181–91.

9. Fox MW, Onofrio BM. The natural history and management of symptomatic and asymptomatic vertebral hemangiomas. J Neurosurg 1993;78:36–45.

10. Constans JP, de Divitiis E, Donzelli R, et al. Spinal metastases with neurological manifestations. Review of 600 cases. J Neurosurg 1983;59:111–8.

11. Levack P, Graham J, Collie D, et al. Don't wait for a sensory level—listen to the symptoms: a prospective audit of the delays in diagnosis of malignant cord compression. Clin Oncol (R Coll Radiol) 2002; 14:472–80.

12. Frankel HL, Hancock DO, Hyslop G, et al. The value of postural reduction in the initial management of closed injuries of the spine with paraplegia and tetraplegia. Paraplegia 1969;7:179–92.

13. Fujita T, Ueda Y, Kawahara N, et al. Local spread of metastatic vertebral tumors: a histologic study. Spine 1997;22:1905–12.

14. Wai EK, Finkelstein JA, Tangente RP, et al. Quality of life in surgical treatment of metastatic spine disease. Spine 2003;28:508–12.

15. Batson OV. The role of the vertebral veins in metastatic processes. Ann Intern Med 1942;16:38–45.

16. Harada M, Shimizu A, Nakamura Y, et al. Role of the vertebral venous system in metastatic spread of cancer cells to the bone. Adv Exp Med Biol 1992; 324:83–92.

17. Yuh WT, Quets JP, Lee HJ, et al. Anatomic distribution of metastases in the vertebral body and modes of hematogenous spread. Spine 1996;21:2243–50.

18. Choong PF. The molecular basis of skeletal metastases. Clin Orthop Relat Res 2003;415:S19–31.

19. Tokuhashi Y. Treatment of metastatic spine tumor. J Jpn Orthop Assoc 2007;81:573–84.

20. Katagiri H, Takahashi M, Inagaki J, et al. Determining the site of the primary cancer in patients with skeletal metastasis of unknown origin: a retrospective study. Cancer 1999;86:533–7.

21. Rougraff BT, Kneisl JS, Simon MA. Skeletal metastases of unknown origin. A prospective study of a diagnostic strategy. J Bone Joint Surg Am 1993;75: 1276–81.

22. Destombe C, Botton E, Le Gal G, et al. Investigations for bone metastasis from an unknown primary. Joint Bone Spine 2007;74:85–9.

23. Boland PJ, Land JM, Sundaresan N. Metastatic disease of the spine. Clin Orthop 1982;162:95–102.

24. Dimar J, Voor M, Zhang Y, et al. A human cadaver model for determination of pathologic fracture threshold resulting from tumorous destruction of the vertebral body. Spine 1998;23:1209–14.

25. Fourney DR, Gokaslan ZL. Spinal instability and deformity due to neoplastic conditions. Neurosurg Focus 2003;14:1–7.

26. Ebihara H, Ito M, Abumi K, et al. A biomechanical analysis of metastatic vertebral collapse of the thoracic spine: a sheep model study. Spine 2004;29:994–9.

27. Olerud C, Jónsson H Jr, Löfberg AM, et al. Embolization of spinal metastases reduces preoperative blood loss: 21 patients operated on for renal cell carcinoma. Acta Orthop Scand 1993;64:9–12.

28. Guzman R, Dubach-Schwizer S, Heini P, et al. Preoperative transarterial embolization of vertebral metastases. Eur Spine J 2005;14:263–8.

29. Lackman RD, Khoury LD, Esmail A, et al. The treatment of sacral giant-cell tumours by serial arterial embolisation. J Bone Joint Surg Br 2002;84:873–7.

30. Boriani S, De Iure F, Campanacci L, et al. Aneurysmal bone cyst of the mobile spine: report on 41 cases. Spine 2001;26:27–35.

31. Ogilvie CM, Torbert JT, Finstein JL, et al. Clinical utility of percutaneous biopsies of musculoskeletal tumors. Clin Orthop Relat Res 2006;450:95–100.

32. Nourbakhsh A, Grady JJ, Garges KJ. Percutaneous spine biopsy: a meta-analysis. J Bone Joint Surg Am 2008;90:1722–5.

33. Hadjipavlou AG, Kontakis GM, Gaitanis JN, et al. Effectiveness and pitfalls of percutaneous transpedicle biopsy of the spine. Clin Orthop Relat Res 2003;411:54–60.

34. Lis E, Bilsky MH, Pisinski L, et al. Percutaneous CT-guided biopsy of osseous lesion of the spine in patients with known or suspected malignancy. AJNR Am J Neuroradiol 2004;25:1583–8.

35. Carrino JA, Khurana B, Ready JE, et al. Magnetic resonance imaging–guided percutaneous biopsy of musculoskeletal lesions. J Bone Joint Surg Am 2007;89:2179–87.

36. Ofluoglu O, Donthineni R. Iatrogenic seeding of a giant cell tumor of the patella to the proximal tibia. Clin Orthop Relat Res 2007;465:260–4.

37. Stener B. Total spondylectomy in chondrosarcoma arising from the seventh thoracic vertebra. J Bone Joint Surg Br 1971;53:288–95.

38. Tomita K, Toribatake Y, Kawahara N, et al. Total en bloc spondylectomy and circumspinal decompression for solitary spinal metastasis. Paraplegia 1994; 32:36–46.

39. Enneking WF, Spanier SS, Goodmann M. System for surgical staging of musculoskeletal sarcoma. Clin Orthop 1980;153:106–20.

40. Heck RK, Stacy GS, Flaherty MJ, et al. A comparison of staging system for bone sarcomas. Clin Orthop 2003;415:64–71.

41. Tomita K, Kawahara N, Baba H, et al. Total en bloc spondylectomy: a new surgical technique for primary malignant vertebral tumors. Spine 1997;22:324–33.

42. Hart RA, Boriani S, Biagini R, et al. A system for surgical staging and management of spine tumors. A clinical outcome study of giant cell tumors of the spine. Spine 1997;22:1773–82.

43. Boriani S, Weinstein JN, Biagini R, et al. Primary bone tumors of the spine. Terminology and surgical staging. Spine 1997;22:1036–44.

44. Tomita K, Kawahara N, Kobayashi T, et al. Surgical strategy for spinal metastases. Spine 2001;26: 298–306.

45. Tokuhashi Y, Matsuzaki H, Oda H, et al. A revised scoring system for preoperative evaluation of metastatic spine tumor prognosis. Spine 2005;30: 2186–91.

46. Ibrahim A, Crockard A, Antonietti P, et al. Does spinal surgery improve the quality of life for those with extradural (spinal) osseous metastases? An international multicenter prospective observational study of 223 patients. J Neurosurg Spine 2008;8:271–8.

Management of Benign Tumors of the Mobile Spine

Alessandro Gasbarrini, MD[a,b],*, Michele Cappuccio, MD[a,b],
Rakesh Donthineni, MD, MBA[c,d], Stefano Bandiera, MD[a,b],
Stefano Boriani, MD[a,b]

KEYWORDS

- Spine • Tumors • Benign • Treatment
- Surgery • Embolization

Primary bone tumors of the mobile spine are very rare. In a series of 1971 patients with musculoskeletal neoplasms in a 17-year period, only 29 patients (1.5%), including 8 children, had primary osseous tumors of the thoracic and lumbar spine.[1] Out of 43,735 primary bone tumors reviewed,[1–6] 1851 (4.2%) were located in the spine above the sacrum. In the treatment of spine metastases, the priority is to preserve mechanical and neurologic function. By contrast, in the treatment of primary tumors, complete local eradication is the main goal, as an oncologically appropriate surgical treatment can substantially improve the prognosis and even be considered a life-saving procedure. However, these procedures can be associated with severe morbidities and sometimes include sacrifice of even important anatomic structures with consequent functional loss.

In deciding the best treatment for primary bone tumors of the spine, the choice of surgery, radiation therapy, chemotherapy, selective arterial embolization, or other medical treatments alone or in combination is based on diagnosis, staging, and a deep understanding of the biology and the behavior of each tumor.

DIAGNOSIS

Histologic diagnosis should always be achieved by biopsy, but clinical, laboratory, and imaging studies are important to direct the diagnosis and select the biopsy technique. Clinical elements are seldom specific. Pain is a very nonspecific complaint, but pain associated with a tumor tends to be progressive, unrelenting, and not closely related to activity. Furthermore, such pain tends to increase during the night. Pain stems from several causes. Tumor growth may cause the bony cortex of the vertebral body to expand, resulting in pathologic fracture and invasion of paravertebral soft tissues. Pain is also associated with acute or chronic compression of the spinal cord, resulting in focal and radicular symptoms of pain or sensory disturbance, and motor weakness leading to paraplegia, bowel dysfunction, and bladder dysfunction.

Swelling and local tenderness were once the common onset symptoms. Today, however, with the availability and use of imaging studies, such as CT and MRI, lesions can be detected before extensive masses form.

Technetium isotope bone scans help to localize single and multiple lesions. Imaging studies (CT and MRI scans) can confirm diagnostic hypotheses, as some patterns are quite distinctive. Angiography shows pathologic vascularity and selective arterial embolization has become an indispensable tool to reduce intraoperative bleeding. The ischemic effect on the tumor mass

[a] Department of Orthopaedics and Traumatology – Spine Surgery Maggiore Hospital, Largo Nigrisoli 2, 40100 Bologna, Italy
[b] Rizzoli Institute, Bologna, Italy
[c] Spine and Orthopaedic Oncology, 5700 Telegraph Avenue, Suite 100, Oakland, CA 94609, USA
[d] Department of Orthopaedics, University of California Davis, Suite 3800, Y Street, Sacramento, CA 95817, USA
* Corresponding author. Department of Orthopaedics and Traumatology – Spine Surgery, Largo Nigrisoli 2, 40100 Bologna, Italy.
E-mail address: boova@libero.it (A. Gasbarrini).

Orthop Clin N Am 40 (2009) 9–19
doi:10.1016/j.ocl.2008.09.009
0030-5898/08/$ – see front matter © 2008 Elsevier Inc. All rights reserved.

provoked by selective arterial embolization can also be considered an adjuvant therapy for local control in selected tumors.

SPECIFIC ENTITIES

Since 1949, we have treated 1077 tumors of the mobile spine. However, for the purposes of analysis using uniform data on diagnosis, staging, and treatment, we prefer to consider only the period from 1997 and 2007. In this period we treated 651 tumors of the mobile spine. These included 226 primary tumors and 141 benign tumors (22% of all tumors) (**Table 1**).

Eosinophilic Granuloma (Langerhans Cell Histiocytosis)

The so-called "eosinophilic granuloma" is the solitary bone occurrence of the Langerhans cell histiocytosis, which usually occurs in children younger than 10 years old. Vertebral involvement is found in 10% to 15% of the cases. Eosinophilic granuloma is a benign, mostly self-limiting condition producing destruction of bone and consisting of an abnormal proliferation of lipid-containing histiocytes from the reticuloendothelial system.

The "coin-on-end" appearance or "vertebra plana" without any evidence of soft tissue mass is pathognomonic of the later stages of vertebral eosinophilic granuloma, and it can be found incidentally after an asymptomatic course (**Fig. 1**).[7]

The initial pattern is a lytic image, which can affect multiple spinal levels, partially or totally destroying the vertebral body, rarely leading to significant pain. Neurologic symptoms are exceptional. It is necessary to rule out infection, a benign tumor, or a malignancy, such as Ewing's sarcoma. Laboratory tests are useful, but the findings on imaging studies of well-marginated borders, maintenance of adjacent intervertebral disc spaces, absence of soft tissue extension are the most important elements to distinguish eosinophilic granuloma from other differential diagnoses.

Osteochondroma (Exostosis)

Osteochondroma is a very common bone hamartoma. Solitary osteochondroma are noninherited malformations. They are painless cartilage-capped bony growths on either a broad base or a stalk, first appearing in relation to the epiphyseal growth plate. After closure of the growth plates, osteochondromas usually stop growing. Vertebral involvement is very rare, occurring mostly in the cervical or upper thoracic spine. A palpable mass is the most prominent symptom. Symptomatic cord compression is possible but very rare.

Osteoid Osteoma

In osteoid osteoma, pain is almost always present and unrelated to activity. Osteoid osteoma is the common cause of painful scoliosis in adolescence.[8] The lumbar spine is the most common location (>50%) followed by the cervical, thoracic, and sacral spine. Night pain in a young patient, relieved by aspirin, can suggest the diagnosis of osteoid osteoma. A very intense technetium isotope scan uptake can localize the lesion and CT scan can confirm the diagnosis. The pathognomonic picture is a small radiolucent area ("nidus") usually about 1.5 cm or smaller. This is mostly (but not exclusively) located in the posterior elements, includes sometimes a small spot of dense bone, and is surrounded by a variable sclerotic area (**Fig. 2**).[9] Such an appearance is noted on the imaging studies (plain radiographs

Table 1
Benign tumors managed at the Rizzoli Institute, from 1997 to 2007*

Specific Entities	n	Sex		Localization			Age (y)			Follow-Up (mo)		
		M	F	C	T	L	Min	Max	Av	Min	Max	Av
Eosinophilic granuloma	7	2	5	2	3	2	9	16	12.2	6	64	30
Osteochondroma	4	1	3	3	/	1	22	36	31.5	12	76	41
Osteoid osteoma	23	16	7	4	10	9	12	39	22.3	6	99	28
Osteoblastoma	25	18	7	7	8	10	10	47	24.5	9	65	33
Aneurysmal bone cyst	11	3	8	6	3	2	5	36	17.9	8	56	22
Giant cell tumor	15	7	8	4	6	5	17	53	33.1	6	113	59

* Of the 141 tumors, some are labeled in the Table, while others (including hemangioma, hemangioendothelioma, and others) are grouped separately as "others."

Abbreviations: Av, average; C, cervical; F, female; L, lumbar; M, male; Max, maximum; Min, minimum; n, number; T, thoracic.

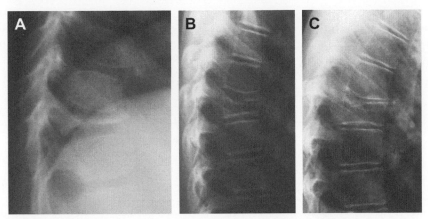

Fig. 1. Eosinophilic granuloma of the thoracic spine with progressive healing and restoration of vertebral height. Vertebra plana at onset (*A*), after 6 months (*B*), and 12 months (*C*) in a young patient.

and CT). Treatment can be performed without a biopsy. MRI is misleading in osteoid osteomas, as in osteoblastomas, due to the extensive edema frequently observed throughout the involved vertebra and related to the reactive zone. On rare occasions, osteoid osteoma may convert to osteoblastoma (**Fig. 3**).

Osteoblastoma

More than 40% of the reported cases of osteoblastoma have been located in the spine,[10,11] mostly arising from the posterior elements. Enneking stage 2 osteoblastoma is histologically indistinguishable from osteoid osteoma and mainly differs in size. Diagnosis is confirmed if its diameter is more than 2 cm (**Fig. 4**). Stage 3 osteoblastoma is a destructive expansive lesion clinically and radiographically similar to other aggressive conditions, such as giant cell tumor.[12] Pathologic bone formation, however, is always

evident, but prominent in stage 2 lesions. As in osteoid osteoma, technetium-99 bone scanning is a reliable screening technique. CT scanning may be the best imaging procedure for defining the location and extent of osteoblastomas with regard to their osseous involvement. CT scans are the best imaging modality for identifying and aiding surgical planning for extirpation and reconstruction. With radiculopathy or myelopathy, MRI may also be considered. When analyzing MRI, be aware of the extensive reactive changes that are enhanced and that can be misleading.

Aneurysmal Bone Cyst

Aneurysmal bone cysts, a pseudotumoral condition commonly found in the spine, occur in younger patients. In 60% of cases, the aneurysmal bone cyst is localized in the posterior elements of the vertebra and occasionally expands into the vertebral body. Plain radiographs show an expansile osteolytic cavity with strands of bone forming a bubbly appearance. The frequently observed "fluid levels" images (**Fig. 5**) are due to the double density of the cyst contents (blood and membranes) and can be considered as pathognomonic of aneurysmal bone cyst ("fluid-fluid" level). The cortex is often eggshell thin and blown out. The lesion is often extremely vascular, but this feature is not often appreciated on angiography even though it is grossly apparent.

Giant Cell Tumors

Giant cell tumors are histologically benign, but their clinical behavior is sometimes unpredictable, with high recurrence rate if not correctly staged and treated. The incidence in the mobile spine (above the sacrum) ranges from 1.4% to 9.4%.[13-16] Giant cell tumors occur in adults and typically follow a fully erosive pattern that usually

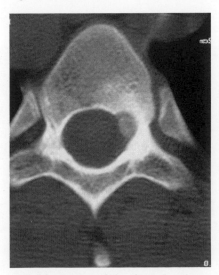

Fig. 2. Osteoid osteoma of the thoracic spine.

A

B

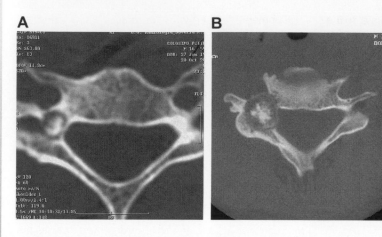

Fig. 3. A rare case of an osteoid osteoma (*A*) evolving into an osteoblastoma (*B*) arising in C5.

occurs in the vertebral body, with well-defined borders in Enneking stage 2 lesions, expanding with indistinct margins eroding the cortex in Enneking stage 3, and forming a soft tissue mass. Classic appearance of giant cell tumors on histology is that of multinucleated giant cells distributed in a background of mononuclear and spindle-shaped cells. Each tumor is highly vascular and, although benign, can be aggressive locally and with a potential to metastasize.[17] From our collection of giant cell tumors of the mobile spine, the order of distribution was thoracic, lumbar, and cervical spine. As in the extremities, there may be aneurysmal cysts within the giant cell tumor.

BIOPSY

The target of a biopsy is to obtain a piece of the tumor representative of the lesion and large enough to allow histologic and ultrastructural analysis as well as immunologic stains. The surgeon must be able to recognize the vital part of the tumor and to discard the necrotic or reactive part. Culture results may also be obtained to rule out infection.

Three traditional forms of spinal biopsy are available to the surgeon: needle/core biopsy, incisional, and excisional.

A number of basic principles should be observed when performing incisional and excisional biopsy to prevent tumor contamination of the surrounding tissue, which is the major risk of biopsy. Transverse incisions and flaps should be avoided; the tumor should be approached in the most direct manner possible. Tissues should be handled carefully, and hemostasis should be meticulous. Bone should not be removed or windowed unless absolutely necessary. Bleeding from exposed bone or from small vessels and injured muscle form a postoperative hematoma that may carry tumor cells beyond the margins of the intended excision and

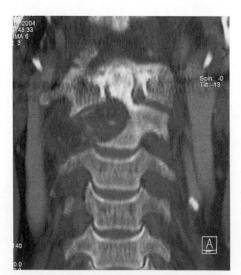

Fig. 4. Osteoblastoma of the cervical spine.

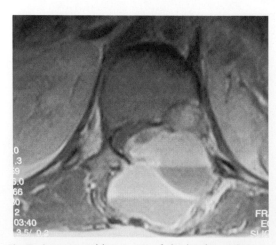

Fig. 5. Aneurysmal bone cyst of the lumbar spine.

contaminate tissues far proximal or distal to the primary lesion. The margin of the soft tissue mass is often the most helpful for diagnosis because the central portions are often necrotic. The surgeon should take care not to crush or distort the specimen, so as to maintain its architecture. Finally, if the definitive excision (with negative margins) is to follow the biopsy under the same anesthesia (frozen section biopsy), it is essential to exchange all instruments used during the biopsy for new. A new sterile field should be draped, and the surgeons should change gowns and gloves before the excision is begun. If fusion is planned, bone graft should be taken through a separate surgical setup.

Transpedicular needle biopsy is an accepted method to obtain fragments of tumor from a vertebral body without violating the epidural space. The pedicle must be perforated carefully so as to avoid breaking of the pedicle, which may result in contamination of the epidural space. A small straight curette is then introduced into the tumor and specimen removed. The soft tissue track can be excised if there is a risk of tumor seeding.

Excisional biopsy can be considered only for conditions whose radiographic pattern is pathognomonic (eg, osteoid osteoma), but most lesions of the spinal column require an incisional or needle biopsy before addressing the tumor for final management.

Needle biopsies are subject to sampling errors and provide small specimens for evaluation. The authors' preferred technique is biopsy with a 16-gauge trocar, performed under CT guidance. The use of the trocar enables the removal of core pieces useful to study tumor histologic architecture. The use of the CT scan makes it possible to reach even small lesions inside the vertebral body.

Intraoperative frozen section evaluation by a pathologist may be performed before the planned excisional procedure when diagnosis is highly probable based on imaging studies and needs confirmation. However, this is not advisable for primary unknown tumors, although very reasonable for unresectable metastases compressing the cord, where diagnosis has to be confirmed during the decompression procedure.

Biopsy is almost always indicated for primary spine tumors. With a combination of the available imaging modalities, the surgeon can confidently diagnose (eg, osteoid osteoma, aneurysmal bone cyst, or in selected cases of chondrosarcoma) and safely perform the definitive surgical procedure at one sitting. This reduces the risks of a biopsy, including the need to excise the bipsy track, and facilitating the tumor excision with the appropriate oncological margins.

ONCOLOGICAL STAGING

The oncological staging proposed by Enneking and colleagues[18] defines the biological behavior of primary tumors and has proven effective in finding a relationship between tumor aggressiveness, type of surgical resection (intralesional, marginal, wide, or radical) and outcome in terms of survival and recurrence rate for limb lesions. This staging system divides benign tumors into three stages—S1 (latent, inactive), S2 (active), and S3 (aggressive)—and localized malignant tumors into four stages (IA, IB, IIA, IIB); I and II for the low and high-grade tumors, respectively, and A and B for intracompartmental versus extracompartmental extension of the tumor, respectively. It was formerly described for long bone tumors and applied to spinal tumors in some reports.[19–23]

BENIGN TUMORS

The first stage of benign tumor (S1) (**Fig. 6**A) includes asymptomatic lesions, bordered by a true capsule, which is usually seen as a sclerotic rim on plain radiographs. These tumors do not grow, or only grow very slowly. No treatment is required, unless palliative surgery is needed for

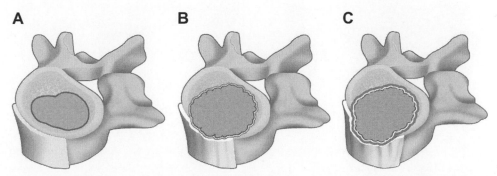

A   **B**   **C**

Fig. 6. The oncological staging proposed by Enneking applied to the vertebrae S1 (*A*), S2 (*B*), and S3 (*C*).

decompression or stabilization. Stage 2 tumors (S2) (**Fig. 6**B) grow slowly, causing mild symptoms. The tumor is bordered by a thin capsule and by a layer of reactive tissue, sometimes found on plain radiographs as an enlargement of the tumor outline. Bone scan is positive. An intralesional excision can be performed with a low rate of recurrence.[21] The incidence of recurrences can be further lowered by local adjuvants (polymethylmethacrylate, embolization, radiation therapy). The third stage of benign tumors (S3) (**Fig. 6**C) includes rapidly growing benign tumors. The capsule is very thin, discontinued, or absent. The tumor invades neighboring compartments, and a wide reactive hypervascularized tissue (pseudocapsule) is often found, sometimes permeated by neoplastic digitations. Bone scan is highly positive, and poorly defined margins are seen on plain radiographs. Meanwhile, CT scan shows extracompartmental extension, and MRI clearly defines a pseudocapsule and its relationship to the neurologic structures. Intralesional excision (curettage), even if augmented by radiation, can be associated with a significant rate of recurrence.[21,24] En bloc excision is the treatment of choice.

SURGICAL STAGING

For the proper application of the above-described grading, a complete preoperative work-up must be performed. To plan surgery properly, the surgeon must have a good grasp of the local anatomy. The first attempt at staging for spine tumors for surgical planning was introduced by Weinstein and McLain.[25] This staging system was subsequently modified in collaboration with the Rizzoli Institute.[26] Now called the WBB (Weinstein, Boriani, Biagini) Staging System (**Fig. 7**),[26] the system has since been subjected to several clinical evaluations.[23,26,27]

According to the WBB Staging System, each vertebra on the transverse plane is divided into 12 radiating zones (1–12 in a clockwise direction) and into five layers (A–E from the prevertebral to the dural involvement) on the transverse plane. The longitudinal extent of the tumor is recorded by identifying the specific vertebrae involved. This system allows for a more rational approach to the surgical planning, provided that all efforts are made to perform surgery along the required margins. The basic concept, a clock-face with radiating zones, accommodates the crucial planning necessary in performing en bloc resections in the presence of the spinal cord/cauda equina around the longitudinal axis of the involved vertebra. To preserve the spinal cord and or cauda equina, the surgeon must resect each sector of the vertebra along the proposed planes. This means an en bloc resection of a vertebral body cannot be performed without first removing the posterior arch. The margins are the pedicles. Conversely, if the tumor occupies an eccentric area, the surgeon is often compelled to remove the healthy contralateral parts of the vertebra, dislocate the dural sac, and perform radiating sections by use of an osteotome and other appropriate instruments along the planned zones.

Terminology

The lack of a logically organized paradigm makes it confusing to evaluate the results of

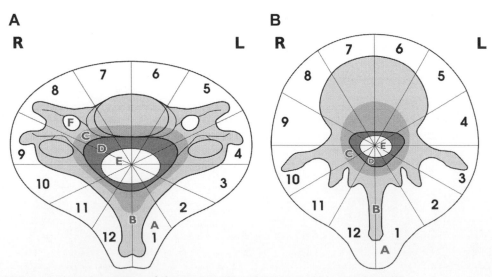

Fig. 7. WBB surgical staging system of the cervical (*A*) and thoracolumbar vertebrae (*B*).

treatment for primary spine tumors. Without a common terminology, difficulties arise in applying surgical principles of the Enneking's oncological staging system[18] to the spine and in comparing the results among institutions. Three terms are often employed: intralesional excision, en bloc excision (resection), and radical resection. An intralesional excision is a piecemeal intralesional removal of the tumor (curettage). En bloc excision (resection) is an attempted en bloc removal of a tumor. According to the gross and histologic findings (evaluation of the tissue margins surrounding the tumor), the en bloc excision is defined as contaminated, marginal, or wide.[18,27]

The term *radical resection* is frequently used just to suggest a complete tumor removal, regardless of the technique used.[28] However, according to the proposed terminology,[18] it means the en bloc removal of the tumor together with the whole compartment of origin. It is obvious that this is possible for a tumor arising in the scapula, or even in the femur, but it is not possible for tumors arising in a vertebra unless the spinal cord is sectioned above and below the levels involved. Even in this dramatic scenario, if the tumor has grown into the epidural space, the term *radical* is not appropriate because the epidural space must be considered an extracompartmental area extending from the skull to the sacrum.

All surgical procedures generally directed toward a functional purpose (cord decompression, fracture stabilization), with or without partial (piecemeal) removal of the tumor, are called "palliative." In general, such procedures are only intended to make a diagnosis, decrease pain, and possibly improve function.

The terms *vertebrectomy* (removal of all the elements of the vertebra), *corpectomy*, and *somectomy* (removal of the vertebral body) have no significance from an oncological viewpoint if they are not specified according to the aforementioned terminology.

GUIDELINES FOR SPECIFIC TREATMENTS
Eosinophilic Granuloma (Langerhans Cell Histiocytosis)

Biopsy is mandatory before any treatment is instituted, unless a completely asymptomatic "vertebra plana" without any soft tissue mass is found. Vertebral reconstitution is greater for younger patients.[29] Spontaneous reconstitution of vertebral height has been attributed to the sparing of areas of endochondral ossification.[30]

The ideal treatment for this disease affecting the spine has not fully been realized. For acute pain, a short period of bed rest followed by an orthosis or body jacket often provides symptomatic relief. Local steroid injection has been successfully performed (**Fig. 8**). In patients with neurologic deficits, biopsy and decompression is a reasonable option.[31]

Multifocal occurrence is a sign of systemic disease involving the skeletal system alone or the skeletal system and visceral organs. In the case of multifocal occurrence, the patient must be referred to pediatric oncologist for steroids and chemotherapy.

Osteochondromas

When malignant transformation is suspected, biopsy is indicated and must include the cartilage component. Tumor excision should include the perichondral soft tissue cover and all cartilage extending to normal cortical bone. Tumor excision is recommended for patients complaining of pain and dysfunction caused by pressure on adjacent soft tissues, such as nerves or blood vessels. Adjuvant treatments are not effective.

Osteoid Osteoma

Long-term administration of nonsteroidal anti-inflammatory drugs (NSAIDs) can be as effective as excision for treatment of osteoid osteomas, and without the morbidity associated with surgery, especially in patients in whom operative treatment would be complex or might lead to disability. Pain

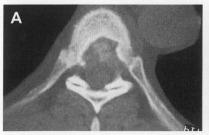
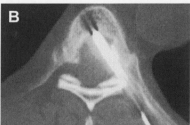
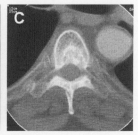

Fig. 8. Eosinophilic granuloma of T10 (*A*) treated with local injection of steroid (*B*). Result at 6 months (*C*).

treated with anti-inflammatory agents can take 30 to 40 months to fully resolve.[32] Because there have been no reports of malignant transformation or metastases, nonoperative treatment remains a viable option, but we need to be aware of the adverse effects of NSAIDs and the possibility that the lesion is an osteoblastoma. Radiation therapy is not necessary and actually may be harmful. Surgical treatment can produce almost immediate pain relief in more than 95% of the cases. On the other hand, incomplete excision is often followed by recurrence of pain. If the lesion does recur, additional attempts at complete excision are recommended. Early diagnosis and complete excision frequently lead to full recovery. Painful scoliosis that develops as a result of an osteoid osteoma is often relieved after excision of the benign lesion if it has not been present for more than 15 months. Lesions that exist for more than 15 months often cause fixed deformities, and raise the concern for lack of correction after excision of the benign tumor.[8] However, in our experience at the Rizzoli Institute, resolution of the deformity is common after excision. Of 16 osteoid osteomas of the spine with associated scoliosis (94% of the cases), deformities in 12 improved or disappeared, and 4 remained unchanged, following the excision of the benign tumor, irrespective of symptom duration.

Recently, we have successfully treated five cases of spinal osteoid osteomas using minimally invasive treatments, either with the use of video endoscopy or a microscope. On one patient we used radiofrequency coagulation. We are convinced this was a safe procedure as the lesion was located in the outer regions (sector 9-10, layer B-C) of the spine, away from important structures that could have been damaged by radiofrequency coagulation.

Osteoblastomas

Osteoblastomas are slowly growing lesions that are locally expansive and destructive, and can often be cured by complete surgical resection. In the vertebrae, intralesional curettage is often the only possible technical solution. However, the authors recommend selecting treatment according to the oncologic staging,[18] as this will likely reduce the recurrence rate significantly. The reported rate of recurrence in the literature is about 10%.[19] Radiation therapy remains controversial and has been reported by some investigators to be ineffective.[12,33] Malignant transformation, spinal cord necrosis, and aggravation of spinal cord compression have been reported.[34,35] The authors believe that radiation therapy should be used as an adjuvant to intralesional excision in stage 3 tumors not suitable for en bloc excision.

Aneurysmal Bone Cysts

For aneurysmal bone cysts, selective arterial embolization is the treatment with the best cost-to-benefit ratio and is indicated when diagnosis is certain on preoperative imaging, when technically feasible and safe, and when neither pathologic fracture nor neurologic involvement are identified (Fig. 9).[36–38]

Complete curettage is the preferred technique (possibly preceded within 48 hours by selective arterial embolization) in cases of pathologic/impending fracture, in cases with neurologic involvement, in anterior or anterolateral locations (sectors 5–8) when selective arterial embolization is not indicated, and in local recurrences after at least two selective arterial embolization procedures.

En bloc marginal excision for posteriorly located aneurysmal bone cysts (sectors 4–9) if selective arterial embolization is not indicated or after local recurrence.[20]

Radiation therapy for these lesions has a limited role and is sometimes associated with poor results,[20] but can be used as an adjuvant postoperatively if chosen. Also, radiation has an adverse effect on growth in children with potential late deformities, as well as having potential late effects on the spinal cord (ie, myelopathy, myelitis, sarcomas).[39,40] The required excision is frequently

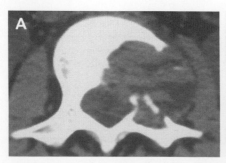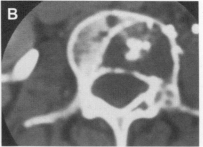

Fig. 9. Aneurysmal bone cyst of L2 (*A*) and 1 year after selective arterial embolization (*B*).

extensive and, with the potential late effects of radiation, instrumented fusion must be considered as part of the procedure with long-term outcomes in mind.

Giant Cell Tumor

Due to the axial location, giant cell tumors of the spine may present at a more advanced stage when compared with those of the extremities and are more challenging surgically. Oncological and surgical staging is helpful for the decision-making process and is based on CT and MRI scans, once histologic diagnosis is made. Selective arterial embolization decreases intraoperative bleeding and is therefore mandatory before intralesional excision. Because local recurrences have a high risk of morbidity from complications related to the tumor and to the surgical management, the initial treatment has to be appropriately tailored. Prolonged disease-free survivals have been reported after curettage and radiotherapy, although some patients require two or more additional procedures because of local recurrence.[41,42] En bloc excision, when feasible, is curative (**Fig. 10**).[23]

In our experience and as indicated in several publications, stage 2 tumors of the spine have much lower recurrence rates compared with stage 3 tumors. As such, wide excision appears to be the choice of treatment for stage 3 tumors, with intralesional complete (extracapsular) excision attempt for the stage 2 lesions.[2,23,41]

Radiation therapy could be an option as adjuvant after complete excision. The 10-year success rate of radiation alone is 69%, compared to 83% for radiation given postoperatively, a difference that is, however, not statistically significant.[43] A high-grade sarcoma occurs in 5% to 15% of cases treated by radiation treatment. On the other hand, giant cell tumors can produce pulmonary metastases without clear biologic relation to their radiographic aggressiveness. These metastases occasionally may regress spontaneously. Some have been controlled by marginal excision. They can be lethal in 25% of cases.

Late recurrences can occur into the fifth year after the final treatment. The risk of these recurrences necessitates local and distant (lung) vigilance with the appropriate imaging studies.

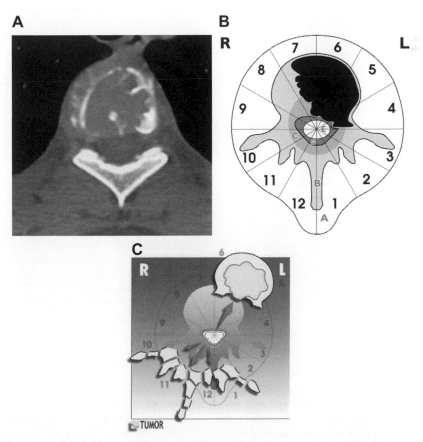

Fig. 10. Giant cell tumor of T10 (*A*) and preoperative planning (*B, C*) for an en bloc resection.

SUMMARY

In determining the most appropriate surgery for obtaining the appropriate margin for any tumor, and therefore for deciding the extent of surgical en bloc or intralesional excision, clinicians must know the biological behavior of the different tumor types. To better identify this behavior, Enneking and colleagues, developed a staging system that was accepted for successful management of extremity tumors.

A surgical staging system is also required for planning the surgical procedure to achieve such margins.[21] The combination of the Enneking staging system and WBB staging systems should aim to:

- help surgeons avoid high-morbidity surgery when not necessary (eg, in stage 2 benign or in metastatic tumors);
- achieve the appropriate margin by correctly guiding the performance of en bloc resections in selected cases;
- enable comparison of outcome data from different institutions.

In deciding how to treat primary tumors of the spine, potential complications have to be taken into consideration because management of such complications can prove to be more difficult than managing the tumor itself. The initial attempt at eradication may be the most important and the best opportunity to reduce the risk of complications and to simplify the management of complications, as well as to ensure local control. Repeat attempts are often difficult and associated with more complications. The ability to combine the best surgical and nonsurgical treatments can affect not only the immediate care of the patient but also long-term survival. Don't perform a biopsy if you are not prepared to perform the definitive treatment. Referral to a center that treats spine tumors is prudent.[44]

REFERENCES

1. Dahlin DC. Bone tumors. General aspects and data on 6221 cases. Springfield (IL): Charles C. Thomas; 1978.
2. Campanacci M. Tumors of bone and soft tissues. Berlin: Aulo Gaggi, Bologna; Springer Verlag; 1990.
3. Huvos AG. Bone tumors. Diagnosis, treatment and prognosis. Philadelphia: Saunders; 1991.
4. Mirra JM, Picci P, Gold RM. Bone tumors. Clinical, radiologic and pathologic correlation. Philadelphia/London: LEA & Febiger; 1989.
5. Schajowicz F. Tumors and tumor like lesions of bone and joints. Berlin: Springer Verlag; 1981.
6. Wilner D. Radiology of bone tumors and allied disorders. Philadelphia: WB Saunders; 1990.
7. Nesbit ME, Kieffer S, D'Angio GJ. Reconstitution of vertebral height in histiocytosis X: a longterm follow-up. J Bone Joint Surg Am 1969;51A:1360–8.
8. Pettine KA, Klassen RA. Osteoid osteomas and osteoblastomas of the spine. J Bone Joint Surg Am 1986;68A:354–61.
9. Afshani E, Kuhn JP. Common causes of low back pain in children. Radiographics 1991;11:277–87.
10. Amacher AL, Eltomey A. Spinal osteoblastoma in children in adolescence. Childs Nerv Syst 1985;1: 29–32.
11. Marsh BW, Bonfiglio M, Brady LP, et al. Benign osteoblastoma: range of manifestations. J Bone Joint Surg Am 1975;57A:1–9.
12. McLeod RA, Dahlin DC, Beabout JW. The spectrum of osteoblastoma. AJR Am J Roentgenol 1976;126: 321–35.
13. Goldenberg RR, Campbell CJ, Bonfiglio M. Giant-cell tumor of bone: an analysis of two hundred and eighteen cases. J Bone Joint Surg Am 1970;52A: 619–24.
14. Sanjay BK, Sim FH, Unni KK, et al. Giant-cell tumours of the spine. J Bone Joint Surg Br 1993; 75B:148–54.
15. Larsson S-E, Lorentzon R, Boquist L. Giant-cell tumor of bone: a demographic, clinical and histopathological study of all cases recorded in the Swedish Cancer Registry for the years 1958 through 1968. J Bone Joint Surg Am 1975;57A:167–73.
16. Shankman S, Greenspan A, Klein MJ, et al. Giant cell tumor of the ischium: a report of two cases and review of the literature. Skeletal Radiol 1988; 17:46–51.
17. Donthineni R, Boriani L, Ofluoglu O, et al. Metastatic behaviour of giant cell tumour of the spine. Int Orthop 2008. May 7 [Epub ahead of print].
18. Enneking WF, Spanier SS, Goodman M. A system for surgical staging of musculoskeletal sarcoma. Clin Orthop 1980;153:106–20.
19. Boriani S, Capanna R, Donati D, et al. Osteoblastoma of the spine. Clin Orthop 1992;278:37–45.
20. Boriani S, De Iure F, Campanacci L, et al. Aneurysmal bone cyst of the mobile spine. Report on 41 cases. Spine 2001;26:27–35.
21. Campanacci M, Boriani S, Giunti A. Giant cell tumors of the spine. In: Sundaresan SN, Schmidek HH, Schiller AL, Rosenthal DI, editors. Tumors of the spine. Diagnosis and clinical management. Philadelphia: WB Saunders; 1990. p. 163–72.
22. Boriani S. Subtotal and total vertebrectomy for tumours. In: Surgical techniques in orthopedics and traumatology 55-070-A. Paris: Editions Scientifiques et Medicales Elsevier; 2000.
23. Hart RA, Boriani S, Biagini R, et al. A system for surgical staging and management of spine tumors.

A clinical outcome study of giant cell tumors of the spine. Spine 1997;22:1773–82.

24. Healy JH, Ghelman B. Osteoid osteoma and osteo-blastoma: current concepts and recent advances. Clin Orthop 1986;204:76–85.

25. Weinstein JN, McLain RF. Primary tumors of the spine. Spine 1987;12:843–51.

26. Boriani S, Weinstein JN, Biagini R. Spine update. A surgical staging system for therapeutic planning of primary bone tumors of the spine. A contribution to a common terminology. Spine 1997;22:1036–44.

27. Boriani S, Weinstein JN. Differential diagnosis and surgical treatment of primary benign and malignant neoplasms. In: Frymoyer JW, editor. The adult spine: principles and practice. 2nd edition. Philadelphia: Lippincott-Raven Publishers; 1997. p. 951–87.

28. Fidler MW. Radical resection of vertebral body tumours. A surgical technique used in ten cases. J Bone Joint Surg Br 1994;76B:765–72.

29. Ippolito E, Farsetti P, Tadisco C. Vertebra plana. Long term follow-up in five patients. J Bone Joint Surg Am 1984;66A:1364–8.

30. Seimon LP. Eosinophilic granuloma of the spine. J Pediatr Orthop 1981;1:371–6.

31. Green NE, Robertson WW Jr, Kilroy AW. Eosinophilic granuloma of the spine with associated neural deficit. Report of three cases. J Bone Joint Surg Am 1980;62A:1198–202.

32. Kneisl J, Simon M. Medical management compared with operative treatment for osteoid osteoma. J Bone Joint Surg Am 1992;72A:179–85.

33. Jackson RP. Recurrent osteoblastoma. Clin Orthop 1978;131:229–33.

34. Conrad E, Olszewski A, Berger M, et al. Pediatric spine tumors with spinal cord compromise. J Pediatr Orthop 1992;4:454–60.

35. Merryweather R, Middlemiss JH, Sanerkin NG. Malignant transformation of osteoblastoma. J Bone Joint Surg Am 1980;62A:381–4.

36. DeRosa G, Graziano G, Scott J. Arterial embolization of aneurysmal bone cyst of the lumbar spine. J Bone Joint Surg Am 1990;72A:777–80.

37. Capanna R, Albisinni U, Picci P, et al. Aneurysmal bone cyst of the spine. J Bone Joint Surg Am 1985;67A:527–31.

38. Hay MC, Patterson D, Taylor TK. Aneurysmal bone cysts of the spine. J Bone Joint Surg Br 1978;60B:406–11.

39. Palmer JJ. Radiation myelopathy. Brain 1972;95:109–22.

40. Tillman BP, Dahlin DC, Lipscomb PR, et al. Aneurysmal bone cyst: an analysis of ninety five cases. Mayo Clin Proc 1968;93:478–95.

41. Di Lorenzo N, Spallone A, Nolletti A, et al. Giant cell tumors of the spine: a clinical study of six cases, with emphasis on the radiological features, treatment, and follow-up. Neurosurgery 1980;6:29–34.

42. Stener B, Jensen E. Complete removal of three vertebrae for giant cell tumor. J Bone Joint Surg Br 1971;53B:278–87.

43. Miszczyk L, Wydmanski J, Spindel J. Efficacy of radiotherapy for giant cell tumor of bone: given either postoperatively or as sole treatment. Int J Radiat Oncol Biol Phys 2001;49:1239–42.

44. Mankin HJ, Mankin CJ, Simon MA. The hazards of the biopsy, revisited. Members of the Musculoskeletal Tumor Society. J Bone Joint Surg Am 1996;78A:656–63.

Primary Malignant Tumors of the Spine

Narayan Sundaresan, MD[a],*, Gerald Rosen, MD[b],
Stefano Boriani, MD[c]

KEYWORDS
- Malignant tumors spine • Chordoma • Chondrosarcoma
- Osteosarcoma • Ewing's sarcoma

The last two decades have witnessed dramatic changes in the approach to tumors of the spine for several reasons.[1–4] Improvement in surgical approaches to the entire vertebral column have made it technically feasible to resect tumors involving the spine at all levels, and the development of third- and fourth-generation instrumentation systems has allowed surgeons to reconstruct entire vertebral segments after surgery. Improvement in the radiologic diagnosis of spine tumors because of the widespread availability of MRI and CT has greatly enhanced the ability of surgeons to visualize tumors in their entirety, plan the proper approach, and assess results of therapy. The introduction of positron emission tomography (PET)-CT scan has further altered treatment paradigms in cancer management. In a recent analysis of the National Oncologic PET registry, change in treatment/management was the major impact of 35% of patients evaluated. It is current standard of care to stage all patients with bone and soft-part sarcoma using PET scans to monitor treatment response and conduct surveillance to detect recurrence.[5] Exciting advances in molecular biology and therapy also offer the promise for treatment not thought feasible before.[6–8] Despite these advances, treatment of spinal tumors is still largely not standardized, and most clinical studies are retrospective reviews of nonuniform treatment modalities spanning several decades.

The field of spinal oncology might be credited properly to the pioneering work of Bertil Stener[9,10] in Goteborg, Sweden. In a series of articles, he described the surgical techniques of en bloc resection of chordomas of the sacrum and chondrosarcomas involving the spine. In an effort to bring uniformity to the field of spine oncology, Boriani and colleagues[11] proposed a staging system for spine tumors based on a system originally developed by Enneking for bone and soft-part sarcomas involving the extremities.

Surgical procedures are classified by the tissue planes and manner of removal.[12–14] "Curettage" and "intralesional" are terms that describe the piecemeal removal of the tumor. Surgeons often characterize a procedure as radical when the tumor capsule was violated by curettage, and we believe that the use of such terms should be avoided. "En bloc" indicates an attempt to remove the whole tumor in one piece, together with a layer of healthy tissue. The specimen is then submitted for careful histologic studies to further define the procedure as intralesional, marginal, or wide. The term "intralesional" is appropriate if the surgeon has cut within the tumor mass; "marginal" is appropriate if the surgeon has dissected along the pseudo-capsule, the layer of reactive tissue around the tumor; and "wide" is appropriate if the plane of surgical dissection is outside the pseudo-capsule, thus removing the tumor with a continuous shell of healthy tissue. This wide en

[a] Mount Sinai Medical School, 1148 Fifth Avenue, New York, NY 10128, USA
[b] Cancer Center, St Vincent's Hospital, 325 W. 15th Street, New York, NY 10001, USA
[c] Department of Orthopaedics and Traumatology–Spine Surgery, Ospedale Maggiore 'C. A. Pizzardi', Largo Nigrisoli 1–40100 Bologna, Italy
* Corresponding author.
E-mail address: drnsundaresan@gmail.com (N. Sundaresan).

Orthop Clin N Am 40 (2009) 21–36
doi:10.1016/j.ocl.2008.10.004
0030-5898/08/$ – see front matter © 2008 Elsevier Inc. All rights reserved.

bloc procedure can be called excision or resection. These terms are too widely used and interchanged for them to be separated. To avoid confusion and compare results, it is essential to distinguish the longer, more difficult, and risky removal of the whole tumor in one piece (en bloc) from a simple intralesional procedure, although this sometimes means the piecemeal removal of the whole vertebra. Intralesional resection of malignant tumors may provide functional palliation and pain relief, but it results in a high incidence of local recurrence.

In this article, we review the current state-of-the-art in primary malignant tumors of the spine. Although various histologic conditions may be encountered in the spine, malignant tumors can broadly be categorized into low-grade and high-grade tumors. Low-grade tumors include chordoma and chondrosarcoma; high-grade tumors include osteosarcoma and other sarcomas, Ewing's sarcoma, and lymphomas. A special category is plasmacytoma, which frequently arises within the spine but later disseminates into multiple myeloma. From an anatomic perspective, low-grade malignant tumors are subdivided into stage 1A (the tumor remains inside the vertebra) and stage 1B (tumor invades paravertebral compartments). No true capsule is associated with these lesions, but a thick pseudo-capsule of reactive tissue often is penetrated by small, microscopic islands of tumor. In these cases a resection performed along the pseudo-capsule often leaves residual foci of active tumor; megavoltage radiation or proton beam therapy often is used as an adjunct to reduce the risk of recurrence. The treatment of choice—if feasible—is a wide en bloc excision.

High-grade malignancies are defined as stages IIA and IIB. The neoplastic growth is so rapid that the host has no time to form a continuous reactive tissue layer. There is continuous seeding with neoplastic nodules (satellites). These tumors also can have neoplastic nodules at some distance from the main tumor mass (skip metastases). These malignancies generally are seen on plain radiographs as radiolucent and destructive and in many cases are associated with a pathologic fracture; CT scanning and MRI give the most detailed views of the transverse and longitudinal extent of these tumors and may confirm the absence of a reactive tissue margin. Invasion of the epidural space is rapid in stage B, particularly in small-cell tumors (Ewing's sarcoma, lymphomas), and is characterized by infiltrating tumor spread beyond the cortical border of the vertebra with no gross destruction. The margin of the en bloc excision must be wide at the very least, because it is not possible to achieve a radical margin in the spine. Adjuvant courses of radiation and chemotherapy (according to the tumor type) must be considered for local control and to prevent distant spread. Stages IIIA and IIIB describe the same lesions as IIA and IIB, but with distant metastasis.

SURGICAL STAGING

Surgical staging is appropriate only after the diagnosis has been established and oncologic staging has been determined. In the transverse plane, the vertebra is divided into 12 radiating zones (numbered 1–12 in a clockwise order) and into five layers (A–E, from the paravertebral extraosseous region to the dural involvement). The longitudinal extent of the tumor is deduced by recording the spine segments involved (**Fig. 1**). CT scanning, MRI, and sometimes angiography of the tumor are the imaging techniques needed to describe the transverse and longitudinal expansion of these tumors. It is the authors' view that this system allows a more rational approach to the surgical planning, provided that all efforts are made to perform surgery along the required margins.

PLANNING OF SURGICAL PROCEDURES

There are three major methods for performing en bloc excisions in the thoracolumbar spine: vertebrectomy, sagittal resection, and resection of the posterior arch. The term "vertebrectomy," which is used to describe removal of the entire tumor in one piece together with portions of the posterior elements, is also termed "spondylectomy."

Vertebrectomy (spondylectomy) involves marginal/wide en bloc excision of the vertebral body (**Fig. 2**). En bloc tumor excision of the vertebral body can be performed with appropriate margins if the tumor is confined to zones 4 to 8 or 5 to 9, which means that it is centrally located and that at least one pedicle is free from tumor. The procedure can be performed in two stages or in one stage. The posterior approach (with patient in the prone position) involves excision of the posterior elements, which enables the annulus fibrosus and the posterior longitudinal ligament to be sectioned. It also allows careful hemostasis of the epidural venous plexus to be achieved and posterior stabilization to be performed. The anterior approach (transpleural thoracotomy, retroperitoneal abdominal, or thoracoabdominal approach) allows the ligature of segmental vessels (at the lesional level, above and below), proximal and distal discectomies (or the section by chisel through the

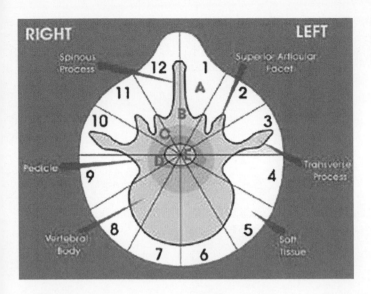

neighboring vertebrae according to the preoperative planning), and the en bloc removal of the vertebral body and anterior reconstruction. The main advantages of performing the vertebrectomy through a bilateral approach are easier ligation of the segmental vessels and dissection of the tumor from the anterior elements entirely under direct vision, which help achieve a better margin when the tumor has expanded anteriorly.

EPIDEMIOLOGY

According to the American Cancer Society, approximately 2380 new cases of bone cancer and 10,390 cases of soft-part sarcomas are diagnosed in the United States each year.[15] Of these cases, approximately 5% involve the spine. The incidence of primary spinal neoplasms has been estimated at 2.5 to 8.5 per 100,000 population per year. Some bone tumors have a special predilection for the vertebral column (eg, osteoblastoma), whereas others (chordoma) occur exclusively in the spine. Tumors of the lymphoid system (eg, plasmacytoma and myeloma) are generally considered in the discussion of spine tumors, although they are tumors of the lymphoreticular system. As a general rule, two important clinical features need to be considered in evaluating the potential malignancy of a lesion in the spine: age and location. More than 75% of lesions located in the vertebral body are malignant, whereas only one third of lesions in the posterior elements are malignant. Second, more than two thirds of all lesions seen in children younger than age 18 are benign, whereas this figure is reversed in adults.

Useful information regarding the relative frequency of the various primary malignancies is available from large national registries and the cancer surveillance (SEER) programs. Dorfman and Czerniak[16,17] analyzed data on 2627 primary malignant tumors of bone collected in the SEER program during the period from 1973 to 1987. Osteosarcoma was the most frequently diagnosed sarcoma of bone (35.1%), followed by chondrosarcoma (25.8%), Ewing's sarcoma (16.0%), chordoma (8.4%), and malignant fibrous histiocytoma, including fibrosarcoma (5.6%). Important racial differences in the spectrum of tumors have been noted in several studies: osteosarcoma is more common in the Chinese and Japanese populations as compared with the white population, whereas chondrosarcoma is less common.[18] In the United States, chordomas and Ewing's sarcoma are seen almost exclusively in the white population.

In a more recent analysis, Damron and colleagues[19] looked at the survival and epidemiologic data from the National Cancer database of the American College of Surgeons. Survival data were reported on cases with a minimum 5-year follow-up from 1985 to 1998. The relative 5-year survival rate was 53.9% for osteosarcoma, 75.2% for chondrosarcoma, and 50.6% for Ewing's sarcoma. In the Leeds tumor registry, which focuses on spine tumors, primary malignant tumors of the spine constituted only 4.6% of the cases registered between 1958 and 2000.[20] The most common malignant spine tumors (based on clinical presentation) were multiple myeloma and plasmacytoma. The second most common tumor was chordoma, being most prevalent in the cervical and sacral regions. The third most common was osteosarcoma. The mean age at presentation was 42 years. Pain was the most common presenting symptom, with it being more common and intense in patients with malignant tumors (96%) versus benign tumors

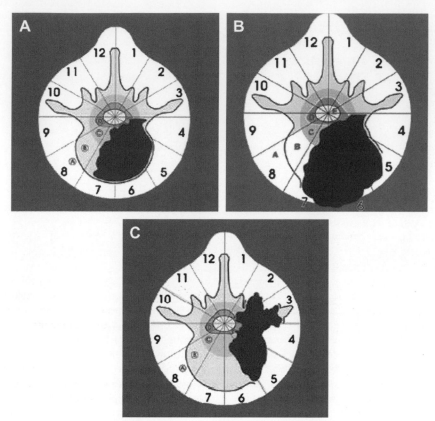

Fig. 2. (*A–C*) En bloc tumor excision of the vertebral bodies can be performed with appropriate margins if the tumor is confined to zones 4–8 or 5–9, with one pedicle that is not involved by tumor.

(76%). Neurologic involvement (cord compression) occurred in 52% of malignant tumors and generally indicated a poorer prognosis.

RADIOLOGY

Most patients with spine tumors are evaluated because of pain or evolving neurologic deficit. Accurate assessment of the spinal segments involved, including staging studies to determine the extent of systemic disease, should be as complete as possible. The major advantages of CT are its wide availability and relative low cost in comparison to MRI. Adequate imaging requires the use of image manipulation using appropriate window width and levels. Currently, CT-guided systems are also used for intraoperative navigation and correct placement of pedicle screws. To a large extent, evaluation of spinal tumors has been revolutionized by MRI. This modality allows tumor assessment in multiplanar dimensions, allows assessment of the entire spine, and detects early marrow invasion and multifocal involvement with great precision. Proper imaging sequences are necessary for full assessment of the tumor.

In patients with hypervascular tumors, spinal angiography may be indicated to diminish tumor vascularity by preoperative embolization and demonstrate the location of critical arteries, such as the artery of Adamkiewicz.[21] Various therapeutic agents are currently used for embolization, of which the most popular is Ivalon (polyvinyl alcohol foam) in particles ranging from 150 to 500 microns in diameter. Reducing intraoperative blood loss has a major impact not only on morbidity but also on the extent of tumor resection that is feasible. Of the primary spine tumors, notoriously vascular lesions include giant cell tumors, hemangiomas, and aneurismal bone cysts, which also should be embolized. In contemporary practice, it is also customary to obtain PET scans as part of the staging process and to monitor the effects of therapy.

BIOPSY

In malignant tumors of bone, it is common to perform a needle biopsy before definitive surgery. Poorly planned biopsies increase the local risk of recurrence by tumor dissemination along fascial planes and the biopsy tract. Biopsies are divided into three different categories: needle biopsy, open incisional biopsy, and excisional biopsies. For tumors limited to the posterior elements, such as osteoblastoma or aneurysmal bone cysts, an excisional biopsy is diagnostic and therapeutic. The most common indication for biopsy is the confirmation of suspected metastatic disease. It is particularly useful in establishing the diagnosis of round cell tumors (eg, Ewing's sarcoma or lymphoma) in which initial chemotherapy is most likely. In other primary malignant tumors, such as osteosarcoma, in which delayed definitive surgery is indicated, needle biopsy may provide the diagnosis so that prompt chemotherapy may be started. Finally, in patients undergoing radiation therapy, biopsy may be indicated to document recurrence; however, the most frequent adverse outcome is a nondiagnostic biopsy. This is particularly true of densely blastic lesions, necrotic tumors, or vascular lesions that may yield insufficient tissue for diagnosis. In experienced hands, the accuracy rate ranges from 80% to 90%.[22–24] In our experience, however, needle biopsy of the spine fails to provide the correct diagnosis or is nondiagnostic in 25% of patients. If an open incisional biopsy is decided on, several fundamental surgical principles should be observed. The incision should be planned so that it can be excised at a definitive operation. Meticulous surgical techniques and homeostasis are essential. Postoperative hematomas carry the potential to disseminate tumor cells along fascial planes. Bone windows should be small and carefully planned so that pathologic fractures do not result, and they must be packed with gelfoam and bone wax. It has been estimated that improper planning of the biopsy and inadequate handling of the tissue is seen in a considerable proportion of patients treated in smaller hospitals, which may adversely affect outcome.[25]

SPECIFIC TUMOR TYPES
Chordomas

Chordomas are rare primary tumors of bone that are thought to arise from the notochord. They constitute between 1% and 4% of bone tumors and are traditionally considered slow growing, locally invasive neoplasms with little tendency to metastasize. Recent data from the Surveillance, Epidemiology, and End Results (SEER) program revealed an annual incidence of 0.08 per 100,000 population, more common occurrence in men (1.0) than women (0.6), and rare in black patients and patients younger than age 40.[26] Within the axial skeleton, 32% were cranial, 32.8% were spinal, and 29.2% were sacral. Younger age and female sex were associated with a higher likelihood of cranial presentation. Although the biologic activity of chordomas varies considerably, more aggressive behavior is usually seen in the younger age group.[27,28]

Nonspecific low back pain is the presenting feature of sacral lesions. In addition to pain, approximately 40% of patients describe symptoms of rectal dysfunction, including obstipation or constipation, tenesmus, or bleeding from associated hemorrhoids. A palpable tumor on rectal examination can be felt in almost every patient. Symptoms are generally of shorter duration in patients with tumors involving the true vertebrae. Almost all patients present with neck or back pain, often with a radicular component. More than two thirds may present with weakness or neurologic deficit, although a minority may have symptoms from the anterolateral soft tissue mass.[29] CT scans demonstrate the bony and soft tissue components of the tumor with ease. More than 90% of sacral tumors have large presacral and posterior extensions of tumor. The soft tissue mass generally has a uniform density, but in 35% of cases irregular lucencies may indicate necrosis. Although the term "calcification" is frequently used to describe the mottled densities seen in the sacrum, it would be more appropriate to use the term "calcific debris."

The use of MRI imaging to evaluate low back pain has greatly revolutionized the diagnosis of chordoma. The combination of sagittal, coronal, and axial imaging clearly outlines the entire tumor extent, especially in the T2-weighted sequences. Soft tissue tumor extensions are especially shown well with long TR and TE (T2-weighted) images, and the presence or absence of a tissue plane between the tumor and rectum is easily seen. There is a characteristic tendency for the tumor to invade the perineurium of spinal nerves and for recurrences to present as high signal intensities on the T2-weighted images.

Grossly, chordomas are lobulated, gray, partially translucent, glistening, cystic, or solid masses that resemble cartilage tumors or occasionally a mucin-producing carcinoma. The consistency varies from firm and focally ossified or calcified tissue to extremely soft, myxoid, gelatinous, or even semifluid material. These tumors seem to be well circumscribed because of a pseudo-capsule formation within soft tissue. In all sacral tumors, intact and elevated periosteum forms the anterior pseudo-capsule of the tumor. In the bone itself, the tumor appears to be multifocal, invading between trabeculae without a clear margin of reactive bone. Microscopically, the tumor is characterized by a distinct, lobular architecture that is formed by the physaliphorous (soap bubble) cells with ample vacuolated cytoplasm and by the "signet ring" type; in between the cells, fibrous septae are incomplete and densely infiltrated by lymphocytes. This tumor may show a wide range in its histologic appearance and pattern. In addition to the areas showing physaliphorous cells, an occasional tumor may show a typical spindle cell sarcoma arrangement or a round cell pattern, whereas others may show an epithelial arrangement.

After treatment with radiation therapy, areas of spindle cell sarcoma formation may be seen. Immunoperoxidase staining is useful in distinguishing chordoma from adenocarcinoma and cartilage tumors. Chordomas are usually positive for keratin and S-100 protein, whereas cartilage tumors are keratin negative and adenocarcinomas are S-100 negative. Naka and colleagues[28] investigated the biologic differences between skull base and non–skull base chordomas; non–skull base chordomas affected more elderly patients and demonstrated a higher MIB-1 labeling index. Apoptosis also was more common in elderly patients and correlated with the appearance of cell necrosis. In recurrent tumors, mitoses and a higher MIB-1 labeling index was seen.[29] Current data also confirm the propensity of these tumors to metastasize; in our series, 30% of patients developed metastases, and this range is consistent with that reported by Berg and colleagues and others.

Currently, newer surgical techniques have improved local control and significantly reduced the likelihood of local recurrence, which in turn is associated with an increased risk of metastases and tumor-related deaths. Bergh and colleagues[30–32] noted that larger tumor size, inadequate surgical margins, tumor necrosis, and the performance of invasive diagnostic procedures outside of a tumor center all were adverse prognostic factors.

Currently, the proper treatment of sacral and vertebral chordomas should be en bloc resection, with the intent to achieve clear margins.[33–37] In patients with sacral tumors, en bloc resection can be performed either by posterior sacrectomy or by using a combined anterior-posterior approach. Some data suggest that anterior- posterior approaches are more likely to result in satisfactory tumor-free margins, but we believe that this decision should be based on the tumor characteristics (ie, extent of presacral soft tissue mass and superior extent of bone involvement of the sacrum). Because bladder, bowel, and sexual functions are mediated through the second through fourth sacral nerves, patients must be warned that the functional effects of bladder, bowel, and sexual loss may be prerequisites to achieving satisfactory margins. For tumors extending to the first sacral or lumbosacral junction, total sacrectomy may be indicated. This procedure clearly has the potential for significant blood loss, and reconstruction and stabilization across the lumbosacral junction may be necessary.

For chordomas that arise in the vertebral body, the true bony and anterolateral soft tissue extent should be defined (**Fig. 3**). En bloc resection of the involved vertebra and tumor should be performed in all cases of vertebral chordoma whenever feasible. This concept is generally accepted as optimum treatment.[38–40] To perform an en bloc resection, the surgical approach should be staged. Generally, we favor an initial posterior approach to stabilize the spine and disconnect the posterior elements, at which time the dural is mobilized and separated from the pseudo-capsule of the tumor anteriorly. The second stage is an anterior en bloc vertebrectomy, followed by reconstruction. We favor the use of a titanium cage filled with autologous bone or recombinant BMP-2. In the cervical spine, management of the vertebral artery is part of the surgical decision-making process. For ipsilateral involvement,

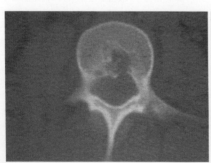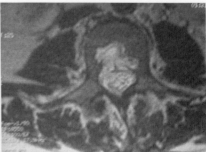

Fig. 3. Radiologic images of chordoma of the lumbar spine potentially curable by en bloc resection. Corresponding CT and MR images identify tumor extent in this patient, who is a long-term survivor.

en bloc resection can be accomplished by endo-vascular trapping of the involved segment with balloons.

Conventional external irradiation is of limited or no value in the treatment of this tumor. Although postoperative radiation therapy RT was routinely used after biopsy or subtotal resection, recur-rences within the first 5 years are common. Before adjunctive treatment is undertaken, it is preferable to refer patients to centers where the expertise ex-ists to complete the resection before irradiation.

Despite its relative lack of response, external ir-radiation is still offered by most radiation oncolo-gists as palliative treatment for subjective pain control and potentially delay time to recurrence.[41] In recent years, it has become customary to use highly conformal higher doses with sparing of critical adjacent structures through the use of combined photon/proton beam therapy, intensity-modulated radiation therapy using linear accelera-tors, or hypofractionation and radiosurgery. Hug and others suggested that an increased response might be seen by combining both photon and high energy proton beam therapy, thus delivering doses radiobiologically equivalent to 70 to 80 Gy.[42–45] The single most important advantage of proton beam therapy is the superior dose distribu-tion produced by the Bragg peak. This combina-tion improves the dose distribution compared with more conventional external beam therapy. High doses can be delivered to critical areas such as the base of the skull and the cervical spine, with the reduced risk of necrosis of the cen-tral nervous system. In most of the reports of par-ticle beam therapy, failures are more common with residual gross disease.[46]

The data on the use of proton beam therapy are still controversial. The chordoma literature ana-lyzed by Brada and colleagues[47] consists of five photon studies, including 100 cases and three pro-ton studies that included 302 cases. Local control and 5-year survival rates were better in the proton series (25% versus 63% and 44% versus 81%). These are not randomized comparisons, and a sur-gical series reported 65% local control in patients, only 20% of whom had any radiotherapy at all. The proton protagonists contend that they have treated the worst cases, but these results cannot be accepted as proof of benefit on the basis of classical health technology assessment criteria. It is important to resect all gross disease before us-ing adjuvant therapy. All data suggest that the cu-rative efforts are best accomplished during the initial attempt, and salvage efforts after recurrence are less likely to be successful.

Despite our current best efforts, the 5-year disease-free survival rate is approximately 65%; late failures are common in chordomas, so survival data at 5 years are likely to be mis-leading. Chordomas are also notorious for seed-ing along the surgical tracts, seen especially after intralesional surgery. Chordomas are resis-tant to chemotherapy. Most patients are referred only after maximum radiation therapy has been given or for treatment of metastatic disease. Re-ports in the literature have suggested occasional subjective and objective responses to chemo-therapy. In patients with dedifferentiated fea-tures or sarcomatous elements, it may be worthwhile to use adriamycin–cisplatin or ifosfa-mide–adriamycin– platinum combinations, such as those used for high-grade spindle cell sarco-mas.[48] In the past, it was not uncommon to en-counter progressive cellularity, spindle cell transformation, and even malignant evolution into malignant fibrous histiocytoma.

The most exciting development in the treatment of recurrent disease has been the demonstration that chordomas respond to molecular targeted agents against the tyrosine kinase and angiogene-sis pathway. Casali and colleagues[49–53] showed that chordomas respond to imatinib (Gleevac) in a small series of patients. We noted long-term sta-ble responses with the use of tarceva (Erlotinib) and irissa (Gefitinib).[54] Because the results of treating recurrent or residual chordoma are poor, some have suggested that proton beam therapy be used as primary therapy even before definitive surgical resection.

Chondrosarcoma

Chondrosarcoma is a malignant tumor in which the basic neoplastic tissue is fully developed carti-lage without tumor osteoid being directly formed by a sarcomatous stroma. Myxoid changes, calci-fication, or ossification may be present. These tu-mors constitute 10% of bone tumors but are exceedingly rare in the spine. Chondrosarcoma may arise de novo in previously normal bone or re-sult from sarcomatous transformation of pre-exist-ing benign cartilage tumor. Repeated surgical excisions after recurrences often precede malig-nant transformation. As with other primary tumors of bone, men are at higher risk than women. The mean age of presentation is appropriately 40 years, with patients ranging from the first to the ninth decades of life. Histologically, tumors may be divided into three grades (low, intermediate, and high) of increasing malignancy. Additional variations include histologic subtypes, such as mesenchymal chondrosarcoma, clear cell chon-drosarcoma, or dedifferentiated chondrosarcoma. The most common presenting feature of chondrosarcoma is pain, associated with neurologic deficit. In the spine, tumors can present as a destructive lesion within the spine or, more commonly, as a paraspinal mass with calcification (**Fig. 4**). Lesions larger than 8 to 10 cm in diameter and bone destruction are features that support the diagnosis of malignancy. In at least 10% of tumors there is a progression toward more anaplasia with local recurrence.

In all patients, treatment should involve complete surgical excision.[55–57] In the case of axial tumors, this may not always be possible. Although chondrosarcomas are resistant to conventional irradiation, the use of particle beam therapy has proved promising. The radiation oncology group at the Massachusetts General Hospital has been using a combination of proton and photon beam therapy to treat primary osseous tumors of the spine, including chordomas and chondrosarcomas. Local control is better achieved in chondrosarcomas in comparison to chordomas.

Osteosarcoma and Other Spindle Cell Sarcomas (Malignant Fibrous Histiocytoma)

Osteosarcoma is the most frequent malignant condition of bone, with an incidence of approximately 5.6 per 1 million children younger than age 15. The peak frequency is during the adolescent growth spurt, and there is no sex- or race-based predilection. Ionizing radiation contributes to the development of some osteosarcomas. Patients with hereditary retinoblastoma have a high risk of second cancers, 50% of which are osteosarcomas. Osteosarcoma can arise in patients with Paget's disease of bone, enchondromatosis, hereditary multiple exostoses, and fibrous dysplasia. Less than 5% of osteosarcomas arise in the axial skeleton. Most patients present with pain and neurologic deficit related to tumor extension into the spinal cord. Plain radiographic findings

may be variable. In the spine, a combination of osteolytic, sclerotic, or mixed patterns may be seen (**Fig. 5**). Pathologic fractures also may occur, and in 90% of cases, the vertebral body is predominantly involved.

The MRI appearance depends heavily on the extent of mineralization: nonmineralized tumor has relatively low signal intensity on T1-weighted images and a bright signal on T2-weighted images. Mineralized tumors may appear dark on all sequences. Radioisotopes using technetium and thallium are particularly helpful in demonstrating either skip or satellite lesions. The use of PET scans is probably the most accurate staging study, however, and serial PET scans are used to monitor effects of therapy. Grossly, the tumor has a reddish, gritty, granular quality because of bone production. All osteosarcomas, despite their classification as to subtype, have as their common feature the production of bone (osteoid) by neoplastic osteoblasts. For simplicity, four divisions may be found, which describes the predominant cell type: osteogenic, chondroblastic, fibroblastic, and secondary osteosarcoma.

Histologically, all osteosarcomas have disorganized, haphazardly arranged spicules or masses of woven bone in a rich vascular stroma. The malignant osteoblasts spring from the background stroma; there is no prominent osteoblastic palisading about the bone spicules. Foci of hemorrhage or necrosis are common features. In all spindle cell and cartilage-producing or giant cell tumors, a diligent search should be made for foci of bone production. If bone production is not evident in a spindle cell malignancy, the tumor may be designated a malignant fibrous histiocytoma or fibrosarcoma based on its overall morphology. The treatment of osteosarcoma of the extremities has been greatly improved by the introduction of multiagent chemotherapy.[58] If the diagnosis of osteogenic sarcoma is established by biopsy,

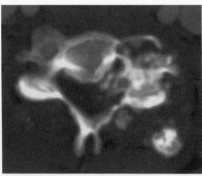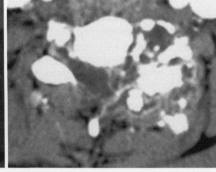

Fig. 4. Chondrosarcoma of the cervical spine. Axial CT images that include bone and soft tissue windows show paraspinal, intraspinal, and intraforaminal extension of tumor, which is heavily calcified.

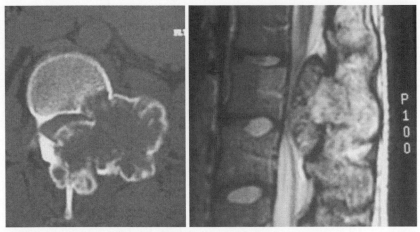

Fig. 5. Axial CT scan and sagital T2-weighted MRI scan of lumbar osteosarcoma.

staging studies are indicated to determine the presence of metastases. In many centers, definitive surgery should be delayed so that early systemic (neoadjuvant) chemotherapy can be instituted. The rationale for early chemotherapy is based on three premises: (1) There is a high likelihood of systemic micrometastases. (2) Regression of the primary tumor makes more effective and less mutilating surgery possible, and in case of spinal lesions, intralesional surgery can be performed with less risk of systemic dissemination. (3) The histologic effects of chemotherapy can be observed in the resected primary specimen, which then allows appropriate planning of future chemotherapy. The amount of necrosis and the persistence of viable tumor cells are also important prognostic factors.

Currently, the only effective treatment for osteosarcoma is total spondylectomy or wide local excision,[59] which should be performed after neoadjuvant chemotherapy has been used to minimize the possibility of local recurrence. In our view, conventional external radiation therapy should not be used except for palliative treatment because these tumors are highly resistant to standard doses of external photon beam radiation. Ozaki and colleagues[60] recently reviewed the results of 22 patients with osteosarcoma of the axial spine (15 with sacral and 7 involving true vertebra). Six patients presented with metastatic disease at onset. Only 12 patients underwent surgery (2 with wide excision, 3 with marginal, and 7 with intralesional). Eight patients received irradiation. The overall median survival was 23 months, with 3 patients surviving longer than 6 years without disease. Patients with metastatic disease at onset, larger tumors, and sacral location had a poorer prognosis. Delaney and colleagues[61] reviewed

the results of external irradiation (photon and/or proton beam) in 41 patients (8 with spinal lesions). The local control rate was 78% for patients undergoing gross total resection, 77% for patients undergoing subtotal resection, and 40% for patients undergoing biopsy only. No definite dose-response rate was seen, although there was a higher local control rate in those receiving doses of 55 Gy or more. They concluded that radiation therapy was more likely to be effective in treating microscopic or minimal residual disease after surgery.

Osteosarcoma also occurs as a sequela of external irradiation in the pediatric population, especially in patients treated for Ewing's sarcoma. Although the incidence of this is less than 5%, it does factor in the debate regarding surgery versus radiation therapy for achieving local control.[62]

Ewing's Sarcoma and Peripheral Neuroectodermal Tumor

Ewing's sarcoma is the prototype of the small, round cell neoplasm of childhood and represents approximately 30% of primary bone tumors in this age group. Ewing's sarcoma is the second most common cancer of bone in children and adolescents, with an incidence of 2.1 per 1 million children in the United States.[63] Occasionally, it may occur at an extraskeletal site.[64] It occurs most often in the second decade of life and is uncommon in children of African or Asian descent. Its cause is unknown. In contrast to osteosarcoma, Ewing's sarcoma does not seem to be caused by exposure to radiation. Currently, with aggressive multimodality treatment, approximately 50% to 60% of patients with localized tumors achieve long-term, relapse-free survival. Approximately

80% of reported cases occur within the first two decades of life. Most patients present with pain and swelling and systemic symptoms, including fever, which may lead to mistaken diagnosis of infection. In spinal lesions, early onset of neurologic symptoms with cord compression is common.[65,66] The sacrum is a common site for axial tumors, where they may grow to a large size before onset of pain. Pelvic lesions may present as a neurogenic bladder. The only reliable blood marker is serum lactic dehydrogenase, which should be monitored closely as an indicator of tumor burden. Radiographic features include a mottled, moth-eaten appearance of irregular bone destruction with poorly defined margins. In the sacrum, the destroyed bone may be replaced with a ground-glass or "cracked ice" appearance.

Approximately 20% of patients present with gross metastatic disease, but the incidence of micrometastases is high. Evaluation for metastatic disease should include chest CT and bone scan and bone marrow aspiration and biopsy. If bone scanning reveals additional suspicious lesions, attempts should be made to obtain histologic verification. Because chemotherapy has considerable potential for cardiac, renal, and hepatic toxicity, assessment of these organs should be included in the pretreatment evaluation.

Ewing's sarcoma encompasses a group of small, round cell malignancies of childhood that include peripheral neuroectodermal tumor of bone, Askin's tumor, and other round cell tumors of childhood. It is believed that Ewing's sarcoma and peripheral neuroectodermal tumor share a common origin from a precursor neural cell. Cytogenetic studies have shown that a fusion protein with enhanced or aberrant transcriptional activity is present in all cases of Ewing's sarcoma, in which unique translocations -t(11;22)(q24.1-q24.3;q12.2) and t(21;22)(22.3;q12.2) fuse the EWSR1 gene on band 22q12.2 to a gene encoding a member of the ETS family of transcription factors.[67] In 85% of cases, this transcription factor is FLI1 on band 11q24.1-q24.3 and ERG on band 22q22.3 in 10%. These chimeric transcription factors possess a potent transactivation domain that induces the transcription of various genes whose expression is required for tumor growth. These tumors also share a consistent pattern of proto-oncogene expression, (ie, high levels of c-*myc*, c-*myb*, and c-*mil*/c-*raf* RNA and a lack of N-*myc* amplification). The differential diagnosis of round cell tumors includes lymphoma, neuroblastoma, and embryonal rhabdomyosarcoma and cannot always be distinguished at the light microscope level. Electron microscopy and immunohistochemistry(CD 99/MIC-2) along with cytogenetic and molecular genetic studies should be part of the initial biopsy evaluation.

Systemic chemotherapy should be the initial treatment of Ewing's sarcoma.[68] Currently, with multimodality treatment, more than half the patients with localized tumors can be cured. There is also considerable debate over the methods used for local control (ie, surgery versus radiation). The third Intergroup Study of Ewing's sarcoma evaluated the addition of etoposide–ifosfamide to the four-drug regimen in a randomized trial and reported a significant improvement in survival among patients with localized disease. The survival rate at 3 years was 80% for patients who received the six-drug regimen as compared with 56% for the patients who received the four-drug regimen. Neither regimen improved survival among the 25% of patients who had metastatic disease at diagnosis.[69,70] A fourth Intergroup Study is currently evaluating dose intensity among patients with localized disease in a randomized trial of a five-drug regimen (vincristine, doxorubicin, cyclophosphamide, ifosfamide, and etoposide) that is given for either 30 or 48 weeks.

Patients with Ewing's sarcoma who have metastatic disease at diagnosis remain a therapeutic challenge. Only about one fifth have not experienced relapse at 5 years. Attempts to improve the outcome in this group by intensifying treatment through the use of myeloablative therapy and stem-cell transplantation have met with limited success. Older age remains an adverse prognostic factor despite the addition of ifosfamide and etoposide. The presence of metastatic disease at onset and large primary tumor size remain the most important prognostic factors, however, which suggests a biologic subset of tumors that is more resistant to chemotherapy. Recent studies have shown that several genetic alterations have been associated with a poorer prognosis in Ewing's sarcoma, such as EWS/FL11 fusion transcript structures, p16/p14 ARF deletion, or p 53 mutations. These genetic alterations indicate resistance to current chemotherapeutic regimens.[71–73] Local control rates with radiation therapy as the primary modality have varied from 55% to 90%. Factors that influence local control include size larder than 8 to 10 in and pelvic or axial location.

Classic radiation therapy dose recommendations include 40 to 45 Gy to the whole field or involved bone followed by a booster dose using a coned-down field to deliver 50 to 60 Gy to the tumor.[74–76] Although the concept of intensive systemic chemotherapy followed by local radiation therapy is considered standard treatment, the role of surgery in local control continues to be debated. In cases of spinal or sacral origin, the presenting feature is generally one of spinal or cauda equina compression. Decompression and tissue diagnosis are usually performed before establishing the diagnosis of Ewing's sarcoma; the long-term result of this strategy is a high incidence of postlaminectomy kyphosis or deformity. Even with intensive systemic chemotherapy and local irradiation, there is a failure of local control in 20% to 25% of patients; thus, surgical eradication of the primary site by en bloc resection is an important consideration in centers with the expertise to perform such surgery. In our view, surgical resection to eradicate local disease is indicated, because obtaining negative margins confers a survival benefit by obtaining superior local control.[77,78]

A major clinical concern in the intensive treatment of Ewing's sarcoma is the development of a second malignancy related to treatment. Dunst and colleagues[79] analyzed the incidence of second malignancies in the German Ewing's Sarcoma Studies CESS 81 and 86. The risk of developing a myelodysplastic/acute myeloid leukemia was 2%, whereas the risk of developing a solid tumor was 5% at 10 years.

Multiple Myeloma and Plasmacytoma

Multiple myeloma is the major malignancy of plasma cells; the feature of osteolytic bone destruction or diffuse osteoporosis with or without fractures distinguishes myeloma from related lymphoid malignancies. It is the second most common hematologic cancer after non-Hodgkin's lymphoma, with an annual prevalence of more than 50,000 patients in the United States alone.[80] Clinically, the disease is characterized by malignant plasma cells in the bone marrow and monoclonal immunoglobulins in the serum or urine or both in 99% of patients.

In approximately 5% of patients, the disease may manifest as a solitary plasmacytoma of bone, with a frequent site being the vertebral column.[81–83] Although most plasmacytomas of bone represent a form fruste of myeloma, in others the disease may remain truly localized with long-term disease-free survival from local radiation therapy alone. In general, patients with solitary plasmacytoma are younger and have greater male predominance, and only two thirds show evidence of a secreting paraprotein. The median survival in patients with multiple myeloma is 28 months, whereas the median survival of patients with solitary plasmacytoma exceeds 60 months. If a paraprotein is secreted, the quantitative levels are generally lower and disappear after local treatment.[84,85] Bone marrow aspirates should show

less than 5% of plasma cells, and most patients generally have preservation of uninvolved immunoglobulins. Because solitary plasmacytoma or myeloma frequently presents with spinal cord compression, serum protein and immune electrophoresis should be performed in all cases of pathologic vertebral compression fractures of the spine in which an obvious primary malignancy is not evident. Decompression of the spinal cord is frequently required because patients present with paraparesis. This technique can be accomplished by posterior stabilization and transpedicular vertebrectomy from a posterior approach.

In patients with solitary plasmacytoma of the spine, long-term remission can be expected with local treatment alone. In our experience, more than two thirds of tumors in these patients evolve into multiple myeloma. The addition of spinal MRI to staging studies has shown a high incidence of marrow abnormalities at other sites, however, which suggests the diagnosis of multiple myeloma.[86,87] Currently, early initial management of these patients includes institution of bisphosphonate therapy and thalidomide/dexamethasone combination treatment if paraproteins are present in the blood or urine.

A substantial proportion of patients with clinically obvious myeloma develop progressive pain and disability from segmental instability or compression fractures after irradiation. A major advance in our therapeutic armamentarium is the use of percutaneous or open kyphoplasty/vertebroplasty to prevent vertebral collapse and relieve pain and disability. The responses to kyphoplasty are so immediately gratifying, with pain improvement in more than 80% of patients, that most radiation oncologists recommend it as a therapeutic maneuver before external radiation therapy or radiosurgery.[88,89]

The persistence or reappearance of paraproteins should be taken as a possible indicator of evolution into myeloma, although this may take place with no rise in abnormal paraproteins. For almost 50 years, the standard of treatment for myeloma was purely palliative, using the drug combination melphalan and prednisone. Standard chemotherapy rarely produced complete remissions. For younger patients, high-dose chemotherapy followed by autologous bone marrow transplantation represented the only promising treatment option.[90,91]

Within the past 5 years there has been a significant paradigm shift in the initial management and continued treatment of patients with multiple myeloma. First a clearer understanding of the mechanisms of bone destruction in myeloma (**Fig. 6**) and the use of bisphosphonates to reduce the morbidity

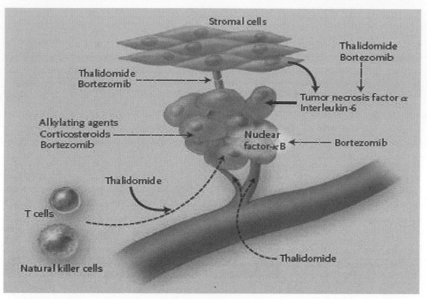

Fig. 6. Therapeutic targets and mechanism of action of drugs in multiple myeloma. (*From* Kyle RA, Rajkumar SV. Multiple myeloma. N Engl J Med 2004;351:1868; with permission.)

of bone resorption clearly had a major impact on treatment.[92,93] Several recent additions to the systemic treatment of myeloma have completely altered the treatment paradigms: the introduction of agents such as thalidomide /dexamethasone and proteosome inhibitors such as bortezomib (Velcade) offers multiple options for individualized treatment.[94–99] Although the use of bisphosphonates has greatly ameliorated the bone pain and osteopenia that were major causes of morbidity in myeloma, newer agents that directly inhibit RANK ligand (Denosumab) are in clinical trials and just on the horizon. These exciting advances have clearly expanded the possibilities for cure in myeloma. These exciting advances must be tempered by the fact that this is still a deadly disease, with a 10% death rate in the early stages.[100]

Primary Lymphomas

Malignant lymphomas account for 10% of all cancers in patients younger than age 15. Approximately 60% of lymphomas in children are non-Hodgkin's lymphoma, and occasionally, lymphomas may arise in bone.[101] Spinal cord compression may result from soft tissue tumor within the epidural space without apparent bone involvement—the so-called "epidural lymphoma." Most patients are within the fifth or sixth decades of life. Between 5% and 25% of non-Hodgkin's lymphomas arise at extranodal sites, and primary lymphoma of bone constitutes 5% of all bone tumors. The spinal cord may be compressed by two separate mechanisms:

tumors may originate in the vertebra or in retroperitoneal nodes and secondarily involve the epidural space. In patients who present with spinal cord compression, urgent decompression may be necessary. If the diagnosis of lymphoma is suspected, fresh tissue should be sent for marker studies, immunoperoxidase testing, and electron microscopy. Proper clinical staging includes the performance of bone scans, CT evaluation of the chest and abdomen, and bone marrow biopsy.

For many years, the most popular staging system was the Ann Arbor staging system; tumors that arose from a vertebra would be staged as 1E (denoting single extranodal site) or stage IV if other sites of involvement were noted. The staging also took into account the presence or absence of constitutional symptoms such as fever, night sweats, or weight loss (designated A or B). Recently, other important factors have been found to be of prognostic value, including maximal diameter of tumor, specific site of extranodal origin, performance status, and serum lactic dehydrogenase levels. Patients with diffuse large cell or immunoblastic non-Hodgkin's lymphoma that involves the epidural space require central nervous system prophylaxis.

If the spinal cord has been decompressed satisfactorily by laminectomy, we currently recommend the use of systemic chemotherapy before radiation therapy, because most patients have occult stage IV disease. Truly localized lymphoma in the epidural space is rare. Because most patients have non-Hodgkin's lymphoma, chemotherapy regimens that incorporate cytoxan, adriamycin, oncovin, and prednisone (CHOP) are most appropriate. Local radiation therapy should be deferred until several cycles of chemotherapy have been completed.

SUMMARY

There has been substantial progress in the understanding of the basic biology, therapeutics, and surgical management of primary malignant tumors of the spine. The cure rate (or disease-free progression at 5 years) has reached a plateau at 50% to 70%, underscoring the need for more improvement. Despite the impressive cure rate in childhood sarcomas, long-term morbidity in terms of cardiac, pulmonary, endocrine, and psychologic deficits have to be taken into account, as should the possibility of increased risk of second malignancies related to therapy.

REFERENCES

1. Sundaresan N, Schiller A, Schmidek HH, et al. Tumors of the spine: diagnosis and management. Philadelphia: WB Saunders; 1990.
2. Sundaresan N, Boriani S, Rothman A, et al. Tumors of the osseous spine. J Neurooncol 2004;69: 273–90.
3. Lewis VO. What's new in musculoskeletal oncology. J Bone Joint Surg Am 2007;89: 1399–407.
4. Weber KL. What's new in musculoskeletal oncology. J Bone Joint Surg Am 2005;87: 1400–10.
5. Hillner BE, Siegel BA, Liu D, et al. Impact of positron emission tomography/computed tomography and positron emission tomography (PET) alone on expected management of patients with cancer: initial results from the national oncologic PET registry. J Clin Oncol 2008;26:2155–61.
6. Croce CM. Oncogenes and cancer. N Engl J Med 2008;358:502–11.
7. O'Connor JPB, Jackson A, Asselin MC, et al. Quantitative imaging biomarkers in the clinical development of targeted therapeutics: current and future perspectives. Lancet Oncol 2008;9:766–76.
8. Ludwig JA, Weinstein JN. Biomarkers in cancer staging; prognosis and treatment selection. Nat Rev Cancer 2005;5(11):845–56.
9. Stener B. Musculoskeletal tumor surgery in Goteborg. Clin Orthop Relat Res 1984;191:8–20.
10. Stener B. Complete removal of vertebrae for extirpation of tumors: a 20-year experience. Clin Orthop Relat Res 1989;245:72–82.
11. Boriani SR, Weinstein JN, Biagini R. Spine update: primary bone tumors of the spine. Spine 1997;22: 1034–6.
12. Sundaresan N, Digiacinto GV, Krol G, et al. Spondylectomy for malignant tumors of the spine. J Clin Oncol 1989;7:1485–91.
13. Boriani S, Biagini F, Delure S, et al. En bloc resections of bone tumors of the thoracolumbar spine. Spine 1996;21:1927–31.
14. Tomita K, Kawahara N, Baba H, et al. Total en bloc spondylectomy: a new surgical technique for primary malignant vertebral tumors. Spine 1997;22: 324–33.
15. American Cancer Society. Facts and figures. 2008. Available at: http://www.americancancersociety.org. Accessed November 19, 2008.
16. Dorfman HD, Czerniak B. Bone cancers. Cancer 1995;75:203–10.
17. Dorfman H, Czerniak B. Bone tumors. St. Louis (MO): Mosby; 1998.
18. Guo W, Xu W, Huvos AG, et al. Comparative frequency of bone sarcomas among different racial groups. Chin Med J 1999;112:1101–4.
19. Damron TA, Ward WG, Stewart A. Osteosarcoma, chondrosarcoma, and Ewing's sarcoma: National Cancer Data Base Report. Clin Orthop Relat Res 2007;459:40–7.
20. Kelley SP, Ashford RU, Rao AS, et al. Primary tumors of the spine: a 42 year old survey from the Leeds Regional Bone Tumor Registry. Eur Spine J 2007;16(3):405–9.
21. Berenstein A, Lasjaunias P. Surgical neuroangiography: endovascular treatment of spine and spinal cord lesions. New York: Springer-Verlag; 1992.
22. Ghelman BM, Lospinuso D, Levine D, et al. Percutaneous computed tomography guided biopsy of the thoracic and lumbar spine. Spine 1991;16: 736–9.
23. Ozsarkak O, DeShepper AM, Wang X, et al. CT guided percutaneous needle biopsy in spine lesions. JBRBTR 2003;86:294–6.
24. Dupuy DE, Rosenberg AE, Punyaratabandhu T, et al. Accuracy of CT-guided needle biopsy of musculo-skeletal neoplasms. American Journal Roentgenology and Therapeutics 1998;171:759–62.
25. Mankin HJ, Mankin CJ, Simon MA. The hazards of biopsy revisited. J Bone Joint Surg Am 1996;78: 656–63.
26. McMaster ML, Goldstein AM, Bromley CM, et al. Chordoma: incidence and survival patterns in the United States 1973–1995. Cancer Causes Control 2001;12:1–11.
27. Eriksson B, Gunterberg B, Kindblom LG. Chordoma: a clinicopathologic and prognostic study of a Swedish national series. Acta Orthop Scand 1981;52: 49–58.

28. Naka T, Boltze C, Samii A, et al. Skull base and non skull base chordomas: clinicopathologic and immunohistochemical study with special reference to nuclear pleomorphism and proliferative ability. Cancer 2003;98:1934–41.

29. Kilgore S, Prayson RA. Apoptotic and proliferative markers in chordomas: a study of 26 tumors. Ann Diagn Pathol 6:222–8.

30. Sundaresan N, Huvos A, Krol G, et al. Surgical treatment of spinal chordomas. Arch Surg 1987;122:1479–81.

31. Bergh P, Kindblom LG, Gunterberg B, et al. Prognostic factors in chordoma of the sacrum and mobile spine: a study of 39 patients. Cancer 2000;88:2122–34.

32. McPherson CM, Suki D, McCutcheon IE, et al. Metastatic disease from spinal chordoma: a 10-year experience. J Neurosurg Spine 2006;5:277–8.

33. Fuchs B, Dickey ID, Yaszemski MJ, et al. Operative management of sacral chordoma. J Bone Joint Surg Am 2005;87:2211–6.

34. Wuisman P, Lieshout O, Sugihara S, et al. Total sacrectomy and reconstruction: oncologic and functional outcome. Clin Orthop 2000;381:192–203.

35. York JE, Kaczaraaj A, Abi-Said D, et al. Sacral chordoma: 40 year experience at a major cancer center. Neurosurgery 1999;44:74–9.

36. Fourney DR, Rhines LD, Hentschel SJ, et al. En bloc resection of primary sacral tumors: classification of surgical approaches and outcome. J Neurosurg Spine 2005;3:111–22.

37. Hulen CA, Temple HT, Fox WP, et al. Oncologic and functional outcome following sacrectomy for sacral chordoma. J Bone Joint Surg Am 2006;88:1532–9.

38. Bosma JJ, Pigott TJ, Pennie BH, et al. En bloc removal of the lower lumbar vertebral body for chordoma: report of two cases. J Neurosurg 2001;94:284–91.

39. Leitner Y, Shabat S, Boriani L, et al. En bloc resection of a C4 chordoma: surgical technique. Eur Spine J 2007;16:2238–42.

40. Currier BL, Papagelopoulos PJ, Krauss WE, et al. Total en bloc spondylectomy of C5 vertebra for chordoma. Spine 2007;32:294–9.

41. Tai PT, Craighead P, Bagdon F. Optimization of radiotherapy for patients with cranial chordoma: a review of dose-response ratios for photon techniques. Cancer 1995;75:749–56.

42. Hug EB, Fitzek MM, Liebsch NJ, et al. Locally challenging osteo- and chondrogenic tumors of the axial skeleton: results of combined proton and photon radiation therapy using three-dimensional treatment planning. Int J Radiat Oncol Biol Phys 1995;31:467–76.

43. Hug EB, Slater JD. Proton radiation therapy for chordomas and chondrosarcomas of the skull base. Neurosurg Clin N Am 2000;11:627–38.

44. Munzenrider JE, Liebsch NJ. Proton therapy for tumors of the skull base. Strhlenther Onkol 1999;175:57–63.

45. Noel G, Feuvret L, Dhermain F, et al. Chordomas of the base of the skull and upper cervical spine. 100 patients irradiated by a 3D conformal technique combining photon and proton beams. Cancer Radiother 2005;9:161–74.

46. Schulz-Ertner D, Karger CP, Feuerhake A, et al. Effectiveness of carbon ion radiotherapy in the treatment of skull-base chordomas. Int J Radiat Oncol Biol Phys 2007;68:449–57.

47. Brada Michael, Pijls-Johannesma Madelon, Ruysscher Dirk De. Proton therapy in clinical practice: current clinical evidence. J Clin Oncol 2007;25(No 8):965–70.

48. Hanna SA, Tirabosco R, Amin A, et al. Briggs dedifferentiated chordoma: a report of four cases arising de novo. J Bone Joint Surg Br 2008;90(5):652–6.

49. Casali PG, Stacchiotti S, Sangalli C, et al. Chordoma. Curr Opin Oncol 2007;19:367–70.

50. Stacchiotti S, Ferrari S, Ferraresi V, et al. Imatinib mesylate in advanced chordoma: a multicenter phase II study. J Clin Oncol 2007;25(Suppl 18):10003 [abstract].

51. Weinberger PM, Yu Z, Kowalski D, et al. Differential expression of epidermal growth factor receptor, c-Met, and HER2/neu in chordoma compared with 17 other malignancies. Arch Otolaryngol Head Neck Surg 2005;131:707–11.

52. Hof H, Welzel T, Debus J. Effectiveness of cetuximab/gefitinib in the therapy of a sacral chordoma. Onkologie 2006;29:572–4.

53. Tamborini E, Miselli F, Negri T, et al. Molecular and biochemical analyses of platelet-derived growth factor receptor (PDGFR) B, PDGFRA, and KIT receptors in chordomas. Clin Cancer Res 2006;12:6920–8.

54. Park L, Delaney TF, Liebsch NJ, et al. Sacral chordomas: impact of high-dose proton/photon-beam radiation therapy combined with or without surgery for primary versus recurrent tumor. Int J Radiat Oncol Biol Phys 2006;65:1514–21.

55. York JE, Berk RH, Fuller GN, et al. Chondrosarcoma of the spine: 1954–1997. J Neurosurg 1999;90:73–8.

56. Boriani S, De Iure F, Bandiera S, et al. Chondrosarcoma of the mobile spine: report of 22 cases. Spine 2000;25:804–12.

57. Bergh P, Gunterberg B, Meis-Kindblom JM, et al. Prognostic factors and outcome of pelvic, sacral, and spinal chondrosarcomas: a center based study of 69 cases. Cancer 2001;91:1201–12.

58. Sundaresan N, Rosen G, Huvos A, et al. Combined treatment of osteosarcoma of the spine. Neurosurgery 1988;23:714–9.

59. Kawahara N, Tomita K, Fujita T, et al. Osteosarcoma of the thoracolumbar spine: total en bloc spondylectomy. A case report. J Bone Joint Surg Am 1997;79:453–8.

60. Ozaki T, Flege S, Liljenqvist U, et al. Osteosarcoma of the spine: experience of the cooperative osteosarcoma study group. Cancer 2002;94(4): 1069–77.

61. Delaney TF, Park L, Goldberg SI, et al. Radiotherapy for local control of osteosarcoma. Int J Radiat Oncol Biol Phys 2005;61:492–8.

62. Koshy M, Paulino AC, Mai WY, et al. Radiation-induced osteosarcoma in the pediatric population. Int J Radiat Oncol Biol Phys 2005;63:1169–74.

63. Arndt CAS, Crist WM. Common musculoskeletal tumors of childhood and adolescence. N Engl J Med 1999;341:342–52.

64. Kennedy JG, Eustace S, Caulfield R, et al. Extraskeletal Ewing's sarcoma: case report and review of the literature. Spine 2000;25:1996–9.

65. Grubb MR, Bradford LC, Pritchard DJ, et al. Primary Ewing sarcoma of the spine. Spine 1994;19: 309–13.

66. Marco RAW, Gentry JB, Rhines LD, et al. Ewing's sarcoma of the mobile spine. Spine 2005;7:769–73.

67. Frohling S, Dohner H. Chromosomal abnormalities in cancer. N Engl J Med 2008;359:722–34.

68. Rosen G, Caparros B, Mosende C, et al. Curability of Ewing's sarcoma and consideration for future therapeutic trials. Cancer 1978;41:888–99.

69. Grier HE, Krailo MD, Tarbell NJ, et al. Addition of ifosfamide and etoposide to standard chemotherapy for Ewing's sarcoma and primitive neuroectodermal tumor of bone. N Engl J Med 2003;348: 694–701.

70. Evans RG, Nesbit ME, Gehan EA, et al. Multimodal therapy for the management to localized Ewing's sarcoma of pelvic and sacral bones: a report from the second intergroup study. J Clin Oncol 1991;9:1173–80.

71. Zoubek A, Dockhorn-Dworniczak B, Delattre O, et al. Does expression of different EWS chimeric transcripts define clinically distinct risk groups for Ewing tumor patients? J Clin Oncol 1996;14: 1245–51.

72. de Alava E, Antonescu CR, Panizo A, et al. Prognostic impact of P53 status in Ewing's sarcoma. Cancer 2000;89:783–92.

73. Huang HY, Illei PB, Zhao Z, et al. Ewing sarcoma with p53 mutation or p16/p14ARF homozygous deletion: a highly lethal subset associated with poor chemotherapy response. J Clin Oncol 2005;23: 548–55.

74. La TH, Meyers PA, Wexler LH, et al. Radiation therapy for Ewing's sarcoma: results from memorial Sloan-Kettering in the modern era. Int J Radiat Oncol Biol Phys 2006;64:544–50.

75. Schuck A, Ahrens A, Von Schorlemer I, et al. Radiotherapy in Ewing tumors of the vertebra: treatment results and local relapse of the CESS 81/86 and EI-CESS 92 trials. Int J Radiat Oncol Biol Phys 2005; 63:1562–7.

76. Rock J, Kole M, Fang-Fang Y, et al. Radiosurgical treatment for Ewing's sarcoma of the lumbar spine. Spine 2002;27:471–5.

77. Scully SP, Temple HT, O'Keefe RJ, et al. Role of surgical resection in pelvic Ewing's sarcoma. J Clin Oncol 1995;13:2336–41.

78. Bacci G, Longhi A, Briccoli A, et al. The role of surgical margins in treatment of Ewing's sarcoma family tumors: experience of a single institution with 512 patients treated with adjuvant and neoadjuvant chemotherapy. Int J Radiat Oncol Biol Phys 2006; 65:766–72.

79. Dunst J, Ahrens S, Paulussen M, et al. Second malignancies after treatment for Ewing's sarcoma: a report of the CESS Studies. Int J Radiat Oncol Biol Phys 1998;42.379–84.

80. Kyle RA, Rajkumar SV. Multiple myeloma. N Engl J Med 2004;351:1860–73.

81. Dimopoulos M, Goldstein J, Fuller L, et al. Curability of solitary bone plasmacytoma. J Clin Oncol 1992;10:587–90.

82. Knowling M, Harwood A, Bergasagel D. A comparison of extramedullary plasmacytoma with multiple and solitary plasma cell tumors of bone. J Clin Oncol 1983;1:255–62.

83. Liebross RH, Ha CS, Cox JD, et al. Solitary bone plasmacytoma: outcome and prognostic factors following radiotherapy. Int J Radiat Oncol Biol Phys 1998;41(5):1063–7.

84. Ozsahin M, Tsang RW, Poortmans P, et al. Outcomes and patterns of failure in solitary plasmacytoma: a multicenter rare cancer network study of 258 patients. Int J Radiat Oncol Biol Phys 2006; 64(1):210–7.

85. Wilder RB, Ha CS, Cox JD, et al. Persistence of myeloma protein for more than one year after radiotherapy is an adverse prognostic factor in solitary plasmacytoma of bone. Cancer 2002;94(5): 1532–7.

86. Moulopoulos LA, Varma DG, Dimopoulos MA, et al. Multiple myeloma: spinal MR imaging in patients with untreated newly diagnosed disease. Radiology 1992;185(3):833–40.

87. Lecouvet FE, Vande Berg BC, Michaux L, et al. Stage III multiple myeloma: clinical and prognostic value of spinal bone marrow MR imaging. Radiology 1998;209(3):653–60.

88. McDonald RJ, Trout AT, Gray LA, et al. Vertebroplasty in multiple myeloma: outcomes in a large patient series. AJNR Am J Neuroradiol 2008;29(4):642–8.

89. Hentschel SJ, Burton AW, Fourney DR, et al. Percutaneous vertebroplasty and kyphoplasty performed

at a cancer center: refuting proposed contraindications. J Neurosurg Spine 2005;2(4):436–40.

90. Child JA, Morgan GJ, Davies FE, et al. High dose chemotherapy with hematopoietic stem cell rescue for multiple myeloma. N Engl J Med 2003;348: 1875–83.

91. Attal M, Harousseau JL, Facon T, et al. Single versus double autologous stem-cell transplantation for multiple myeloma. N Engl J Med 2003;349:2495–502.

92. Edwards CM, Zhuang J, Mundy GR. The pathogenesis of bone disease of multiple myeloma. Bone 2008;42:1007–13.

93. Berenson JR, Hillner BE, Kyle RA, et al. American Society of Clinical Oncology clinical practice guidelines: the role of bisphosphonates in multiple myeloma. J Clin Oncol 2002;17:3719–36.

94. Richardson P, Anderson K. Thalidomide and dexamethasone: a new standard of care for initial therapy in multiple myeloma. J Clin Oncol 2006;24(3): 334–6.

95. Hicks LK, Haynes AE, Reese DE, et al. A meta-analysis and systemic review of thalidomide for patients with previously untreated multiple myeloma. Cancer Treat Rev 2008;34:442–52.

96. Rajkumar SV, Rosiñol L, Hussein M, et al. Multicenter, randomized, double-blind, placebo-controlled study of thalidomide plus dexamethasone compared with dexamethasone as initial therapy for newly diagnosed multiple myeloma. J Clin Oncol 2008;26(13):2171–7.

97. Utecht KN, Kolesar J. Bortezomib: a novel chemotherapeutic agent for hematologic malignancies. Am J Health Syst Pharm 2008;65(13): 1221–31.

98. Katzel JA, Hari P, Vesole DH. Multiple myeloma: charging toward a bright future. CA Cancer J Clin 2007;57:301–18.

99. San-Miguel J, Harousseau JL, Joshua D, et al. Individualizing treatment of patients with myeloma in the era of novel agents. J Clin Oncol 2008;26: 2761–6.

100. Augustson Bradley M, Begum Gulnaz, Dunn Janet A, et al. Drayson early mortality after diagnosis of multiple myeloma: analysis of patients entered onto the United Kingdom Medical Research Council Trials between 1980 and 2002. Medical Research Council Adult Leukaemia Working Party. J Clin Oncol 2005;23((36):9219–26.

101. Loeffler JS, Tarbell NJ, Kozakewich H, et al. Primary lymphoma of bone in children: analysis of treatment results with adriamycin, prednisone, oncovin (APO) and local radiation therapy. J Clin Oncol 1986;4(4):496–501.

Algorithms and Planning in Metastatic Spine Tumors

Yasuaki Tokuhashi, MD*, Yasumitsu Ajiro, MD,
Masashi Oshima, MD

KEYWORDS

- Prognosis evaluation system
- Metastatic spine tumor • Surgical indication
- Treatment modality • Decision making

Metastatic spine tumors cause the loss of the supporting function of the spine through vertebral destruction or invade and compress the spinal cord or cauda equine. As a result, metastatic spine tumor causes severe pain, paralysis, or impairment of activities of daily living (ADL).[1–4] Also, because the finding of metastatic foci in the spine suggests a generalized disorder, life expectancy and treatment options have many limitations. For this reason, treatment is primarily symptomatic, and the major goals in selecting therapeutic modalities are to relieve pain, prevent paralysis, and improve ADL.[2–4] Among the various treatment modalities, surgery should be considered in the initial steps.[1–3] Furthermore, surgery can achieve long-term local control in selected cases. This article discusses the selection of treatment for metastatic spine tumors and, in particular, the indications for surgical treatment.

PRINCIPLES OF THERAPEUTIC STRATEGY FOR METASTATIC SPINE TUMORS

If a metastatic spinal lesion is diagnosed in a patient who has a history of cancer, a recurrence should be suspected, although it must be confirmed histologically.[5] Multidisciplinary treatment is necessary for metastatic spine tumors, and if possible the recruitment of the previously treating oncologist should be attempted.[5,6] Even if there are temporary improvements in symptoms, the goal of the treatments should be for the longer

term, and the possibility of relapse and worsening of the general condition should be considered.

If the primary lesion is unknown, treatment for pain and paralysis and a prompt search for the primary lesion must be performed simultaneously.[5,6] In decreasing order of incidence, spinal metastases arise from primary lung, prostate, kidney, liver, gastric, and colon cancers in males and from primary breast, lung, uterine, thyroid, and gastric cancers in females.[7] Most patients who have spinal metastases from digestive tract cancers have a history of treatment for such cancers. On the other hand, the primary tumor sometimes is not identified. In such cases, it is important to perform chest, abdomen, and pelvis CT and serum tumor markers looking for possible lung cancer and kidney cancer in males, prostate cancer in elderly men, and breast cancer and lung cancer in females.[7,8] Simultaneously, the possibility of blood dyscrasia, such as multiple myeloma or malignant lymphoma, should be investigated.[5–7] If the primary cancer is unknown, the new focus (single or multiple) should be biopsied. When the primary lesion has been identified, treatment modalities should be evaluated with the oncologist. Treatment modalities for metastatic spine tumors include hormonal therapy or chemotherapy as systemic therapies and radiotherapy, bracing, or surgery as local therapies. Treatment should be selected in collaboration with oncologists and radiotherapists by evaluating the pathology of the cancer, its sensitivity to adjuvant

Department of Orthopaedic Surgery, Nihon University School of Medicine, 30-1 Oyaguchi-kamimachi, Itabashi-ku, Tokyo, 173-8610, Japan
* Corresponding author.
E-mail address: ytoku@med.nihon-u.ac.jp (Y. Tokuhashi).

Orthop Clin N Am 40 (2009) 37–46
doi:10.1016/j.ocl.2008.09.002

treatments, and the patient's general condition and expected survival. The decision process and treatments should be prompt and flexible to accommodate the urgency.[2–7,9,10]

SURGICAL INDICATIONS FOR METASTATIC SPINE TUMORS

Currently, common indications for surgery are[1–3]

- Pain and/or paralysis caused by spinal instability
- Pain and/or paralysis caused by spinal cord invasion of tumor
- Pain caused by radioresistant cancer
- Sustained pain resisting conservative treatment
- Long-term local control in patients who have localized lesions and a life expectancy of at least 1 year

Harrington's classification for evaluating surgical indications is well known.[1,8] This classification consists of five categories:

1. No significant neurologic involvement
2. Involvement of bone without collapse or instability
3. Major neurologic impairment (sensory or motor) without significant involvement of bone
4. Vertebral collapse with pain resulting from mechanical causes or instability but with no significant neurologic compression
5. Vertebral collapse or instability combined with major neurologic impairment

Harrington argued that categories 1, 2, and 3 should be regarded as indications for conservative treatment and that categories 4 or 5 require surgical intervention.[8] Patients in category 3 sometimes undergo surgical intervention because of a greater risk of neurologic degradation or unchanging paralysis.[11] Thus, bone involvement has been considered an important factor in evaluating indications for surgery.

Indication one: pain and/or paralysis caused by spinal instability.

Even today, surgery is considered the most effective treatment for pain and paralysis caused by spinal instability, because patients can attain immediate relief not provided by other treatment modalities.[1,2] There is, however, no clear evidence supporting this indication for surgery.

Kostuik's[12] six-column concept has been used often for the evaluation of spinal instability. Kostuik divided the vertebra into six segments, four segments that are cross-sections of vertebral bodies and two segments comprised of posterior

elements, and proposed that spinal instability can occur when the tumor occupies three or more segments and is severe when five or more segments are involved. He also proposed that instability is present when angular collapse of the vertebral body is 20° or greater (**Fig. 1**).[12] This classification is a useful general guideline, but it is not always applicable, because a tumor may invade three or more segments without causing symptoms.

Indication Two: Involvement of Bone Without Collapse or Instability

In patients experiencing pain and/or paralysis caused by invasion of the spinal cord by tumor, recovery has been considered impossible unless significant decompression is performed within 24 hours after the establishment of complete paralysis.[1–3] Therefore, emergency surgery (formerly laminectomy and now usually posterior decompression and stabilization) has been performed. In patients who have very rapidly progressing paralysis (ie, progressively worsening ambulatory incapacity deteriorating each day to complete paralysis), surgery might alleviate the paralysis temporarily, but the paralysis often recurs or deterioration resumes within a few days to 1 to 2 weeks after surgery.[13] Emergency radiotherapy also has been reported to be effective.[10] For this reason, spinal cord paralysis is no longer regarded as an absolute indication for emergency surgery, but surgery may still be the treatment of choice because of limited availability of emergency radiotherapy or other considerations. The effectiveness of direct decompression by surgical resection has been demonstrated by a randomized, controlled study comparing radiotherapy alone with radiotherapy plus surgery.[14]

Indication Three: Pain Caused by Radioresistant Cancer

Pain caused by radioresistant cancer generally has been excluded as an indication for surgery, because radiotherapy is widely considered to be effective in 80% to 90% of cancers and has long been considered the first choice for treating spinal metastasis of cancer.[2,10] Recently, however, as the sensitivity to adjuvant treatments has begun to be considered in selecting treatment, pain caused by radioresistant cancer has become an important indication for surgery,[5,7,9] particularly in kidney cancers, which now are treated by debulking surgery followed by interferon therapy or radiotherapy.

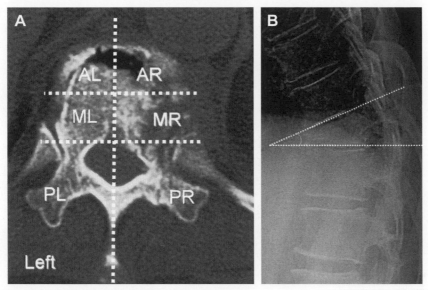

Fig. 1. Evaluation of spinal instability in patients with spine tumor. (*A*) Kostuik and colleagues[12] thought that the spine was stable if no more than two of the six segments were destroyed and was unstable if three or more segments were destroyed. (*B*) They thought that the spine was also unstable if the angular deformity caused by vertebral collapse was more than 20°. AL, anterior left; AR, anterior right; ML, middle left; MR, middle right; PL, posterior left; PR, posterior right.

Indication Four: Sustained Pain Resisting Conservative Treatment

Because of recent improvements in pain-control techniques, including narcotic analgesics, surgery now is performed less often than in the past when the only indication is sustained pain resisting conservative treatment.

Indication Five: Long-Term Local Control

In practice, very few patients fit the indication of long-term local control, because these must have localized lesions and a life expectancy of at least 1 year. Excellent levels of ADL and local control have been achieved in patients who survived for a long period after en bloc resection, however.[5,9,15,16] Therefore, patient selection is more important in this indication than in any of the other indications.

LIMITATIONS OF SURGERY FOR METASTATIC SPINE TUMORS

Surgery may not be the optimal choice for all patients who fit the indications for surgery, because the procedure itself involves significant morbidity. Surgery cannot be recommended unless the patient selection criteria discussed in the next sections are fulfilled.[5,17]

General Condition

Because patients who have spinal metastases experience considerable postsurgical morbidity,

a thorough evaluation of the patient's general condition before and after surgery is important. A reasonably healthy presentation that enables the patient to undergo general anesthesia safely and a positive attitude toward the goals of treatment (eg, will to live) are minimum requirements.[17]

Life Expectancy

The estimated duration of survival of patients who have spinal metastases depends on overall tumor load and rapidity of progression rather than simply on the local disease. Therefore, the natural course of the primary cancer is a very important factor. The predicted prognosis that considers the effects of other therapeutic options, including sensitivity to adjuvant treatments, is particularly important, whether surgery is selected or not.[1–3,5,9,13,18]

Currently, surgery generally can be considered as part of the treatment plan if the patient's predicted survival is 3 to 6 months or longer.[1–3,5,9]

Other Selection Criteria

Therapeutic effects, including improvements in ADL are mild in (1) patients without paralysis who respond to oral narcotic analgesics; (2) patients who are highly responsive to radiotherapy; (3) patients showing very rapid progression or severe paralysis of Frankel's A type or B. In these patients, the progression of paralysis does not stop despite transient recovery or, in patients with severe

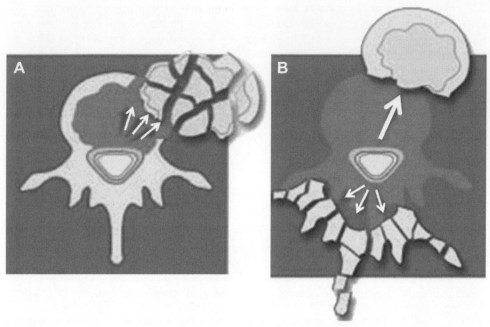

Fig. 2. Excisional procedure for metastatic spine tumor There are two type of excision: (A) intralesional excision or debulking, which is more-or-less complete removal of the tumor piece-by-piece, and (B) en bloc resection, in which the tumor is removed in a single piece. Resection can be along the outer surface of the pseudocapsule (marginal resection) or further out, removing a continuous layer of healthy tissue (wide resection). (*From* Gasbarrini A, Cappuccio M, Mirabile L, et al. Spinal metastases: treatment evaluation algorithm. Eur Rev Med Pharmacol Sci 2004;8:269; with permission.)

paralysis, there is no recovery after surgery.[13,19] Patients in these categories are not regarded as good candidates for surgery.[5,13]

SURGICAL PROCEDURES FOR METASTATIC SPINE TUMORS AND THEIR SELECTION

Surgical procedures for metastatic spine tumors can be classified as excisional procedures (ie, complete resection of the involved vertebrae or the tumor, followed by reconstruction of the vertebrae using spinal instruments or implants) (**Fig. 2**),[7] and palliative procedures (ie, posterior decompression and stabilization using spinal instrumentation for alleviation of pain or paralysis) (**Fig. 3**).[7]

Excisional procedures include those aimed piecemeal resection of the tumor, such as intralesional excision or debulking (see **Fig. 2**A),[7] and those aimed at en bloc resection of the involved vertebrae (see **Fig. 2**B).[7] The former procedures often are performed with an anterior approach for tumors in the cervical spine, but an anterior, posterior, or combined approach can be used for tumors in the thoracic and lumbar spine. The en bloc resections, which involve removal of the tumor as a single piece, include marginal resection (ie, resection along the outer layer of the

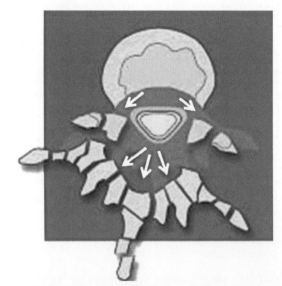

Fig. 3. Posterior decompression and stabilization is the most common palliative procedure for metastatic spine tumor. This procedure aims at decompression of the spinal cord and cauda equine and stabilization of the unstable spine. This procedure does not necessarily involve a direct approach to the tumor. (*From* Gasbarrini A, Cappuccio M, Mirabile L, et al. Spinal metastases: treatment evaluation algorithm. Eur Rev Med Pharmacol Sci 2004;8:269; with permission.)

Table 1

Evaluation system for the prognosis of metastatic spine tumors (revised in 1999)[a]

Predictive Factor	Score
General condition (performance status)	
Poor (PS 10%–40%)	0
Moderate (PS 50%–70%)	1
Good (PS 80%–100%)	2
Number of extraspinal bone metastases foci	
≥ 3	0
1–2	1
0	2
Number of metastases in the vertebral body	
≥ 3	0
2	1
1	2
Metastases to the major internal organs	
Unremovable	0
Removable	1
No metastases	2
Primary site of the cancer	
Lung, osteosarcoma, stomach, bladder, esophagus, pancreas	0
Liver, gall bladder, unidentified	1
Other	2
Kidney, uterus	3
Rectum	4
Thyroid, breast, prostate, carcinoid tumor	5
Palsy	
Complete (Frankel A, B)	0
Incomplete (Frankel C, D)	1
None (Frankel E)	2

Abbreviation: PS, Karnofsky's performance status.

[a] Criteria for predicted prognosis: total score 0–8 = < 6 months' survival; total score 9–11 = ≥ 6 months' survival; total score 12–15 = ≥ 1 year's survival.

From Tokuhashi Y, Matsuzaki H, Oda H, et al. A revised scoring system for preoperative evaluation of metastatic spine tumor prognosis. Spine 2005;30(19):2189; with permission.

pseudocapsule of the tumor) and wide resection (ie, resection of the tumor with a layer of healthy tissue as a margin). En bloc resection should be considered particularly in patients who have involvement of a single vertebra with a good prognosis or who have hypervascularized lesions.[7,9] The palliative procedure consists of posterior decompression by laminectomy and, if possible, excision of as much of the tumor as possible and posterior

stabilization using instrumentation. This procedure does not necessarily involve a direct approach to the tumor. It is selected for patients who have thoracic or lumbar lesions and a poor prognosis and is performed most frequently as an emergency operation for metastatic spine tumors.

These surgical procedures are selected according to the localization or spread of the lesion and the patient's life expectancy. Excisional procedures aimed at long-term local control are recommended if the lesion involves a single vertebra (or occasionally two neighboring vertebrae) and if the predicted survival period is 1 year or longer. On the other hand, palliative procedures usually are selected for multivertebral metastases involving two or more vertebrae or single vertebral metastases in a patient who has a predicted survival period of less than 1 year.

PREDICTING THE PROGNOSIS OF METASTATIC SPINE TUMORS

The predicted prognosis before treatment is important and difficult, because it helps determine the treatment modalities (especially surgical procedures).[1,2] The natural course of the primary cancer is the most important factor affecting the prognosis.[3–6] Primary cancers are classified according to the tumor-node-metastasis staging system (TNM staging), and the approximate prognosis after treatment of the primary lesion can be predicted in most cancers; however, unlike the recurrence of symptoms after treatment of the primary lesion, the appearance of symptoms caused by spinal metastasis has not been sufficient to estimate the survival period. Surgical interventions for spinal metastases involve risks and complications, however, so predicting the prognosis after surgery is indispensable for surgeons. In addition, functional recovery (ie, level of ADL) provided by various treatment modalities also is affected markedly by the expected survival period.[16,18,19]

Various evaluation systems have been devised for predicting prognosis.[9,20–29] Initially, staging using bone scintigraphy was reported. Citrin and colleagues[20] and Swenerton and colleagues[21] used the number of bone metastases. Yamashita and colleagues[22] developed a method based on the distribution of bone metastases; however, there was no direct relationship between the extent of bone metastases and the survival time, and the presence or absence of metastases to major internal organs was reported to have a greater effect on the survival time than the distribution of bone metastases.[22] There also were limitations in the evaluation of the survival period according to a single parameter, such as the pathology of the primary lesion or the presence or absence of metastasis to major internal organs. Therefore, some scoring systems for the preoperative evaluation of the prognosis of patients who have metastatic spine tumors[9,24–29] were proposed. These scoring systems consists of multiple clinical factors that affect the survival time and are relatively easy to evaluate.

SCORING SYSTEM FOR PREOPERATIVE EVALUATION OF METASTATIC SPINE TUMOR PROGNOSIS (TOKUHASHI SCORE)

The scoring system for the preoperative evaluation of prognosis of metastatic spine tumor consists of six factors thought to affect the duration of survival: the patient's general condition, the number of extraspinal bone metastatic foci, the number of metastases in the vertebral body, metastases to the major internal organs, the primary site of the cancer, and the degree of paralysis. The predicted prognosis is based on the total score of the prognostic criteria (**Table 1**).[23–27] The six parameters are relatively simple to evaluate and are clinically convenient.

The authors retrospectively evaluated the prognostic criteria, according to which a total score of 8 or less indicates a survival period of less than 6 months, a score of 9 to 11 indicates a survival period of 6 months or longer, and a score of 12 or higher indicates a survival period of 1 year or longer. Using these criteria, the authors have selected conservative treatment or palliative surgical treatment for patients who have a total score of 8 or less and excisional surgical treatment for patients who have a single vertebral involvement with a total score of 12 or higher and even for patients who have with a total score of 9 to 11, depending on the condition of the lesion (**Fig. 4**).[5,26,27] When the reliability of these criteria was evaluated retrospectively in 246 patients, the survival period was less than 6 months in 85.3% of those who had a total

score between 0 and 8, 6 months or longer in 73.1% of those who had a total score of 9 to 11, and 1 year or longer in 95.4% of those who had a total score of 12 to 15. Each prognostic criterion was in agreement with the survival period in a high percentage of patients, and it was reported that the rate of consistency was 82.5% in all 246 patients (**Table 2**) (**Fig. 5**).[27] This scoring system has been used internationally, and many authors have confirmed its usefulness.[19,30,31] Various investigators have developed prognostic methods based on similar scoring systems and reported the usefulness of these systems.[9,28,29]

SURGICAL STRATEGY FOR SPINAL METASTASES (TOMITA SCORE)

Because each parameter of the scoring system for preoperative evaluation of metastatic spine tumor prognosis (Tokuhashi score)[24,25] is not weighted using a statistical indicator such as the hazard ratio, Tomita and colleagues devised a new scoring system by excluding the "state of paralysis" from these parameters to adjust the system to subdivided and diversified options of surgical procedure.[9] The scoring system of Tomita and colleagues consists of three items: grade of the primary tumor, visceral metastases to vital organs (lungs, liver, kidneys, and brain), and bone metastases, including the spine. The strategy was to select the optimal treatment based on the total score of three items, according to the hazard ratio calculated from retrospective data (**Fig. 6**). This strategy indicated wide or marginal excision, such as total en bloc spondylectomy and spinal reconstruction for patients who had a total score of 2 or 3; intralesional excision (piecemeal excision, thorough debulking, if possible, total en bloc spondylectomy as a marginal excision) for a patients who had a total score of 4 or 5; palliative surgery, such as spinal cord decompression with spinal stabilization, for patients who had a total score of 6 or 7; and

Table 2
Distribution of the total score and the survival period

Total Score	Survival Period		
	< 6 Months	6 Months to 1 Year	> 1 Year
0–8 (n = 156)	133 (85.3%)	16	7
9–11 (n = 67)	18	29	20 (73.1%)[a]
12–15 (n = 23)		2	21 (95.4%)

[a] The 73.1% refers to the combination of the 29 and the 20 survivors in this row.

From Tokuhashi Y, Matsuzaki H, Oda H, et al. A revised scoring system for preoperative evaluation of metastatic spine tumor prognosis. Spine 2005;30(19):2190; with permission.

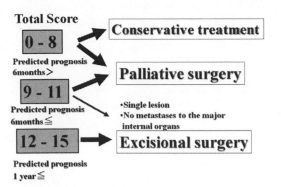

Fig. 4. Strategy for treatment of spinal metastases. (*From* Tokuhashi Y, Matsuzaki H, Oda H, et al. A revised scoring system for preoperative evaluation of metastatic spine tumor prognosis. Spine 2005;30(19): 2188; with permission.)

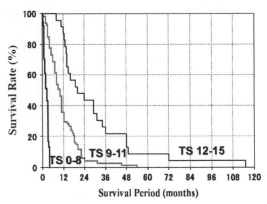

Fig. 5. Kaplan-Meier curves of the survival period after treatment for patients who have a total Tokuhashi score of 0 to 8, 9 to 11, or 12 to 15. (*From* Tokuhashi Y, Matsuzaki H, Oda H, et al. A revised scoring system for preoperative evaluation of metastatic spine tumor prognosis. Spine 2005;30(19):2189; with permission.)

conservative therapy with supportive care for patients who had a total score of 8 to 10. In patients treated with wide or marginal excision (ie, total en bloc spondylectomy or en bloc corpectomy), the mean total score was 3.3 (range, 2–5; n = 28), and the mean survival period was 38.2 months (range, 6–84 months). In patients treated with intralesional excision, such as piecemeal subtotal excision or thorough debulking, the mean total score was 5.0 (range, 3–7; n = 13), and the mean survival period was 21.5 months (range, 4–60 months). In patients treated with palliative spinal cord decompression, the mean score was 7.5 (range, 5–10; n = 11), and the mean survival period was 10.1 months (range, 3–23 months). Nine patients who had a mean score of 9.2 (range, 8–12) received terminal care; their mean survival period was 5.3 months (range, 1–12 months) (**Fig. 7**).[9]

Whether paralysis affects the prognosis remains controversial. Spiegel and colleagues[32] and Enkaoua and colleagues[30] report negative results, but Sioutos and colleagues[33] present positive results. Tokuhashi and colleagues[34] also evaluated

the weighting of various factors according to the hazard ratio by preparing a Cox's proportional hazard model from retrospective data, including paralysis. Ironically, however, there was no significant difference in the rate of consistency between the final category as a result of a Cox's proportional hazard model and the original category. Further accumulation of cases is considered necessary.

A scoring system that combines various factors considered to affect prognosis is undoubtedly useful for a general prediction of the survival period (eg, "within or more than 6 months" or "within or more than 1 year"). With any method proposed to date, however, the correlation between the predicted and actual survival period was unavoidably low in the intermediate-score group compared with the high-scoring and low-scoring groups, and further improvements in the system or the development of new approaches are awaited.

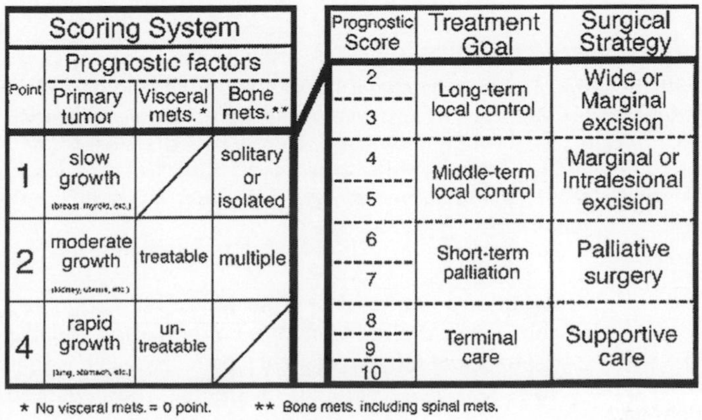

Scoring System				Prognostic Score	Treatment Goal	Surgical Strategy
Prognostic factors						
Point	Primary tumor	Visceral mets.*	Bone mets.**			
				2	Long-term local control	Wide or Marginal excision
				3		
1	slow growth (breast, thyroid, etc.)		solitary or isolated	4	Middle-term local control	Marginal or Intralesional excision
				5		
2	moderate growth (kidney, uterus, etc.)	treatable	multiple	6	Short-term palliation	Palliative surgery
				7		
4	rapid growth (lung, stomach, etc.)	untreatable		8	Terminal care	Supportive care
				9		
				10		

* No visceral mets. = 0 point.   ** Bone mets. including spinal mets.

Fig. 6. Surgical strategy for spinal metastases. The treatment modality is determined by the prognostic score, which is the sum of three parameters: (1) grade of malignancy (eg, slow growth: breast, prostate, thyroid; moderate growth: kidney, uterus; or rapid growth: lung, liver, stomach, colon, unknown primary), (2) visceral metastases to vital organs (lung, liver, kidney, and brain), and (3) bone metastases, including the spine. (*From* Tomita K, Kawahara N, Kobayashi T, et al. Surgical strategy for spinal metastases. Spine 2001;26(3):299; with permission.)

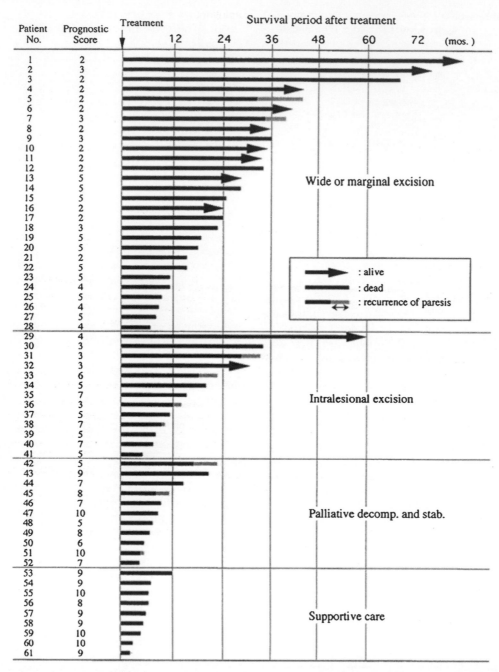

Fig. 7. Survival periods of each patient treated with the surgical strategy for spinal metastases. Twenty-eight patients were treated oncologically with wide or marginal excision. Thirteen patients were treated with intralesional excision (eg, piecemeal subtotal excision, eggshell curettage, or through debulking). Eleven patients were treated with palliative decompression and stabilization. Nine patients were treated with terminal supportive care. (*From* Tomita K, Kawahara N, Kobayashi T, et al. Surgical strategy for spinal metastases. Spine 2001;26(3):302; with permission.)

ALGORITHM FOR TREATMENT OPTIONS FOR SPINAL METASTASES

Gasbarrini and colleagues[7] admitted the usefulness of these scoring systems for predicting prognosis and treatment selection but suggested that using the same numerical scale for variable factors that differ in clinical significance is a weakness of these scoring systems. They warned against reducing the choice of treatment modalities by using an overly simplistic mathematical score and proposed selecting a treatment by using an algorithm for each patient (**Fig. 8**). They also suggested that the sensitivity of the tumor histotype to adjuvant treatments is the most important factor for the treatment selection.

According to their algorithm (see **Fig. 8**), after the diagnosis of spinal metastases, the first consideration is whether surgery under general anesthesia is possible, given the patient's general condition. If surgery is difficult, the sensitivity of the tumor to adjuvant treatments is evaluated. If the tumor does not respond to any treatment, pain relief is the only treatment option for these patients.

If surgery is possible, the likelihood of recovery from the neurologic injury is evaluated according its severity (Frankel's classification) and the time from the onset (because the possibility of recovery is low if the injury is severe and long-standing). If the paralysis is judged to be permanent, effective adjuvant treatments are reevaluated. On the other hand, if the patient has acute incomplete spinal cord palsy, emergency surgery is selected. If paralysis is absent or mild, promising adjuvant treatments are tried first. If the histotype of the tumor is not sensitive to adjuvant treatments, surgical treatment (an excisional procedure for a single lesion and palliative decompression and stabilization for multiple lesions) is selected. If surgery is not possible, the goal of treatment is pain relief only.

If there is no paralysis, and the histotype of tumor responds to adjuvant treatments, spinal instability (actual or impending pathologic fracture) is evaluated. According to the severity of spinal instability, the decision whether to treat the patient with adjuvant treatment alone or with palliative decompression and stabilization is made. Resection of the tumor may be performed en bloc with a wide margin or through debulking. En bloc removal is indicated for hypervascularized tumors such as metastases from kidney cancer and from sarcoma or for cases in which this type of operation is easy to perform.

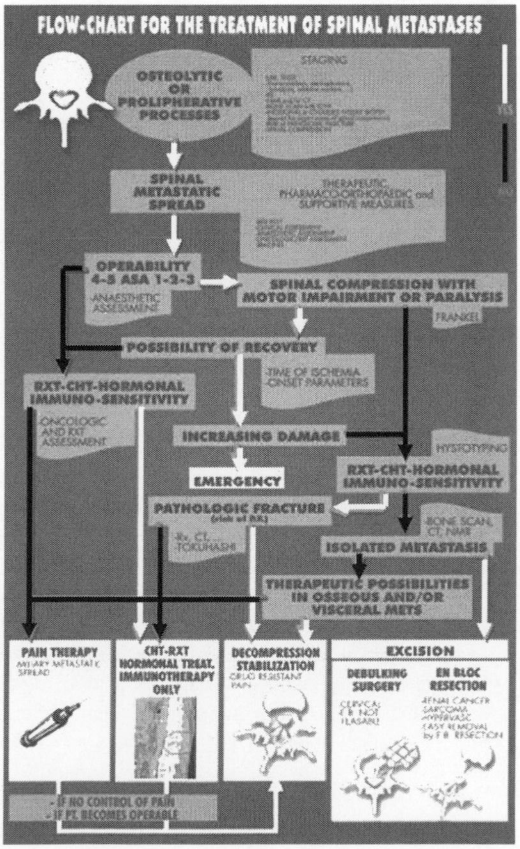

SUMMARY

Metastatic spine tumors are not rare and cause major impairment of patients' functions and ADL. The choice of the most suitable treatment is of crucial importance for patients who may be severely disabled by spinal metastases. Surgical treatment, from which immediate pain relief, alleviation of paralysis, and improvement in ADL can be anticipated, has great significance in the orthopedic management of symptoms and local control of this disease. Surgical interventions for spinal metastatic tumor may be extensive, however, and carry significant risks. In addition, the functional prognosis (ie, ability to perform ADL) associated with various treatment modalities is affected markedly by the actual survival period. Therefore, the orthopedic surgeon must evaluate the survival time, observe the appropriate indications for surgical treatment, and select the most suitable surgical procedure.

Spine surgeons should play an active role in the treatment of metastatic spine tumors.

Fig. 8. Algorithm and flow-chart for the treatment of spinal metastases. (*From* Gasbarrini A, Cappuccio M, Mirabile L, et al. Spinal metastases: treatment evaluation algorithm. Eur Rev Med Pharmacol Sci 2004;8:272; with permission.)

REFERENCES

1. Harrington KD. Current concept review, metastatic disease of the spine. J Bone Joint Surg 1986;68-A: 1110–5.
2. Kaneda K, Takeda N, Taneichi H, et al. Treatment for spinal metastases. Monthly Book Orthopaedics 1995;8:25–34.
3. Aboulafia AJ, Levine AM. Musculoskeletal and metastatic tumors. In: Farden DF, Garfin SR, Abidol JJ, et al, editors. Orthopaedic knowledge update: spine

2. Rosemont (IL): The American Academy of Orthopaedic Surgeons; 2002. p. 411–30.

4. Wai EK, Finkelstein JA, Tangente RP, et al. Quality of life in surgical treatment of metastatic spine disease. Spine 2003;28:508–12.

5. Tokuhashi Y. Treatment of metastatic spine tumor. Journal of the Japanese Orthopaedic Association 2007;81:573–84.

6. Katagiri H, Takahashi M, Inagaki J, et al. Determining the site of the primary cancer in patients with skeletal metastasis of unknown origin; a retrospective study. Cancer 1999;86:533–7.

7. Gasbarrini A, Cappuccio M, Mirabile L, et al. Spinal metastases: treatment evaluation algorithm. Eur Rev Med Pharmacol Sci 2004;8:265–74.

8. Harrington KD. Orthopaedic surgical management of skeletal complications of malignancy. Cancer Supplement 1997;80:1614–27.

9. Tomita K, Kawahara N, Kobayashi T, et al. Surgical strategy for spinal metastases. Spine 2001;26:298–306.

10. Shirato H, Hashimoto S. Forefront of radiotherapy for spinal tumors. Spine & Spinal Cord 1999;12:507–13.

11. Siegel T, Siegal T. Current considerations in the management of neoplastic spinal cord compression. Spine 1989;14:225–6.

12. Kostuik JP, Weinstein JN. Differential diagnosis and surgical treatment of metastatic spine tumors. In: Frymoyer JW, Ducker TB, Hadler NM, et al, editors. The Adult Spine. New York: Raven Press; 1991. p. 861–88.

13. Tokuhashi Y, Nemoto Y, Matsuzaki H. Surgery for metastatic spine tumor at present. Orthopaedic Surgery and Traumatology 2003;46:663–9.

14. Patchell RA, Tibbs PA, Regine WF, et al. A randomized trial of direct decompression surgical resection in the treatment of spinal cord compression caused by metastasis. Lancet 2005;366:643–8.

15. Sundaresan N, Rothman A, Manhart K, et al. Surgery for solitary metastases of the spine, rationale and results of treatment. Spine 2002;27:1802–6.

16. Tokuhashi Y, Koga A, Ajiro Y, et al. Strategy for metastatic spine tumor using scoring system for preoperative evaluation of prognosis. The Journal of the Japanese Spine Research Society 2006;17:240.

17. Tateishi A. Philosophy of treatment for bone metastases. Monthly Book Orthopaedics 1995;8:9–15.

18. Tang V, Harvey D, Dorsay JP, et al. Prognostic indicators in metastatic spinal cord compression: using functional independence measure and Tokuhashi scale to optimize rehabilitation planning. Spinal Cord 2007;45:671–7.

19. Eriks IE, Angenot ELD, Lankhorst GJ. Epidural metastatic spinal cord compression: functional outcome and survival after inpatient rehabilitation. Spinal Cord 2004;42:235–9.

20. Citrin DL, Hougen C, Zweibel W, et al. The use of serial bone scans in assessing response of bone metastases to systemic treatment. Cancer 1981;47:680–5.

21. Swenerton KD, Legha SS, Smith T, et al. Prognostic factors in metastatic breast cancer treated with combined chemotherapy. Cancer Res 1979;39:1552–62.

22. Yamashita K, Ueda T, Komatsubara Y, et al. Breast cancer with bone-only metastases: visceral metastases-free rate in relation to anatomic distribution of bone metastases. Cancer 1991;68:634–7.

23. Karnofsky DA. Clinical evaluation of anticancer drugs: cancer chemotherapy. GANN Monograph 1967;2:223–31.

24. Tokuhashi Y, Kawano H, Ohsaka S, et al. A scoring system for preoperative evaluation of the prognosis of metastatic spine tumor prognosis. Journal of the Japanese Orthopaedic Association 1989; 63:482–9.

25. Tokuhashi Y, Matsuzaki H, Toriyama S, et al. Scoring system for the preoperative evaluation of metastatic spine tumor prognosis. Spine 1990;15:1110–3.

26. Tokuhashi Y, Matsuzaki H, Okawa Akihiro, et al. Indications of operative procedures for metastatic spine tumors, a scoring system for preoperative evaluation of prognosis. J East Jpn Orthop Traumatol 1999;11: 31–5.

27. Tokuhashi Y, Matsuzaki H, Oda H, et al. A revised scoring system for preoperative evaluation of metastatic spine tumor prognosis. Spine 2005;30: 2186–91.

28. Kostuik JP. The development of a pre-operative scoring assessment system of metastatic spine disease. In: Proceedings of the 12th annual meeting of North American Spine Society, New York: 1997. p. 182.

29. Katagiri H, Takahashi M, Wakai K, et al. Prognostic factors and a scoring system for patients with skeletal metastasis. J Bone Joint Surg Br 2005;87: 698–703.

30. Enkaoua EA, Doursonian L, Chatellier G, et al. A critical appreciation of the preoperative prognostic Tokuhashi score in a series of 71 cases. Spine 1997;22:2293–8.

31. Ulmar B, Richter M, Cakir B, et al. The Tokuhashi score: significant predictive value for the life expectancy of patients with breast cancer with spinal metastases. Spine 2005;30:2222–6.

32. Spiegel DA, Sampson JH, Richardson WJ, et al. Metastatic melanoma to the spine. Diagnosis, risk factors, and prognosis in 114 patients. Spine 1995; 20:2141–6.

33. Sioutos PJ, Arbit E, Meshulam CF, et al. Spinal metastases from solid tumors. Analysis of factors affecting survival. Cancer 1995;76:1453–9.

34. Tokuhashi Y, Hashimoto H. Epidemiological study in the prognosis evaluation system for metastatic spine tumor. Journal of Japanese Society of Lumbar Spine Disorders 2002;8:44–52.

Total En Bloc Spondylectomy for Spinal Tumors: Surgical Techniques and Related Basic Background

Norio Kawahara, MD, Katsuro Tomita, MD*, Hideki Murakami, MD,
Satoru Demura, MD

KEYWORDS
- Spinal tumors • Total en bloc spondylectomy
- Oncologic resection

Conventionally, curettage or piecemeal excision of vertebral tumors has been commonly practiced. Nevertheless, clear disadvantages of these approaches include high risk for tumor cell contamination to the surrounding structures and residual tumor tissue at the site attributable to the difficulty in demarcating tumor from healthy tissue. These disadvantages contribute to incomplete resection of the tumor and high local recurrence rates of malignant spinal tumors.[1–3]

Roy-Camille and colleagues,[4,5] Stener,[6–8] Stener and Johnsen,[9] Sundaresan and colleagues,[10] and Boriani and colleagues[11,12] have described total corpectomy or spondylectomy for reducing local recurrence of vertebral tumors, with excellent clinical results. The authors' group has developed a new surgical technique of spondylectomy (vertebrectomy) called "total en bloc spondylectomy" (TES).[2,3,13–17] This technique is different from spondylectomy in that it involves en bloc removal of the lesion, that is, removal of the whole vertebra, body and lamina, as one compartment.[1]

The surgical technique of TES has been remarkably improved based on adequate knowledge and consideration of the surgical anatomy, physiology, and biomechanics of the spine and spinal cord.[18] Review of the developmental process of this operation leads to recognition of the tips, pitfalls, and solutions.

SURGICAL INDICATION FOR TOTAL EN BLOC SPONDYLECTOMY

The TES technique was designed to achieve oncologic complete tumor resection en bloc, including the main and satellite microlesions in a vertebral compartment, so as to avoid local recurrence. The following pathologic findings are primary candidates: primary malignant tumor (stage I or II), aggressive benign tumor (stage III), and isolated metastasis with a long life expectancy (see surgical strategy; **Figs. 1** and **2**).[18,19]

From the viewpoint of tumor growth (see surgical classification; **Fig. 3**), TES is recommended for type 3, 4, and 5 lesions and is relatively indicated for type 1, 2, and 6 lesions. A type 1 or 2 lesion can still be a candidate for radiotherapy, chemotherapy, corpectomy, or hemivertebrectomy. TES is not recommended for type 7 lesions. Systemic treatment or hospice care may be the treatment of choice for these lesions.[2,3,18]

PREOPERATIVE EMBOLIZATION
Triple-Level Embolization

Preoperative embolization of bilateral segmental arteries at three levels (ie, embolization of bilateral segmental arteries of the tumor-laden level and two adjacent vertebrae [one cephalad and one

Department of Orthopedic Surgery, Graduate school of Medical Science Kanazawa University, School of Medicine, Kanazawa University, 13-1 Takaramachi, Kanazawa, 920–8641, Japan
* Corresponding author.
E-mail address: seikei@pop01.kanazawa-u.ac.jp (K. Tomita).

Orthop Clin N Am 40 (2009) 47–63
doi:10.1016/j.ocl.2008.09.004
0030-5898/08/$ – see front matter © 2008 Elsevier Inc. All rights reserved.

orthopedic.theclinics.com

Surgical Strategy for Primary Spinal Tumors

Surgical Staging	Contamination/ Residual tumor	Surgical margin	Spinal cord Salvage Surgery
Benign tumor :			
1. Latent			**Don't touch!**
2. Active	OK / OK	*intralesional*	**Debulking (piecemeal)**
3. Aggressive	OK / No	*intralesional or marginal*	**Thorough excision (piecemeal / en bloc)**
Malignant tumor :			
I. Low grade	No / No	*marginal or wide*	*Total en bloc excision*
II. High grade	No / No		
III. with metastases	No / No	*(radical : impractical)*	

Fig. 1. Surgical strategy for primary spinal tumors. (*From* Tomita K, Kawahara N, Murakami H, et al. Total en bloc spondylectomy for spinal tumors: improvement of the technique and its associated basic background. J Orthop Sci 2006;11(1): 3–12; with permission.)

caudal]) is tried within 48 hours before the operation (**Fig. 4**).[18]

Embolization is performed under local anesthesia in all cases. Arterial access is established using an intravascular sheath placed within the common femoral artery. After the aortic runoff, selective angiograms of segmental arteries supplying the targeted tumor and adjacent vertebrae (typically, one level above and below the lesion) are obtained. Embolization coils or pieces of gelatin sponge are used for proximal embolization of the segmental arteries lateral to the vertebral bodies, and polyvinyl alcohol particles are used for peripheral embolization of the posterior branches of the segmental arteries to block the backward flow. The segmental artery(s) that supply the anterior spinal artery are not embolized. This original embolization method has dramatically reduced intraoperative blood loss in TES compared with before using this method at the authors' hospital.

Surgical Strategy for Spinal Metastases

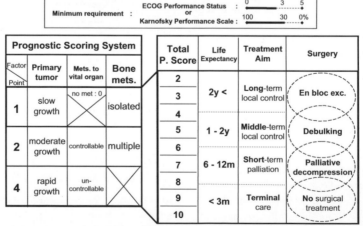

Fig. 2. Surgical strategy for spinal metastases: points for each primary tumor. **1 point = slow growth** Breast cancer,* Thyroid cancer,* Prostatic cancer, Testicular cancer. **2 points = Moderate growth** Renal cell cancer,* Uterus cancer, Ovarian cancer, Colorectal cancer. **4 points = Rapid growth** Lung cancer, Gastric cancer, Esophageal cancer, Nasopharyngeal cancer, Hepatocellular cancer, Pancreas cancer, etc., Bladder cancer, Melanoma Sarcoma (osteosarcoma, Ewing sarcoma, Leiomyosarcoma, etc.), Primary unknown metastasis, other rare cancer.
* Rare types of the following cancer should be given 4 points as a rapidly growing cancer: 1. Breast cancer, inflammatory type; 2. Thyroid cancer, undifferentiated type; 3. Renal cell cancer, inflammatory type. (*From* Tomita K, Kawahara N, Murakami H, et al. Total en bloc spondylectomy for spinal tumors: improvement of the technique and its associated basic background. J Orthop Sci 2006;11(1):3–12; with permission.)

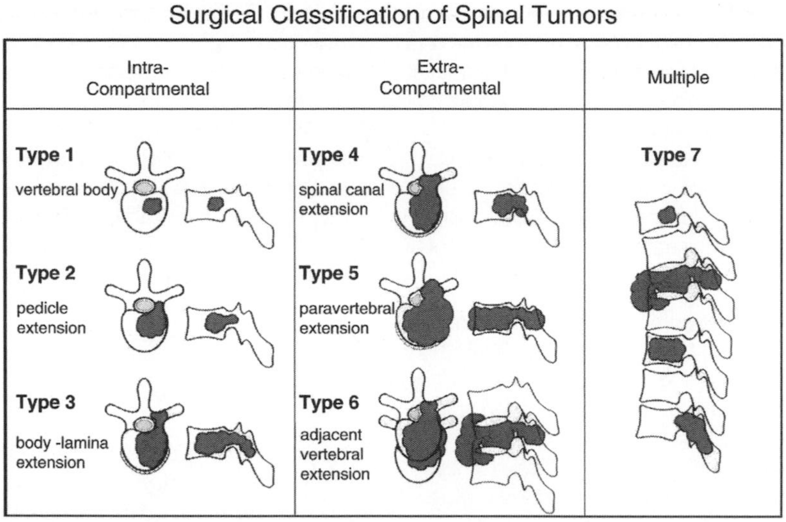

Surgical Classification of Spinal Tumors

Intra-Compartmental	Extra-Compartmental	Multiple
Type 1 vertebral body	**Type 4** spinal canal extension	**Type 7**
Type 2 pedicle extension	**Type 5** paravertebral extension	
Type 3 body -lamina extension	**Type 6** adjacent vertebral extension	

Fig. 3. Surgical classification of spinal tumors. (*From* Tomita K, Kawahara N, Murakami H, et al. Total en bloc spondylectomy for spinal tumors: improvement of the technique and its associated basic background. J Orthop Sci 2006;11(1):3–12; with permission.)

SURGICAL TECHNIQUE OF TOTAL EN BLOC SPONDYLECTOMY

The TES technique consists of two steps, including en bloc resection of the posterior element and en bloc resection of the anterior part to salvage the spinal cord. In some cases, a small part (the pedicle in most cases) becomes intralesional deliberately, but this must be permitted to salvage the spinal cord. The surgical approach is decided on the basis of the degree of tumor development or the affected spinal level(s).[2,3,13,15–17]

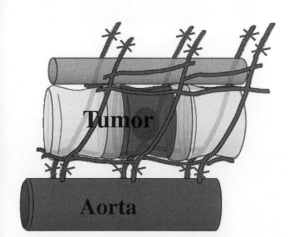

Fig. 4. Triple-level embolization. Preoperative embolization of bilateral segmental arteries at three levels (the tumor-laden level and two adjacent [one cephalad and one caudal] vertebrae) is tried within 48 hours before surgery.

A Single Posterior Approach

We prefer a single posterior approach rather than a posteroanterior combined approach for a TES higher than L3 or L4 when the tumor does not involve major vessels (most tumors of types 1, 2, 3, and 4, and some tumors of types 5 and 6). The main advantage of this is that the spinal cord can be observed carefully throughout the procedure, especially during anterior spinal column osteotomy, corpectomy, and spinal reconstruction by posterior instrumentation.

Step 1: En Bloc Laminectomy (en bloc resection of the whole posterior element of the vertebra)

Exposure. The patient is placed prone over a Relton-Hall four-poster frame to avoid compression of the vena cava. A straight vertical midline incision is made over the spinous processes and is extended three vertebrae above and below the involved segment(s). The paraspinal muscles are dissected from the spinous processes and the laminae and are then retracted laterally. If the patient underwent a posterior route biopsy, the tracts are carefully resected in a manner similar to that used in a limb salvaging procedure. After a careful dissection of the area around the facet joints, a large retractor called the "articulated spinal retractor," which has a uniaxial joint in each limb and was designed for this operative procedure, is applied. By spreading the retractor and detaching the muscles around the facet joints, a wider exposure is obtained. The operative field must be wide enough on both sides to allow dissection under the surface of the transverse processes. In the thoracic spine, the ribs on the affected level and one level below are transected 3 to 4 cm lateral to the costotransverse joint and the pleura is bluntly separated from the vertebra.

To expose the superior articular process of the uppermost vertebra, the spinous and inferior articular processes of the neighboring vertebra are osteotomized and removed with dissection of the attached soft tissues, including the ligamentum flavum.

Introduction of the T-saw guide. To make an exit for the T-saw guide through the nerve root canal, the soft tissue attached to the inferior aspect of the pars interarticularis is dissected and removed using the utmost care so as not to damage the corresponding nerve root. A C-curved malleable T-saw guide is then introduced through the intervertebral foramen in a cephalocaudal direction (**Fig. 5**A). In this procedure, the tip of the T-saw guide should be introduced along the medial cortex of the lamina and the pedicle so as not to injure the spinal cord and the nerve root (see **Fig. 5**A). After passing the T-saw guide, its tip at the exit of the nerve root canal can be found beneath the inferior border of the pars interarticularis. In the next step, a threadwire saw (T-saw [flexible multifilament threadwire saw 0.54 mm in diameter]; Koshiya Co., LTD., Kanazawa, Japan) is passed through the hole in the wire guide and is clamped with a T-saw holder at each end.[20] The T-saw guide is removed, and tension on the T-saw is maintained.

Cutting the pedicles and resection of the posterior element. While tension is maintained, the T-saw is placed beneath the superior articular and transverse processes with a specially designed T-saw manipulator. With this procedure, the T-saw placed around the lamina is wrapped around the pedicle. With a reciprocating motion of the T-saw, the pedicles are cut and the whole posterior element of the spine (the spinous process, the superior and inferior articular processes, the transverse process, and the pedicle) is then removed in one piece (**Fig. 5**B; **Fig. 6**B left and right). The cut surface of the pedicle is sealed with bone wax to reduce bleeding and to minimize contamination by tumor cells. To maintain stability after segmental resection of the anterior column, temporary posterior instrumentation is performed. When one vertebra is resected, two-above and two-below segmental fixation is recommended. If two or three vertebrae are resected, however, more than two-above and two-below segmental fixation is mandatory.

Step 2: En Bloc Corpectomy (resection of the anterior column of the vertebra)

Blunt dissection around the vertebral body. At the beginning of the second step, the segmental arteries must be identified bilaterally. The spinal branch of the segmental artery, which runs along the nerve root, is ligated and divided. This procedure exposes the segmental artery, which is seen just lateral to the cut edge of the pedicle (**Fig. 7**). In the thoracic spine, it is better to sacrifice the corresponding bilateral nerve roots to avoid avulsion nerve root injury. The blunt dissection is done on both sides through the plane between the pleura (or the iliopsoas muscle) and the vertebral body (**Figs. 6**C and **8**). Usually, the lateral aspect of the body is easily dissected with a curved vertebral spatula. The segmental artery should then be dissected from the vertebral body. By continuing dissection of both lateral sides of the vertebral body, the aorta is carefully dissected from the anterior aspect of the vertebral body with a spatula and the surgeon's fingers (see **Fig. 8**B, C). Vascular anatomy around the vertebral body should be thoroughly understood so as to avoid vascular

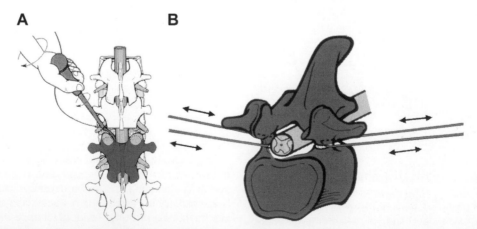

A   **B**

Fig. 5. Operative schema of a pediculotomy. (*A*) Operative schema of introducing the T-saw guide. (*B*) Operative schema of a pediculotomy using a T-saw.

damage (see **Fig. 7**).[21,22] When the surgeon's fingertips meet each other anterior to the vertebral body, a series of spatulas, starting from the smallest size, are inserted sequentially to extend the dissection. A pair of the largest spatulas is kept in the dissection site to prevent the surrounding tissues and organs from iatrogenic injury and to make the surgical field wide enough for manipulating the anterior column.

Passage of the T-saw. T-saws are inserted at the proximal and distal cutting levels of the vertebral bodies, where grooves are made along the desired cutting line using a V-notched osteotome after confirmation of the disc levels with needles.

Dissection of the spinal cord and removal of the vertebra. Using a cord spatula or Penfield dissector, the spinal cord is mobilized from the surrounding venous plexus and ligamentous tissue. The teeth-cord protector, which has teeth on both edges to prevent the T-saw from slipping, is then applied. The anterior column of the vertebra is cut by the T-saw, together with the anterior and posterior longitudinal ligaments (**Fig. 6**C left; **Fig. 9**). After cutting the anterior column, the mobility of the vertebra is again checked to ensure a complete corpectomy. The details of the appropriate procedure are discussed elsewhere in this article (see Figs. **9**B and **6**C right upper and lower) if the spinal cord is compressed by the epidural tumor extension.

The freed anterior column is rotated around the spinal cord and removed carefully to avoid injury to the spinal cord. With this procedure, a complete anterior and posterior decompression of the spinal cord (circumspinal decompression)[23] and total en bloc resection of the vertebral tumor are achieved.

Anterior reconstruction and posterior instrumentation. Bleeding, mainly from the venous plexus within the spinal canal, should be exhaustively arrested. An anchor hole on the cut end of the remaining vertebra is made on each side to seat the graft. A vertebral spacer, such as autograft or fresh or frozen allograft and a titanium mesh cylinder (MOSS-Miami; DePuy Motech, Warsaw, Indiana), is properly inserted between the remaining healthy vertebrae to ensure biologic bony fusion.[24,25] After checking the appropriate position of the vertebral spacer radiographically, the posterior instrumentation is adjusted to compress the inserted vertebral spacer slightly (**Fig. 10**A).[26] If two or three vertebrae are resected, application of the connector device between the posterior rods and anterior spacer is recommended (see Figs. **10**B and **6**E left and right). Finally, a Bard Marlex mesh (Bard, Billerica, Massachusetts) covers the entire anterior and posterior reconstructed areas to establish the compartment for suppressing the bleeding.

ILLUSTRATIVE CASE PRESENTATION

A 40-year-old woman had thoracic metastasis from a sacrum chordoma. She had back pain and gait disturbance attributable to thoracic myelopathy. MRI of the thoracic spine showed that a vertebral tumor of T6 extended to the spinal canal in a craniocaudal direction, severely compressing the spinal cord and also expanding outside the vertebral body (see **Fig. 6**A left and right).

The patient underwent TES by means of a single posterior approach. The T5, T6, and T7 laminae were removed en bloc one by one using a T-saw (see **Fig. 6**B left and right). After dissection around the vertebral bodies, the anterior spinal column was osteotomized at the T4-to-T5 and T7-to-T8 disc levels using T-saw reciprocating motion (see **Fig. 6**C left). The tumor vertebral bodies were pushed away 5 to 10 mm in the ventral direction from the dural tube (see **Fig. 6**C right upper and 8C right lower). The adhesion between the pseudocapsule of the epidural tumor and the anterior aspect of the dural tube was safely dissected using a dissector (see **Fig. 6**C right lower). The tumor vertebrae were removed, including the epidural tumor and paravertebral tumor, with a safe margin (see **Fig. 6**D left and right).

Anterior cage and posterior rods were connected by connector devices to secure spinal stability (see **Fig. 6**E left and right). After the operation, the patient regained ambulation.

Anteroposterior Double Approach

In type 5 or 6 tumors, when they involve major vessels or segmental arteries, anterior dissection followed by posterior TES is indicated (**Fig. 11**). A thoracotomy or extraperitoneal approach is generally required. A vascular surgeon may help to dissect the vessels if needed. A thoracic surgeon can also perform a lobectomy if the lung is invaded. Nowadays, a thoracoscopic or mini-open approach is preferred for anterior dissection.[16]

Anteroposterior double approach is safer for the vessels around the vertebral body than TES by a single posterior approach.

Posterior-Anterior-Posterior Approach

A posterior laminectomy and stabilization, followed by an anterior en bloc corpectomy and placement of a vertebral prosthesis, is indicated in spinal tumors at the lumbar level of L3 to L5 because of the technical challenge presented by the iliac wing and lumbosacral plexus nerves.[16]

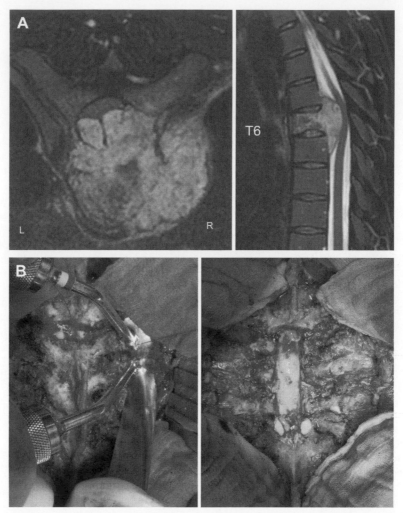

Fig. 6. Thoracic metastasis from a sacrum chordoma in a 40-year-old woman. (*A*) MRI (T2 fat suppression) of the thoracic spine. (*Left*) Axial image of the T6 vertebral level. The vertebral tumor extended to the spinal canal, severely compressing the spinal cord, and also expanded outside the vertebral body. (*Right*) Sagittal image of the thoracic spine. The epidural tumor expanded in the craniocaudal direction from the T6 level. (*B*) En bloc laminectomy. (*Left*) Pediculotomy by T-saw reciprocating motion. The T5, T6, and T7 laminae are removed en bloc one by one. (*Right*) Operative photograph after T5, T6, and T7 en bloc laminectomy. (*C*) En bloc corpectomy. (*Left*) Anterior spinal osteotomy by T-saw reciprocating motion. (*Right upper*) Operative photograph after dissection around the vertebral body from the posterolateral direction. (*Right lower*) Operative photograph after dissection between the pseudocapsule of the epidural tumor and the anterior aspect of the dural tube. The tumor vertebral bodies are pushed away 5 to 10 mm in the ventral direction from the dural tube. An adhesion between the pseudocapsule of the epidural tumor and the anterior aspect of the dural tube was safely dissected using a dissector. The white arrows indicate the osteotomy line of the anterior column. (*D*) Resected specimen of the tumor vertebrae. (*Left*) Posterior aspect of the tumor vertebral bodies. An epidural tumor was removed with a safe margin without violating the pseudocapsule. (*Right*) Right lateral aspect of the tumor vertebral bodies. A paravertebral tumor was removed with a safe margin. (*E*) Postoperative radiograph of the thoracic spine. (*Left*) Anterior-posterior view. Six coils for preoperative embolization are recognized. (*Right*) Lateral view. Anterior cage and posterior rods are connected by connector devices to secure spinal stability. (*From* Kawahara N, et al. Cadaveric vascular anatomy for total en bloc spondylectomy in malignant vertebral tumors. Spine 1996;21:1404; with permission.)

Step 1: posterior approach

The posterior laminectomy and stabilization are the similar to TES by a single posterior approach, as mentioned previously. Basically, lumbar nerves are preserved if they are not involved by the tumor.

Lumbar nerves should be dissected from the vertebral body to their conjunction with the neighboring lumbar nerves. The dural tube is also dissected from the posterior longitudinal ligament or the epidural tumor. Ligamentous tissues between the

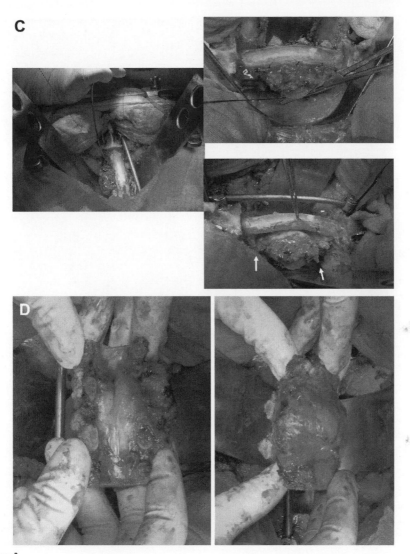

Fig. 6. (*continued*)

dural tube or lumbar nerves and the posterior longitudinal ligaments should be cut off. The psoas muscle should be dissected from the lateral wall of the vertebral body, not violating the tumor margin. The posterior halves of the craniocaudal adjacent discs of the tumor vertebra are excised. If the cutting level of the anterior column is at the vertebral body, the cutting line should be made by a high-speed drill into the posterior half of the vertebral body. An artificial sheet, such as a Gore-Tex Patch (W.L.GORE & ASSOCIATES, INC., Flagstaff, Arizona) is placed between the lumbar nerves and the tumor vertebral body to separate them. The artificial sheet is an operative landmark in the step 2 operation. These procedures are performed in preparation for an en bloc corpectomy by an anterior approach (step 2).

Step 2: anterior approach

An anterolateral extraperitoneal approach is generally indicated above the L4 (or L5) level. The bilateral segmental vessels of the corresponding level(s) are ligated and cut off. Major vessels (the descending aorta and the inferior vena cava) and the psoas muscles are retracted. The anterior halves of the craniocaudal adjacent discs of the tumor vertebra are excised, or the anterior half of the vertebral body is cut off using a high-speed drill at the coincident precutting level of the posterior half of the vertebral body. The tumor vertebral body(ies) is(are) removed en bloc.

An anterior midline transperitoneal approach is indicated at the L5 (or L4) level. Major vessels (the descending aorta, the inferior vena cava, and the common iliac arteries and veins) are dissected from the vertebral body(ies). The anterior

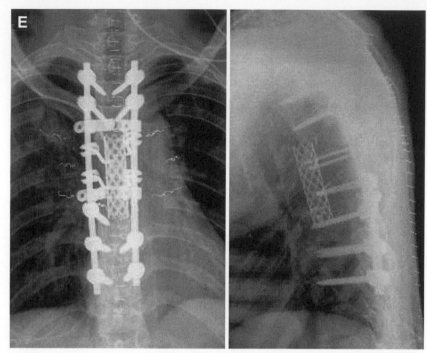

Fig. 6. (*continued*)

halves of the anterior spinal column are cut off at the coincident precutting level of the posterior halves. Specifically, the L5-to-S1 disc is excised from the surgical accesses of the lateral side of the bilateral common iliac vessels and also between the bilateral iliac vessels by retracting the vessels. The tumor vertebral body(ies) is(are) removed en bloc. A vertebral spacer is properly inserted between the remaining healthy vertebrae.

In a type 5 or 6 tumor that adheres to or involves major vessels, a vascular surgeon may be required to dissect the vessels from the tumor vertebra(e).

Step 3: posterior approach

After checking the appropriate position of the vertebral spacer radiographically, the posterior instrumentation is adjusted to compress the inserted vertebral spacer slightly by a posterior approach. If two or three vertebrae are resected, application of the connector device between the posterior rods and anterior spacer is recommended.

ILLUSTRATIVE CASE PRESENTATION

A 38-year-old woman had a giant-cell tumor of the lumbar spine. She had severe lumbar pain. Images revealed that an L4 vertebral tumor largely expanded outside the vertebral body and had grown to the neighboring vertebrae (L3 and L5) (**Fig. 12**A left and right, B). The bilateral common iliac arteries were compressed and shifted to the anterior

direction, and the vena cava inferior was also severely compressed so as to be flattened (see **Fig. 12**A left). The patient underwent TES by a posterior-anterior-posterior double approach.

Step 1: Posterior Approach

After a sequential en bloc laminectomy, the bilateral L3, L4, and L5 lumbar nerves were dissected from the vertebral body to their conjunction with the neighboring lumbar nerves (see **Fig. 12**C left and right). The psoas muscles were dissected from bilateral sides of the L3, L4, and L5 vertebral bodies. The posterior halves of the L2-to-L3 disc were excised, and those of the midlevel of the L5 vertebral body were cut by a drill, followed by posterior stabilization (see **Fig. 12**D left and right).

Step 2: Anterior Transperitoneal Approach

A vascular surgeon helped the authors to dissect major vessels, such as the aorta, bilateral common iliac arteries, inferior vena cava, and right common iliac vein, from the vertebral tumor (see **Fig. 12**E). The left common iliac vein was sacrificed because it was completely involved by the tumor. The anterior halves of the L2-to-L3 disc were excised, and those of the midlevel of the L5 vertebral body were cut by a drill. The tumor vertebral bodies of L3, L4, and the upper half of L5, including the paravertebral tumor, were removed en bloc with a marginal

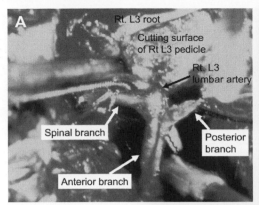

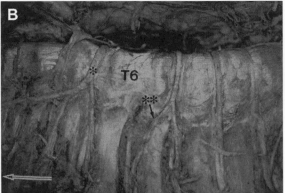

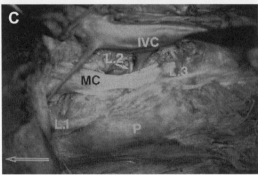

Fig. 7. Vascular anatomy. (*A*) Anatomy of the segmental artery. (*B*) Variations in intercostal arteries in a cadaveric study. The left second, third, and fourth intercostal arteries branch from the fifth intercostal artery (*) anterior to the head of the fifth rib. The left sixth intercostal artery (**) branches as a variant of the seventh intercostal artery. The arrow indicates the cranial direction. (*C*) Right medial crus of the lumbar diaphragm and surrounding vessels in a cadaveric study. The medial crus originates at L2 to L3. IVC, inferior vena cava; MC, right medial crus; P, psoas muscle. L.1, L.2, and L.3 indicate the first, second, and third lumbar arteries. The arrow indicates the cranial direction. (*From* Tomita K, Kawahara N, Baba H, et al. Total en bloc spondylectomy for solitary spinal metastasis. Int Orthop 1994;18:291–8; with permission; and Tomita K, Kawahara N, Murakami H, et al. Total en bloc spondylectomy for spinal tumors: improvement of the technique and its associated basic background. J Orthop Sci 2006;11(1):3–12; with permission.)

margin (see **Fig. 12**F left and right). A titanium mesh cylinder (MOSS-Miami) with autogenous bone graft inside was placed in the vertebral defect (see **Fig. 12**G left and right).

Step 3: Posterior Approach

Spinal reconstruction was finalized. The anterior cage and posterior rods were connected by connector devices to secure spinal stability (see **Fig. 12**H left and right).

POSTOPERATIVE MANAGEMENT

Suction draining is preferred for 4 to 5 days after surgery, and the patient is allowed to start walking 1 week after surgery. The patient wears a thoracolumbosacral orthosis for 3 months until the bony union or incorporation of the artificial vertebral prosthesis is attained.

POSSIBLE SOLUTIONS FOR MAJOR RISKS

How to Reduce Excessive Bleeding

Preoperative triple-level embolization

Intraoperative bleeding is sometimes excessive in patients who have hypervascular spinal tumors in TES surgery. There is no doubt that preoperative embolization of the feeding artery at the affected vertebra is mandatory; nevertheless, this does not seem to be sufficient to stop the bleeding altogether. In a canine study, the authors found that when bilateral segmental arteries at three levels were ligated, blood flow of the middle vertebra was reduced to 25% of that of the control group[27] while maintaining 80% of spinal cord blood flow (SCBF) and spinal cord function was not damaged at all (see **Fig. 4**).[18,28]

In all patients who have thoracic hypervascular spinal tumors of a single level, embolization of segmental arteries supplying the tumor (group A, 18 patients) or embolization of bilateral segmental

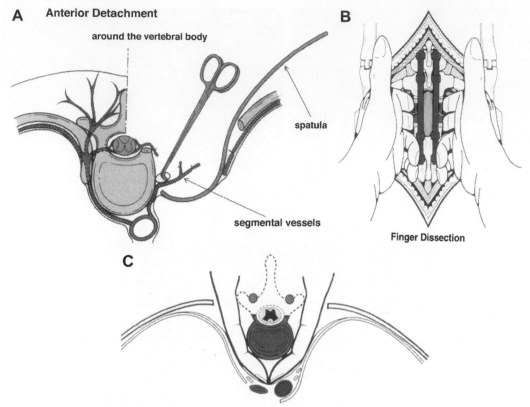

Fig. 8. Anterior dissection around the vertebral body. (*A*) Dissection of the segmental artery using a peanut (cotton ball). (*From* Kawahara N, Tomita K, Murakami H, et al. Total en bloc spondylectomy for spinal metastases. In: Jasmin C, Coleman RE, Coia LR, et al, editors. The textbook of bone metastases. Chichester, West Sussex, England: John Wiley & Sons Ltd; 2005. p. 215–23; with permission.) (*B*) Anterior dissection using fingers. Posterior view. (*C*) Anterior dissection using fingers. Axial view.

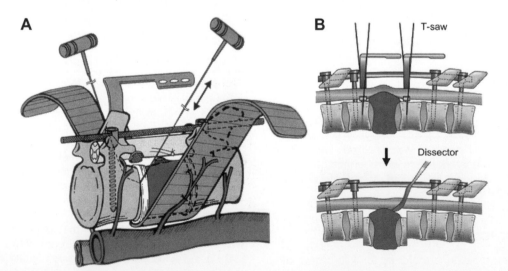

Fig. 9. (*A*) Anterior column osteotomy and removal of the tumor vertebral body(ies). (*B*) How to remove the spinal tumor with epidural extension. (*Upper*) The anterior column is cut at a safe margin approximately 10 mm above and below the epidural tumor using a T-saw. (*Lower*) The tumor vertebral body is pushed away 5 to 10 mm in the ventral direction from the dural tube, which results in spinal cord decompression. An adhesion between the pseudocapsule of the epidural tumor and the anterior aspect of the dural tube is safely dissected using a dissector.

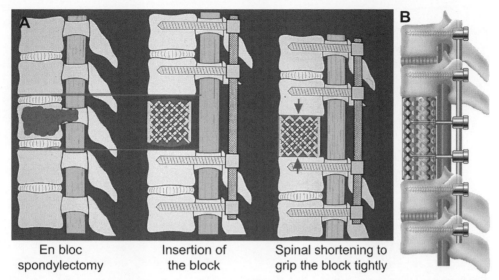

| En bloc spondylectomy | Insertion of the block | Spinal shortening to grip the block tightly |

Fig. 10. Spinal reconstruction. (*A*) Spinal reconstruction. (*B*) Spinal reconstruction for a large defect. If two or three vertebrae are resected, application of the connector device between the posterior rods and anterior spacer is recommended to secure spinal stability.

arteries at three levels (group B, 18 patients) was attempted, and subsequent TES was evaluated. On average, 2.0 segmental arteries were embolized in group A, whereas 5.3 arteries were embolized in group B. No neurologic complications occurred as a result of embolization. The average time of the operation was 8.4 hours (range: 7.4–10.8 hours) in group A and 9.0 hours (range: 6.8–11.5 hours) in group B. This difference was not statistically significant. The average intraoperative blood loss was 2612 mL (range: 1530–5950 mL) in group A and 1406 mL (range: 375–2550 mL) in group B. There was a significant reduction in blood loss ($P<.05$). No comparable incidents have occurred after surgery at the authors' hospital. It should be cautioned that there is a possibility of subacute neurologic degradation after embolization because of the increase in spinal cord compression of the epidural tumor tissue resulting from ischemic edema of the tumor necrosis, although this is rare.

Hypotensive anesthesia

It has become a common practice to manage relatively hypotensive anesthesia (systolic blood pressure: 80–100 mm Hg). This does not influence the spinal cord blood circulation as was once thought.

How to Avoid Damage to the Major Vessels and Segmental Vessels

Blunt dissection of the anterior part of the vertebral body is another risky maneuver in TES by a single posterior approach (see **Fig. 8**). Of

course, careful step-by-step dissection is an important fundamental key, and each anatomic relation between the vertebra and visceral organs, major vessels, segmental artery and its spinal branch should be well acknowledged (see **Fig. 7**).[21,22,29] Based on the authors' anatomic studies on cadavers,[22] it became clear that dissection is less likely to damage the thoracic aorta or azygos vein between T1 and T4. Nevertheless, the segmental artery must be carefully detached and clipped anteriorly in areas caudal to T5 before manipulation of the affected vertebra (see **Fig. 7**B). It might be helpful to consider

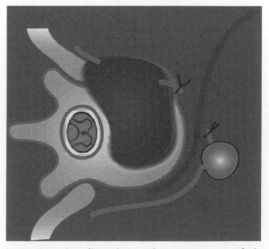

Fig. 11. Anterior dissection and management of the segmental artery by an anterior approach if the arteries are involved by the tumor.

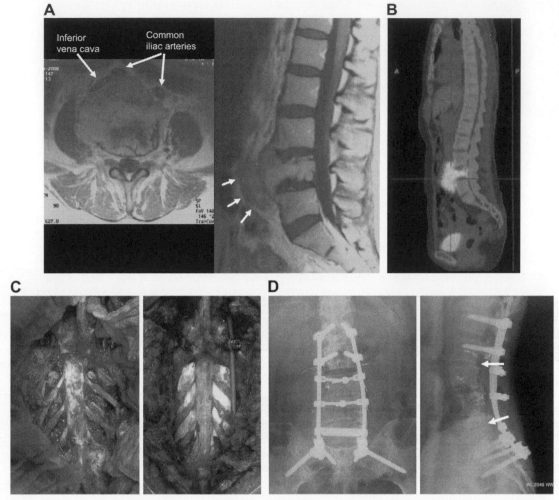

Fig. 12. Giant-cell tumor of the lumbar spine in a 38-year-old woman. (*A*) MRI (T1-gadolinium enhanced). (*Left*) Axial image of the L4 vertebral level. The vertebral tumor largely expanded outside the vertebral body. The bilateral common iliac arteries were compressed and shifted in an anterior direction, and the inferior vena cava was also so severely compressed as to be flattened. (*Right*) Sagittal image of the lumbar spine. The vertebral tumor largely expanded outside the vertebral body (*white arrows*) and grew to the neighboring vertebrae (L3 and L5). (*B*) Positron emission tomography superimposed by CT (sagittal image). (*C*) Operative photograph after dissection of the lumbar nerves. (*Left*) Dissection of lumbar nerves. Bilateral L3, L4, and L5 lumbar nerves were dissected from the vertebral body to their conjunction with the neighboring lumbar nerves. (*Right*) Placement of an artificial sheet between the lumbar nerves and the tumor vertebral body. The artificial sheet serves as an operative landmark in the anterior approach. (*D*) Radiographs after step 1 of the operation (posterior approach). (*Left*) Anterior-posterior view. (*Right*) Lateral view. The white arrows indicate the cutting line of the posterior halves of the anterior column. The upper half was at the L2-to-L3 disc level and the lower half was midlevel of the L5 vertebral body in this patient. (*E*) Anterior dissection of the major vessels. A vascular surgeon helped the authors to dissect major vessels, such as the aorta, bilateral common iliac arteries, inferior vena cava, and right common iliac vein, from the vertebral tumor. The left common iliac vein was sacrificed because it was completely involved by the tumor. (*F*) Resected specimen. (*Left*) Operative photograph of the resected specimen. Tumor vertebral bodies of L3, L4, and the upper half of L5, including paravertebral tumor expanding outside, were removed en bloc with a marginal margin. (*Right*) Radiograph of the resected specimen from an anterior-posterior view. (*G*) Operative photograph after removal of the tumor vertebrae by an anterior approach. (*Left*) Large defect after removal of the tumor vertebrae. The large defect was recognized after removal of the tumor vertebrae. The anterior aspect of the lumbar dural tube and nerves were directly seen from ventral side by retracting major vessels aside. (*Right*) Anterior spinal reconstruction using a cage. A titanium mesh cylinder (MOSS-Miami) with autogenous bone graft inside was placed in the vertebral defect. (*H*) Postoperative radiograph. (*Left*) Anterior-posterior view. (*Right*) Lateral view.

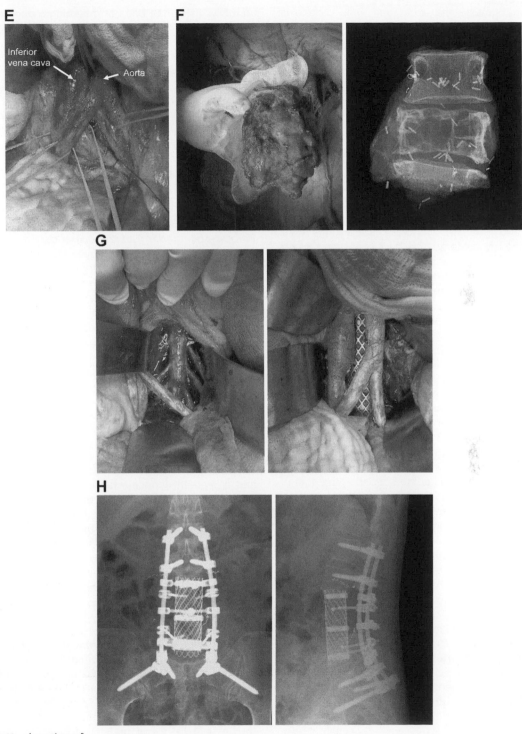

Fig. 12. (*continued*)

Pledget Nescosuture (Alfresa Pharma Corporation, Osaka, Japan) patching over the pinhole of the aorta in case of pulling out the segmental artery. At a lesion of L1 and L2, the diaphragm insertions should be dissected from the vertebral body before the lumbar arteries are dissected because the segmental arteries run between the vertebral body and diaphragm insertion (see **Fig. 7**C). The utmost care is necessary to dissect around the vertebral body in the lumbar spine because the aorta and vena cava exist closely in front of the lordotic spine.

After all structures surrounding the vertebral body are dissected, the following processes are continued under the protection barricade by means of a vertebral spatula (recompartmentalization), which is also useful for less bleeding.

How Many Ligations of Segmental Arteries Occur in Ischemic Spinal Cord Damage, Especially Including the Artery of Adamkiewicz

Possible circulatory compromise after the ligation of the radicular artery is another concern. Woodard and Freeman[30] reported that animals (adult mongrel dogs) prepared by the section of from one to four sets of adjacent nerve roots showed no neurologic deficits or such deficits were extremely transient and that animals with five sets of adjacent nerve roots sectioned frequently showed transient neurologic deficits.[30] The authors also reported that interruption of bilateral segmental arteries at five or more consecutive levels risks producing spinal cord ischemia capable of injuring the spinal cord at a level that does not include the artery of Adamkiewicz.[31]

In the feline model, the authors found that ligation of the artery of Adamkiewicz reduced SCBF by approximately 81% of the control value and that this decrease did not have an effect on spinal cord evoked potentials.[32] Furthermore, using a canine experiment, the authors reported that four or more levels of ligation of bilateral segmental arteries, including the artery of Adamkiewicz, has a risk for producing ischemic spinal cord damage.[33] Summarizing these data, it may be suggested that in animals, bilateral ligation of segmental arteries of less than four levels, even including the artery of Adamkiewicz level, hardly produces a risk for postoperative neurologic degradation as a result of spinal cord ischemia. This is because the blood supply of the spinal cord is protected by three arterial plexus layers: intercanal, dural, and pial arterial. These may compensate the blood supply for ligation of bilateral segmental arteries of less than four segments.[34]

Clinically, the authors have performed the TES procedure in more than 150 patients who had spinal tumors at their university hospital. It was proved by angiography for preoperative embolization that corresponding segmental arteries to TES level(s) included a radiculomedullary artery(ies), which supplied the anterior spinal artery in 14 patients. The TES procedure was of a single segment in 10 patients, two segments in 2 patients, and three segments in 2 patients of these 14 patients.

Actually, there has been no neurologic degradation attributable to spinal cord ischemia in this series of patients who have undergone TES, even including these 14 patients. It may also be suggested that bilateral ligation of segmental arteries of less than four levels is less likely to produce a risk for postoperative neurologic degradation attributable to spinal cord ischemia in humans. Nevertheless, there is still no doubt that it is necessary to inform the patient and family about the possibility of ischemic spinal cord damage during TES and preoperative triple-level embolization.

How to Avoid Spinal Cord Injury

Atraumatic handling of the spinal cord
The spinal cord compressed by the tumor is terribly delicate and fragile. It is common knowledge to avoid mechanical damage to the neural structures, especially shifting aside, twisting, and hanging down or upward of the cord. The authors also learned from spinal cord monitoring during surgery that spinal cord stretching causes irreversible mechanical damage. Too much nerve root traction also damages the cord as a result of the root avulsion mechanism.

T-saw cutting
To cut the vertebral bone sharply while reducing the risk for spinal cord and nerve root damage, the authors designed the T-saw.[20] It is made of multifilament twisted stainless steel wires and has a smooth surface with which to cut bone, with minimal damage to the surrounding soft tissue. Because its diameter is 0.5 mm, the cutting loss is negligible. The T-saw is used in a pediculotomy for en bloc laminectomy and in anterior column osteotomy for en bloc corpectomy. An improved version of this T-saw is now available as the Diamond T-sawR (Medtronic Sofamor Danek, Memphis, Tennessee) for easier cutting of the anterior column.

How to remove the spinal tumor with epidural extension safely to the spinal cord
In the patients with spinal cord compression by epidural tumor extension, it is dangerous to the spinal cord to dissect using a cord spatula or Penfield dissector between the pseudocapsule of the epidural tumor and the adhered anterior aspect of the dural tube because the spinal cord is already compressed by the epidural tumor. To remove the vertebral tumor en bloc safely, including epidural extension, without injuring the spinal cord, the operative procedures are three steps using a posterior approach as follows (see **Fig. 9**B):

1. The anterior column is cut at a safe margin approximately 10 mm above and below the epidural tumor using a T-saw (see Figs. **9**B and **6**C right lower).
2. The tumor vertebral body is pushed away 5 to 10 mm in the ventral direction from the dural tube, which leads to spinal cord decompression (see Figs. **9**B and **6**C right lower).
3. Adhesion between the pseudocapsule of the epidural tumor and the anterior aspect of the dural tube is safely dissected using a dissector. This procedure allows oncologic en bloc vertebral resection without injuring the spinal cord in patients with epidural tumor extension (see **Fig. 6**D left).

The authors have experienced local recurrence in 5 of 97 patients who underwent TES.[18] All local recurrences occurred at the edge of an unsuccessful excised tumor margin, that is, from residual tumor tissue, especially around the epidural area.[18] Therefore, removal of the tumor vertebra en bloc with the epidural tumor, including a sufficiently safe margin as mentioned previously, is expected to decrease of the rate of local recurrence after the TES procedure.

Risk for Tumor Cell Contamination

Tumor cell contamination or tumor tissue residue

Residual tumor tissue and contaminated cells are different entities from the viewpoint of oncologic regrowth.[18] Residual tumor is certain to regrow if it exists, whereas the potential of regrowth is low from contaminated tumor cells. Residual tumor tissue does not remain after TES with an adequate oncologic margin, even if the tumor vertebra is divided into two blocks by the T-saw (anterior and posterior parts). The risk for tumor cell contamination does exists during this process, however.[18]

Rinsing with distilled water and anticancer drug

Contamination might be minimal[35] but is still a possible cause of local recurrence after TES. To eradicate contaminated cancer cells, a new type of local chemotherapy was developed—double rinsing with distilled water and high concentrated cisplatinum.[18,36] In an in vitro experiment, no living tumor cells were detected after tumor cells were exposed to distilled water for 2.5 minutes, followed by high-concentration cisplatinum (0.5 mg/mL) for 2.5 minutes. The reason why this works is that osmosis of the tumor cell membrane is increased by contact with distilled water and the permeability of cisplatinum through the cell membrane into the

cytoplasm of the tumor cells is then accelerated, resulting in the eradication of contaminated tumor cells.[18,36]

Spinal Column Shortening

The posterior instrumentation is adjusted to compress the inserted vertebral prosthesis slightly to secure it in the final step of spinal reconstruction. This process of spinal shortening has two important advantages: (1) it increases the spinal stability of the anterior and posterior spinal column, and (2) it increases SCBF, which is preferable to improve spinal cord function.[26] The safety limits and physiologic effects of spinal shortening on the spinal cord were studied in dogs.[26] Acute spinal column shortening can be characterized into three phases:

- Phase 1: safe range—spinal shortening within one third of the vertebral segment, which is characterized by no deformity of the dural sac or the spinal cord
- Phase 2: warning range—spinal shortening between one third and two thirds of the vertebral segment, which is characterized by shrinking and buckling of the dural sac and no deformity of the spinal cord
- Phase 3: dangerous range—spinal shortening in excess of two thirds of the vertebral segment, which is characterized by spinal cord deformity and compression by the buckled dura

The authors' experiment revealed the interesting and important fact that spinal shortening within the safe range increases SCBF. As mentioned previously, the posterior instrumentation is adjusted to compress the inserted vertebral prosthesis slightly in a final step of spinal reconstruction. This maneuver results in slight spinal shortening from 5 to 10 mm, which is within the safe range of the spinal shortening that also leads to an increase in SCBF. Numerous researchers have demonstrated that reperfusion of SCBF is of paramount importance in the recovery of spinal cord function after spinal cord injuries.[37–42]

In the authors' series, neurologically compromised patients had a significant recovery after circumspinal decompression and shortening of the spinal column in those individuals undergoing TES.[2,3,13] This may be partly attributable to an increase in SCBF achieved by limited (phase 1 and 2) shortening.

ACKNOWLEDGMENT

The authors deeply thank all the doctors in the Department of Orthopaedic Surgery, Kanazawa

University, who have contributed throughout this work.

REFERENCES

1. Fujita T, Ueda Y, Kawahara N, et al. Local spread of metastatic vertebral tumors. A histologic study. Spine 1997;22(16):1905–12.
2. Tomita K, Kawahara N, Baba H, et al. Total en bloc spondylectomy for solitary spinal metastasis. Int Orthop 1994;18:291–8.
3. Tomita K, Kawahara N, Baba H, et al. Total en bloc spondylectomy. A new surgical technique for primary malignant vertebral tumors. Spine 1997;22:324–33.
4. Roy-Camille R, Mazel CH, Saillant G, et al. Treatment of malignant tumor of the spine with posterior instrumentation. In: Sundaresan N, Schmidek HH, Schiller AL, Rosenthal DI, editors. Tumors of the spine. Philadelphia: WB Saunders; 1990. p. 473–87.
5. Roy-Camille R, Saillant G, Bisserie M, et al. Resection vertebrale totale dans la chirurgie tumorale au niveau du rachis dorsal par voie posterieure pure. Rev Chir Orthop 1981;67:421–30.
6. Stener B. Total spondylectomy in chondrosarcoma arising from the seventh thoracic vertebra. J Bone Joint Surg Br 1971;53:288–95.
7. Stener B. Complete removal of vertebrae for extirpation of tumors. Clin Orthop 1989;245:72–82.
8. Stener B. Technique of complete spondylectomy in the thoracic and lumbar spine. In: Sundaresan N, Schmidek HH, Schiller AL, Rosenthal DI, editors. Tumors of the spine. Philadelphia: WB Saunders; 1990. p. 432–7.
9. Stener B, Johnsen OE. Complete removal of three vertebrae for giant cell tumour. J Bone Joint Surg Br 1971;53:278–87.
10. Sundaresan N, Rosen G, Huvos AG, et al. Combined treatment of osteosarcoma of the spine. Neurosurgery 1988;23:714–9.
11. Boriani S, Biagini R, De Iure F, et al. Vertebrectomia lombare per neoplasia ossea: tecnica chirurgica. Chir Organi Mov 1994;79:163–73.
12. Boriani S, Chevalley F, Weinstein JN, et al. Chordoma of the spine above the sacrum. Treatment and outcome in 21 cases. Spine 1996;21:1569–77.
13. Kawahara N, Tomita K, Fujita T, et al. Osteosarcoma of the thoracolumbar spine. Total en bloc spondylectomy. A case report. J Bone Joint Surg Am 1997;79:453–8.
14. Kawahara N, Tomita K, Murakami H, et al. Total en bloc spondylectomy for spinal metastases. In: Jasmin C, Coleman RE, Coia LR, Capanna R, Saillant G, editors. The textbook of bone metastases. Chichester, West Sussex, England: John Wiley & Sons Ltd; 2005. p. 215–23.
15. Kawahara N, Tomita K, Tsuchiya H. Total en bloc spondylectomy: a new surgical technique for malignant vertebral tumors. In: Watkins RG, editor.

16. Murakami H, Kawahara N, Abdel-Wanis ME, et al. Total en bloc spondylectomy. Semin Musculoskelet Radiol 2001;5(2):189–94.
17. Tomita K, Toribatake Y, Kawahara N, et al. Total en bloc spondylectomy and circumspinal decompression for solitary spinal metastasis. Paraplegia 1994; 32:36–46.
18. Tomita K, Kawahara N, Murakami H, et al. Total en bloc spondylectomy for spinal tumors: improvement of the technique and its associated basic background. J Orthop Sci 2006;11(1):3–12.
19. Tomita K, Kawahara K, Kobayashi T, et al. Surgical strategy for spinal metastases. Spine 2001;26: 298–306.
20. Tomita K, Kawahara N. The threadwire saw: a new device for cutting bone. J Bone Joint Surg Am 1996;78:1915–7.
21. Adachi B. Das Arteriensystem der Japaner. Kyoto Tokyo: Maruzen Publishing; 1928.
22. Kawahara N, Tomita K, Baba H, et al. Cadaveric vascular anatomy for total en bloc spondylectomy in malignant vertebral tumors. Spine 1996;21:1401–7.
23. Tomita K, Kawahara N, Baba H, et al. Circumspinal decompression for thoracic myelopathy due to combined ossification of the posterior longitudinal ligament and ligamentum flavum. Spine 1990;15(11):1114–20.
24. Akamaru T, Kawahara N, Sakamoto J, et al. Transmission of the load sharing inside a titanium mesh cage used in anterior column reconstruction after total spondylectomy; a finite element analysis. Spine 2005;30(24):2783–7.
25. Akamaru T, Kawahara N, Tsuchiya H, et al. Healing of autogenous bone in a titanium mesh cage used in anterior column reconstruction after total spondylectomy. Spine 2002;27(13):E329–33.
26. Kawahara N, Tomita K, Kobayashi T, et al. Influence of acute shortening on the spinal cord. An experimental study. Spine 2005;30(6):613–20.
27. Numbu K, Kawahara N, Murakami H, et al. Interruption of bilateral segmental arteries at several levels. Influence on vertebral blood flow. Spine 2004; 29(14):1530–4.
28. Ueda Y, Kawahara N, Tomita K, et al. Influence on spinal cord blood flow and spinal cord function by interruption of bilateral segmental arteries at up to three levels: experimental study in dogs. Spine 2005;30(20):2239–43.
29. Winter RB, Denis F, Lonstein JL, et al. Techniques of surgery: anatomy of thoracic intercostal and lumbar arteries. In: Lonstein JL, Bradford DS, Winter RB, Ogilvie JW, editors. Moe's textbook of scoliosis and other spinal deformities. 3rd edition. Philadelphia: WB Saunders; 1994. p. 196–8.
30. Woodard JS, Freeman LW. Ischemia of the spinal cord. J Neurosurg 1956;13:63–72.

Surgical approach to the spine. 2nd edition. New York: Springer-Verlag; 2003. p. 309–25.

31. Fujimaki Y, Kawahara N, Tomita K, et al. How many ligations of bilateral segmental arteries cause ischemic spinal cord dysfunction? An experimental study using a dog model. Spine 2006;31(21): E781–9.

32. Toribatake Y. The effect of total en bloc spondylectomy on spinal cord circulation. J Jpn Orthop Assoc 1993;67:1070–80 [in Japanese].

33. Kato S, Kawahara N, Tomita K, et al. Effects on spinal cord blood flow and neurologic function secondary to interruption of bilateral segmental arteries which supply the artery of Adamkiewicz: an experimental study using a dog model. Spine 2008; 33(14):1533–41.

34. Yosizawa H. Blood supply of spinal cord and nerve root. Its clinical meaning. J Centr Jpn Orthop Traum 1988;31(1):1–13 [in Japanese].

35. Abdel-Wanis ME, Tsuchiya H, Kawahara N, et al. Tumor growth potential after tumoral and instrumental contamination: an in-vivo comparative study of T-saw, Gigli saw, and scalpel. J Orthop Sci 2001;6: 424–9.

36. Kose H, Kawahara N, Tomita K. Local irrigation with cisplatin following resection of malignant vertebral tumors. J Japan Spine Res Soc 1999; 10(2):358–64 [in Japanese].

37. Carlson GD, Warden KE, Barbeau JM, et al. Viscoelastic relaxation and regional blood flow response to spinal cord compression and decompression. Spine 1997;22:1285–91.

38. Ducker TB, Salcman M, Lucas JT, et al. Experimental spinal cord trauma. II: blood flow, tissue oxygen, evoked potentials in both paretic and plegic monkeys. Surg Neurol 1978;10:64–70.

39. Holtz A, Nystrom B, Gerdin B. Relationship between spinal cord blood flow and functional recovery after blocking weight-induced spinal cord injury in rats. Neurosurgery 1990;26:952–7.

40. Ohashi T, Morimoto T, Kawata K, et al. Correlation between spinal cord blood flow and arterial diameter following acute spinal cord injury in rats. Acta Neurochir (Wien) 1996;138:322–9.

41. Winter RB. Spine update; neurologic safety in spinal deformity surgery. Spine 1997;22:1527–33.

42. Young W, Flamm ES. Effect of high-dose corticosteroid therapy on blood flow, evoked potentials, and extracellular calcium in experimental spinal injury. J Neurosurg 1982;57:667–73.

Biomechanics and Materials of Reconstruction After Tumor Resection in the Spinal Column

Robert P. Melcher, MD, Jürgen Harms, MD*

KEYWORDS

- Spinal tumor • Spinal metastasis • Anterior support
- Posterior tension band • Titanium mesh cage
- Pedicle screw

Surgical treatment of tumors in the muscular-skeletal system often requires extensive resection with safety margins reaching far into adjacent structures. This is often not possible for the surgical treatment of spinal tumors because of the close proximity of important neural and vascular tissue. However, improvement of surgical techniques,[1–3] as well as surgical tools, has resulted in better outcomes.[4,5]

An important aspect of spinal tumor surgery is the reconstruction and stabilization after wide resections of one or multiple spinal segments. With today's available resources and knowledge of biomechanical principles it should be possible to accomplish stable reconstructions in nearly all patients. The benefit of spinal stabilization is early mobilization, particularly in patients with limited survival time because of the nature of their malignancy. This early mobilization allows for resumption or improvement of motor function as well as quality-of-life parameters. In contrast, one should also avoid inadequate and inconsequent reconstruction causing early failure and further deterioration of the patient's conditions that may finally result in life-threatening revision surgery. It is also important to realize that tumor surgery is not always the treatment of choice for patients with an unfavorable prognosis. Especially when performing instrumented surgery of benign tumors in young patients, one should consider the long-term consequences.

We initially review the general biomechanical principles that should be considered in surgical reconstruction of spinal tumors. This will be further clarified by more detailed descriptions for individual spinal regions in the subsequent part of the article.

GENERAL CONSIDERATIONS
Decision Making

The following questions need to be answered as part of the decision-making process defining the most adequate surgical and reconstructive options:

Is complete resection of the tumor feasible? This should be the goal for benign tumor intervention of the spine. Unfortunately, such is not the case with many malignant tumors of the spinal axis. This often includes use of adjuvant treatment options such as chemo and radiation therapy. The dilemma becomes even more challenging in patients with a solitary metastasis, such as in carcinoma of the breast, kidney, or lung. Recent studies have conclusively shown the benefit of initial surgical

Department of Orthopaedics and Spine Surgery, Klinikum Karlsbad-Langensteinbach, Guttmannstrasse 1, 76307, Karlsbad-Langensteinbach, Germany
* Corresponding author.
E-mail address: juergen.harms@kkl.srh.de (J. Harms).

Orthop Clin N Am 40 (2009) 65–74
doi:10.1016/j.ocl.2008.09.005

intervention in patients with neurologic compromise to spinal metastasis.[4,5]

Biomechanical Considerations for Reconstruction

One of the basic prerequisites for biomechanically intact reconstructions is knowledge in principles of load transfer through the so-called central axis organ of the human body.[6] The predominant amount of axial load is transferred anteriorly, whereas only a small quantity runs posterior. These loads change upon flexion and extension of the spine. On principle, the anterior column consists of the vertebral bodies and the intervertebral discs representing the "load-sharing" portion of the spine. The posterior osseous structures in combination with the ligaments and joint capsules reflect the tension band of the construct. One feature that tumor invasion and surgical intervention have in common is the disruption of this antero-posterior balance.

Options for Reconstruction

When the stability of the anterior column is compromised by tumor destruction, surgical options vary quite considerably. They range from percutaneous cement injection to complete vertebral body replacement with interbody spacer. The expectation of such an anterior spacer is to compensate for the load-bearing capacity of the removed vertebra, and indirectly decrease the load to the adjacent segment. To achieve anterior support following tumor resection, autologous or allogeneic tricortical bone blocks of different origin are used as well as individually formed poly-methyl-methacrylat inlays with or without metal reinforcement. Today, a large selection of reinforcement devices made from different metal alloys, carbon fibers, synthetic plastics, or ceramic is on the market. Although most have been initially designed for trauma surgery, they have found their way into tumor surgery. To fit the defect, the spacers are trimmed, stacked, or expanded. Especially in patients with a good prognosis, the spacers should allow for enough room for osseous integration, partially at the endplates of the construct. The association between the required volume of a spacer for providing enough anterior support with prevention of severe subsidence, and its relationship to the outcome of osseous incorporation has been investigated for cervical spine fusion devices by Kandziora and colleagues.[7] In their conclusion, the "volume-related stiffness" was essential for the outcome of a fusion, and this was best accomplished by use of a mesh spacer.

Failures of anterior support after reconstruction in tumor surgery can have multiple factors. They include the following:

- The tendency for dislocation of a graft will increase where the rotational forces in the reconstructed area has not been sufficiently reduced. Graft designs resulting in good primary anchoring at the graft-bone interface can provide further rotational stability, whereas grafts with smooth surfaces will increase the rotational instability.
- Subsidence of the spacer into the adjacent vertebrae is a result of excess stress to the bone, and can be caused by two main sources. They are poor bone quality and mechanical overload owing to incorrect construct design. A surgeon's option for poor bone quality is limited, although augmentation with small amounts of bone cement can possibility increase the stability of the augmented segments and contribute to overall construct stability.
- Fracture or collapse of the anterior device is observed with long bone graft constructs.[8] However, collapse of manufactured devices has also been reported. This is especially true where the weight-bearing capacity of the graft is overestimated or the occurring forces acting on the graft have been underappreciated.
- Despite adequate anterior construct, neglect of the status within the posterior tension band has been problematic. Functional interaction between the pressure-resisting anterior column and a stable posterior tension band provides a high likelihood for spinal stability.[9]

Posterior stabilization techniques have progressed a great deal over the past 30 years. Wiring techniques have been surpassed by hook- or screw-based fixation devices.[10] The latter technique provides a more rigid stabilization and has shorter construct length.

Although advances have been made, complications with posterior instrumentation do exist. They include pullout or breakage of the anchor points or longitudinal connectors, likely because of a mechanical overload of the system.

Since long-term survival rates have improved with many forms of cancer, it should be noted that patients with spinal involvement have a different measurement of success. For patients with long-term survival, it is important that osseous fusion accompany the cancer survival. This can sometimes be accomplished with the first surgery, but may often require a reoperation for the addition of bone graft materials and products.

SYSTEMATIC APPROACH TO THE ANATOMIC REGIONS OF THE SPINE
Reconstruction for Tumors at the Cranio-Cervical Junction

The cranio-cervical junction consists of the occipital bone, the atlas and axis, and a complex ligamentous apparatus. In this composite, the course of the vertebral artery has its own importance, especially with respect to surgery. The cranio-cervical junction combines a sophisticated anatomic make-up allowing for mobility, but at the same time crucial for stability. Pain is the most common presenting complaint with tumor involvement in this area. Because of the relative width of the spinal canal in this area, neurologic disturbances occur at a later stage of the disease, secondary to spinal canal impingement or pathologic fracture. Painful range of motion from head rotation maneuvers is a common manifestation in patients with tumor destruction of a lateral mass of the C1 or C2 lateral masses. Treatment of this painful instability is often surgical stabilization. Resection of the pathologic component is performed via an anterior-lateral approach, whereas stabilization is accomplished posteriorly. Preoperative angiographic evaluation of the vertebral artery is crucial for surgical safety. The load-bearing capacity of the lateral mass strongly depends on the amount of destruction within the bony architecture (**Fig. 1**A). In cases of significant osseous inadequacy, replacement of the destroyed lateral mass can become necessary to restore stability. In our experience, small cylindric titanium mesh cages can be a viable option. However, replacement of the lateral mass will not restore rotational stability and cranio-cervical instrumentation is critical (see **Fig. 1**B, C).

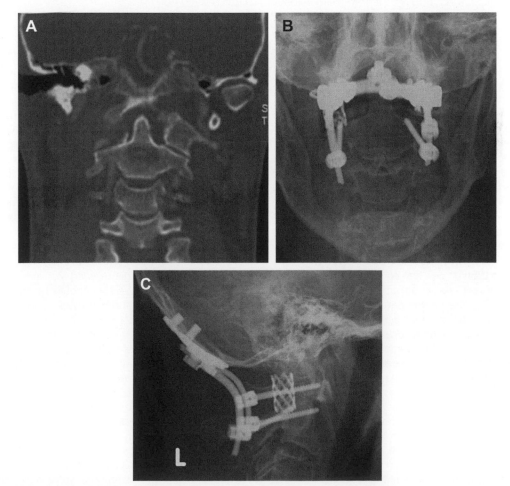

Fig. 1. (*A*) Metastatic destruction of right C1 lateral mass. (*B, C*) Same patient after posterior-only performed stabilization with cage replacing lateral mass of C1 and additional occipito-cervical instrumentation.

For posterior cranio-cervical fixation, rod/plate constructs with screw anchors provide better stability compared with wire fixation.[11] Fixation of these occipital plates is performed in the midline of the occipital bone where the thickest bone can be found.[12] Screw fixation to the upper cervical spine is possible into the lateral mass of C1 and the pedicles or the lamina of C2,[13–15] as well as lateral masses or pedicles of the subaxial spine. Biomechanical studies have shown that the primary stability of a cranio-cervical fixation from C0 to C3 is equivalent when using bilateral plate fixation or occipital plate with a screw-rod connection.[14] However, many surgeons currently prefer the rod/screw system over the plate/screw for a variety of reasons:

- The location of the entry point and also the trajectory for the screw fixation is dictated by the holes in the plate.
- Reduction has to be performed before the plate fixation and it has to be maintained unchanged throughout the entire fixation process.
- Corrections or adjustment of the reduction is very difficult, when plate fixation has been completed.
- Revision surgeries are more laborious with the plate system.

In contrast, a top-loading system allows for individual positioning of every single screw anchor in the best suitable modality. Screw heads are finally connected by the contoured rod. Necessary reduction maneuvers can be performed at any time of the procedure and can be modified without the need to change the position of the screws. The implants by themselves can act as reduction devices. In the case of revision surgery, only the rods have to be removed and further extension of the construct with additional anchors in the mid- and lower cervical or even to the thoracic spine are quite easy.

Tumors of the central part of the axis are commonly detected at an advanced stage. If detected at an early stage, smaller lesions that are strictly limited to a region like the odontoid or the lamina can be excised locally. Reconstruction, if deemed necessary, can be limited to the discussed segment. Resection of the odontoid always creates an atlanto-axial instability requiring C1-C2 fixation.[16]

More frequently we see patients with expanded tumor spread requiring removal of the vertebra's central part. This will result in severe destabilization requiring reconstruction with special implants. **Box 1** shows the indications in patients who required subtotal or total C2 corpectomy and subsequently received such a construct. It consists of

---

Box 1
Indications for C2 resection followed by cage implantation

Primary malignant tumors, n = 17

- 10 Chordoma
- 3 Osteosarcoma
- 1 Synovial sarcoma
- 3 Plasmacytoma

Primary benign tumors, n = 6

- 2 Aneurysmal bone cyst
- 2 Giant cell tumor
- 2 Aggressive hemangioma

Metastasis, n = 11

- 6 Breast
- 2 Prostate
- 1 Renal cell
- 1 Thyroid
- 1 Melanoma

Remaining unclear tumor, n = 1

Spondylitis C2, n = 1

Osteonecrosis, n = 1

---

a central cylindric titanium mesh connected to an anterior T-shaped plate with screw holes for screw fixation to the lateral mass of C1 and the corpus of C3. Critical in this construct are the bilaterally attached small winglike cages, meant to hold the lateral masses of C1 when C2 has been removed. With little spikes at their top surface, additional resistance to rotation is provided. The biomechanical concept behind the design of this implant is to transfer the loads from the two lateral masses of C1 onto the vertebral body of C3 and to control some of the high rotational forces in this area.[17] A posterior stabilization follows such an anterior procedure. Interestingly, owing to our clinical experience, posterior fixation could be limited in most patients to an upper cervical fixation from C1 to C3 or C4 (**Fig. 2**A, B). Preserving the occipito-cervical joint has not resulted in any detectable signs of instability, and moreover, has allowed for physiologic maintenance of functions such as chewing and swallowing. In patients with more extensive tumors reaching to the mid-cervical area, wider exposure via mandibulo-glossotomy can be accomplished (**Fig. 3**).

High mechanical stresses and unique morphology have to be overcome in this region with a solid reconstruction device. Concomitantly, this construct is implanted into an area with a high risk for bacterial contamination and the available tissue layers for coverage are very limited. Therefore,

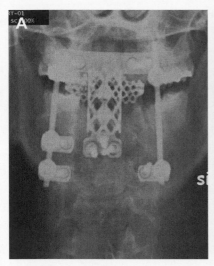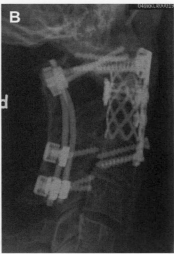

Fig. 2. (*A, B*) AP and lateral x-ray views 10 years after resection of recurrent chordoma of C2.

meticulous preparation of the posterior wall of the oral cavity is crucial. The senior author (J. Harms) has had very good experiences in transoral surgery for tumor and rheumatoid arthritis over the past 20 years with the "double-layer preparation" of the posterior pharyngeal wall.[18] The first layer, consisting of the mucosa, is dissected starting with a far lateral longitudinal and two oblique incisions. This creates a flap of approximately 2.5 × 2.5 mm in an open door–like fashion retracted to the contralateral side. The second layer formed by the longus colli and longus capitis muscles is dissected in a French door–like fashion. This approach allows for a full visualization also to the far lateral aspects of C2 and the vertebral artery. For wound closure, two separate layers with different incision sites are available for a tight seal over the implant.

Tumors of the mid cervical spine are most often located in the anterior column. Once they start to invade the neural foraminae or the spinal canal they tend to become symptomatic. Collapse of the anterior column can result in an acute

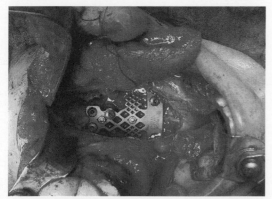

Fig. 3. Intraoperative photograph of radical tumor resection and cage reconstruction before wound closure.

detection of the lesion secondary to pain and/or neurologic sequelae. In tumors requiring resection, the approach is based on the pathology. In isolated cases of small tumors located in the corpus without penetrating the cortical wall and adequately away from the transverse foraminae, complete removal of the tumor without opening the tumor capsule is feasible. Most devices for anterior support are placed between the endplates of the vertebral bodies adjacent to the tumor-affected vertebra. Complete removal of the disc material will increase the stable positioning of the implant and promote osseous integration. Lesions involving a single level can often be treated using an anterior approach alone. For multilevel corpectomy, additional fixation is advisable. Panjabi and colleagues[19] has described excessive screw-vertebra motion caused by fatigue at the lower end of the three-level corpectomy model. One of his suggested solutions to overcome this problem was supplemental posterior fixation, which may decrease screw-vertebra loosening. This positive stabilizing effect of additional posterior instrumentation in a two-level corpectomy model has been demonstrated by Singh and colleagues.[20] Among many clinical reports about successful use of combined fixation after multilevel resection, Acosta and colleagues[21] reported good results after long-term follow-up.

Anterior reconstruction accomplished with structural bone grafts bear the risk of graft fracture and dislocation.[8,22,23]

It has been previously stated that there are a variety of devices available for spinal reconstruction. However, they must fulfill the main prerequisite: to provide and maintain sufficient anterior support. For replacement of multiple levels, lordotic contoured devices are also available.

In cases of reconstruction of malignant tumors with metastases or patients with very limited bone stock (eg, osteopenia), we tend to fill a mesh cage with bone cement, leaving a few millimeters at the ends of the cage cement free. In case of benign or primary malignant tumors without metastasis, the cage can be filled and surrounded by bone graft, where good osseous integration can be expected.[24]

Posterior instrumentation for the mid cervical spine using a screw-based system can be accomplished by positioning of the screws into the lateral mass (facet) or the pedicles. Although pedicle screws are clearly superior in terms of primary stability,[25] not all pedicles are suitable to harbor these screws (**Fig. 4**B). The preference for using pedicle screw or lateral mass fixation depends on the surgeon's training and preferences (see **Fig. 4**B, C).

In tumors affecting the lower cervical and upper thoracic spine, an anterior approach is obstructed by the manubrium sterni. In our experience, classic sternum split as it is performed on routine basis in cardiac surgery, provides an excellent exposure of the upper thoracic spine. Exposures through the sterno-clavicular joints do not provide comparable results, and typically cause long-standing joint discomfort.

For the anterior preparation of expanded tumors, ligation of the left brachiocephalic vein may become necessary. Graft replacement of the vessels, eg, the subclavian, is also feasible. Reconstruction in the case of multiple-level resections in the transition zone of the mobile lordotic cervical region to the more rigid kyphotic thoracic spine needs to reestablish this sagittal contour. This can be best accomplished by an S-like–shaped device (**Fig. 5**). The adequate posterior stabilization from the cervical to the thoracic region as part of the global reconstruction is of paramount importance.

Tumors and metastases of the thoracic spine can often be removed via posterior corpectomy from T2 to T5. This is accomplished via en-bloc spondylectomy with a bilateral costo-transversectomy. Resection and stabilization of anterior-only located tumors may be performed by a ventral-only approach. Thus, maneuvers that may potentially weaken the posterior elements and therefore

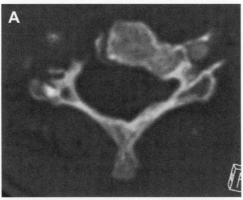

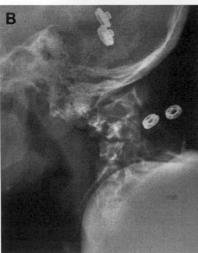

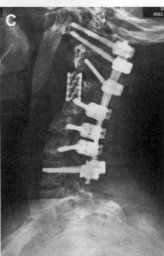

Fig. 4. (*A*) CT scan shows severe mutilation of vertebral body in patient with neuro-fibromatosis. (*B*) Collapse of cervical spine in patient with neurofibromatosis. (*C*) After anterior-posterior reduction and reconstruction using anterior support and posterior screw-rod construct with pedicle screw fixation.

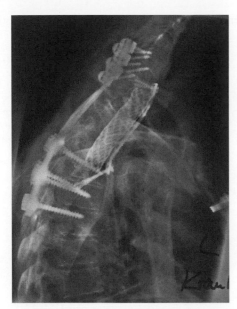

Fig. 5. Patient with 10-year follow-up after resection of giant cell tumor in C7-T2. Anterior approach was performed by sternum split. Implantation of double-contoured cage.

the posterior tension bend must be avoided to prevent progressive kyphosis over the long term. Natural compensatory mechanisms to prevent progressive kyphosis, especially in the upper and mid-thoracic region, are limited and may result in progressive spinal cord injury. Lesions caudal to T5 should be treated via a combined anterior and posterior approach to allow for better visualization of the closely located great vessels. These vessels must be evaluated preoperatively for any signs of adherence of even erosion by the tumor.

Resection of tumors in the thoraco-lumbar junction often leads to biomechanical dilemma. Although many spine surgeons know this area from fracture treatment and are well attuned in performing corpectomy, one should not forget that major resection of the tumor in combination with the suboptimal quality of adjacent levels often result in fracture type C conditions.

Performing the en-bloc spondylectomy in this area represents a complete disruption of the entire column. Therefore stabilization has to be planned as a central part of the intervention to avoid severe intraoperative translation or dislocation. Different reconstruction scenarios after spondylectomy have been studied biomechanically by several investigators. One of the concordant findings is the poor performance of posterior-only constructs compared with constructs using anterior support and posterior instrumentation. To achieve a reasonable stability, posterior constructs would have to span multiple segments.[26,27] However, anterior-only constructs have also failed to provide adequate stability after spondylectomy, even with additional lateral support devices, eg, plates or rods.[9] Disch and colleagues[28] could demonstrate that these additional lateral devices increase primary stability. However, a finite element model published by Akamura and colleagues[29] suggests that the effect of stress shielding by such rigid constructs may become an issue when osseous integration is expected. Posterior instrumentation in circumferential constructs with pedicle screw fixation two segments above and below the resected vertebra created more stable constructs when compared with single-segment screw placement.[28] To accomplish maximum stability but also to preserve lumbar motion segments, fixation of multiple levels in the thoracic spine may be combined with single-level fixation in the lumbar spine. However, additional stability is provided by application of a diagonal-connector (**Fig. 6**A, B). Mechanical testing of different transverse connector options demonstrated an increase of 10% in torsional stiffness when using two transverse connectors bridging the longitudinal rod screw system. However, a diagonal connector (**Fig. 6**A) increased torsional stiffness by 60%. In lateral bending, the increase by two transverse connectors was 32% and 290% for the diagonal connector. (H. Mueller-Storz, PhD, and W. Matthis, unpublished data, 1998).

Another option in providing anterior support is the expandable vertebral body replacement device.[30] These devices with an internal threaded mechanism are expanded cranio-caudally after implantation against the neighboring endplate. The assumption that the device will retain its position by the counteracting elasticity of the spinal tissues demonstrates the poor understanding of the elastic behavior of human tissue. Biomechanical tests have shown that these implants cannot be used as standalone devices and do not provide more stability than nonexpandable devices.[28,31] With additional posterior fixation, the conceptual function of these devices becomes questionable. There may also be a significant financial discrepancy with these cages compared with the traditional "nonexpandable" cages.

Most of the aforementioned principles also apply for the lumbar spine, except for the lumbosacral junction where additional shear forces due to the slope/inclination of the sacral endplate become an important issue. To resist these shear forces, the friction at the oblique footprint of the caudal part of the anterior graft can be increased, for example having small spikes that will increase the primary anchoring properties of the device to the endplate of S1. Posterior instrumentation may be extended to the iliac bone.

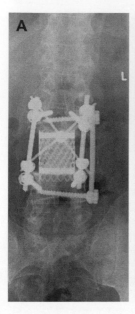

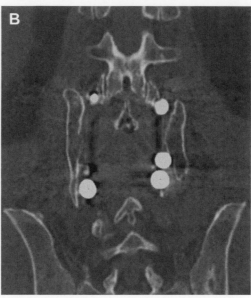

Fig. 6. (*A*) Three-year follow-up after en bloc resection of chordoma in L2. Short posterior construct with additional cross connector stabilization. (*B*) AP CT scan reconstruction demonstrating solid bilateral bone formation 1 year after augmentation with autolog bone graft. Bone graft was added 5 months after tumor removal.

An extremely challenging biomechanical situation with reconstruction occurs in cases of resection of tumors within the upper part of the sacrum. Resections below S2 do not require stabilization. The sacrum has to be regarded as the keystone of the pelvic ring. The vertical load from the spine is transferred through the sacro-iliac joints laterally via the pelvis to the femoral heads. The joint-like interlocking of the sacro-iliac joints is significantly reinforced by a pronounced ligamentous apparatus. Resections affecting sacral areas with proximity to the SI joint will subsequently result in severe instability.[32,33] After partial or complete sacrectomy, restoration of load sharing from the lumbar spine to the iliac bone and the lost tension band of the pelvic ring must be accomplished.[34] Such a construct has to provide enough stability to compensate for the different stresses and strains resulting from standing, walking, sitting, and laying. The reconstructive implant must also leave room for the preserved neural structures. For more than 10 years we have use a combined construct of contoured cages placed between the endplate of L4 or L5 and the iliac bone. The posterior stabilization is provided by a screw rod system between the lower lumbar spine and the ileum with additional posterior cross links. Nearly all of the patients with this type of construct remained ambulatory without the need of any gait assistance (**Fig. 7**A, B).

Final Considerations

One of the early examples of a perfectly performed reconstruction after tumor resection in the spine was published by Stener in 1971 describing a total en bloc spondylectomy in a patient with chondrosarcoma of T7.[2] His approach to the biomechanics of the reconstruction still plays a major role today.

However, today's available devices have improved dramatically. Especially with the progress of anterior support devices[35] and the posterior screw-rod systems, circumferential reconstruction even after resection of multiple spinal segments became a standardized procedure. Immediate postoperative mobilization of the patient is possible in most cases.

Tumor destruction has a negative impact on the mechanical properties of the spine, likely resulting in instability. Surgical tumor removal has a further impact on spinal stability. The surgeon has to analyze the impact of tumor destruction on the biomechanics of the spine as well as the biomechanical consequences of the surgical intervention.

Acknowledging and considering the mechanical properties and the forces to be expected are the basic prerequisite for the correct planning of any reconstruction. The anterior column with its mainly weight-bearing properties has to be adequately reconstructed, but attention has to be paid to the tension bend system of the posterior elements.

In the spinal transition zones, occurrence of higher stresses must be taken into account. The thoracic spine gains some stability from the ribcage. A biomechanically appropriate reconstruction after resection of the sacrum is challenging but possible. Restoration of the spinal sagittal profile of the junction zones is important.

Generally accepted principles of reconstructive spine surgery should also be obeyed in spinal

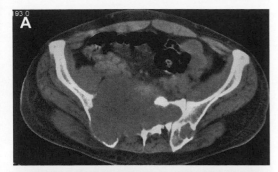

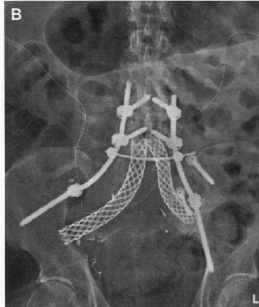

Fig. 7. (A) Massive metastatic destruction of pelvic ring in patient suffering from thyroid carcinoma. (B) Postoperative AP view after reconstruction of the pelvis following tumor resection. Patient 1 year postoperatively able to walk 50 to 100 m without support despite distal paresis from nerve root resection. Good sphincter control.

tumor surgery. This is true not only for patients with benign tumors, but also for patients with malignant tumors undergoing radical tumor resection. Suboptimal outcome with inadequate stabilization resulting in the breakdown of the construct is an avoidable hazard.

Minimal or subtotal resection of the tumor in hope of avoiding instrumentation can also lead to early clinical relapse and spine instability.

In the case of patients with spinal metastases, especially in patients with a median survival time of less than a few months, a thorough review of the risks and benefits regarding surgical intervention must be discussed with the patient. However, once the decision for surgery has been made, a biomechanically sound reconstruction should be performed to help restore or maintain the patient's mobility.

REFERENCES

1. Lièvre JA, Darcy M, Pradat P, et al. Tumeur a cellules géantes du rachis lombaire, spondylectomie totale en deux temps [Giant cell tumor of the lumbar spine; total spondylectomy in 2 stages]. Rev Rhum Mal Osteoartic 1968;35(3):125–30.
2. Stener B. Total spondylectomy in chondrosarcoma arising from the seventh thoracic vertebra. J Bone Joint Surg Br 1971;53(2):288–95.
3. Tomita K, Toribatake Y, Kawahara N, et al. Total en bloc spondylectomy and circumspinal decompression for solitary spinal metastasis. Paraplegia 1994; 32:36–46.
4. Ibrahim A, Crockard A, Antonietti P, et al. Does spinal surgery improve the quality of life for those with extradural (spinal) osseous metastases? An international multicenter prospective observational study of 223 patients. J Neurosurg Spine 2008;8: 271–8.
5. Patchell RA, Tibbs PA, Regine WF, et al. Improvement in quality of life after surgery for spinal metastasis. Direct decompressive surgical resection in the treatment of spinal cord compression caused by metastatic cancer: a randomised trial. Lancet 2005;366:643–8.
6. White AA, Panjabi MM. Clinical biomechanics of the spine. 2nd edition. Philadelphia: Lippincott Williams & Wilkins; 1990.
7. Kandziora F, Pflugmacher R, Schaefer J, et al. Biomechanical comparison of cervical spine interbody fusion cages. Spine 2001;26(17):1850–7.
8. Thompson RC, Pickvance EA, Garry D. Fractures in large-segment allografts. J Bone Joint Surg Am 1993;75:1663–73.
9. Vahldiek MJ, Panjabi MM. Stability potential of spinal instrumentations in tumor vertebral body replacement surgery. Spine 1998;23(5):543–50.
10. Roy-Camille R, Saillant G, Mazel C. Plating of thoracic, thoracolumbar, and lumbar injuries with pedicle screw plates. Orthop Clin North Am 1986; 17(1):147–59.
11. Oda I, Abumi K, Sell LC, et al. Biomechanical evaluation of five different occipito-atlanto-axial fixation techniques. Spine 1999;24(22):2377–82.
12. Ebraheim NA, Lu J, Biyani A, et al. An anatomic study of the thickness of the occipital bone. Implications for occipitocervical instrumentation. Spine 1996;21(15):1725–9.
13. Goel A, Kobayashi S. Craniovertebral and spinal stability. In: Kobayashi S, Goel A, Hongo K, editors. Neurosurgery of complex tumors and vascular lesions. New York: Churchill Livingstone; 1997. p. 339–72.

14. Puttlitz CM, Melcher RP, Kleinstueck FS, et al. Stability analysis of craniovertebral junction fixation techniques. J Bone Joint Surg Am 2004;86(3):561–8.

15. Wang MY. C2 crossing laminar screws: cadaveric morphometric analysis. Neurosurgery 2006;59 (Suppl 1):ONS84–8.

16. Kandziora F, Kerschbaumer F, Starker M, et al. Biomechanical assessment of transoral plate fixation for atlantoaxial instability. Spine 2000;25(12): 1555–61.

17. Jeszenszky D, Fekete TF, Melcher R, et al. C2 prosthesis: anterior upper cervical fixation device to reconstruct the second cervical vertebra. Eur Spine J 2007;16(10):1695–700.

18. Harms J, Schmelzle R. Ventrale transorale Eingriffe. In: Bauer R, Kerschbaumer F, Poisel S, editors. Orthopädische Operationslehre, Wirbelsäule. New York: Thieme; 1991. p. 373–5.

19. Panjabi MM, Isomi T, Wang JL. Loosening at the screw-vertebra junction in multilevel anterior cervical plate constructs. Spine 1999;24(22):2383–8.

20. Singh K, Vaccaro AR, Kim J, et al. Biomechanical comparison of cervical spine reconstructive techniques after a multilevel corpectomy of the cervical spine. Spine 2003;28(20):2352–8.

21. Acosta FL Jr, Aryan HE, Chou D, et al. Long-term biomechanical stability and clinical improvement after extended multilevel corpectomy and circumferential reconstruction of the cervical spine using titanium mesh cages. J Spinal Disord Tech 2008; 21(3):165–74.

22. Wang JC, Hart RA, Emery SE, et al. Graft migration or displacement after multilevel cervical corpectomy and strut grafting. Spine 2003;28(10):1016–21.

23. Jones J, Yoo J, Hart R. Delayed fracture of fibular strut allograft following multilevel anterior cervical spine corpectomy and fusion. Spine 2006;31(17): E95–9.

24. Akamaru T, Kawahara N, Tsuchiya H, et al. Healing of autologous bone in a titanium mesh cage used in anterior column reconstruction after total spondylectomy. Spine 2002;27(13):E329–33.

25. Johnston TL, Karaikovic EE, Lautenschlager EP, et al. Cervical pedicle screws vs. lateral mass screws: uniplanar fatigue analysis and residual pullout strengths. Spine J 2006;6(6):667–72.

26. Oda I, Cunningham BW, Abumi K, et al. The stability of reconstruction methods after thoracolumbar total spondylectomy. An in vitro investigation. Spine 1999;24(16):1634–8.

27. Shannon FJ, DiResta GR, Ottaviano D, et al. Biomechanical analysis of anterior Poly-Methyl-Methacrylate reconstruction following total spondylectomy for metastatic disease. Spine 2004;29(19):2096–102.

28. Disch AC, Schaser KD, Melcher I, et al. En bloc spondylectomy reconstructions in a biomechanical in-vitro study. Eur Spine J 2008;17:715–25.

29. Akamaru T, Kawahara N, Sakamoto J, et al. The transmission of stress to grafted bone inside a titanium mesh cage used in anterior column reconstruction after total spondylectomy: a finite-element analysis. Spine 2005;30(24):2783–7.

30. Ernstberger T, Kögel M, König F, et al. Expandable vertebral body replacement in patients with thoracolumbar spine tumors. Arch Orthop Trauma Surg 2005;125:660–9.

31. Khodadadyan-Klostermann C, Schaefer J, Schleicher P, et al [Expandable cages: biomechanical comparison of different cages for ventral spondylodesis in the thoracolumbar spine]. Chirurgia 2004;75(7):694–701.

32. Gunterberg B, Romanus B, Stener B. Pelvic strength after major amputation of the sacrum. An exerimental study. Acta Orthop Scand 1976;47(6):635–42.

33. Ronald R, Hugate RR, Dickey ID, et al. Mechanical effects of partial sacrectomy when is reconstruction necessary? Clin Orthop Relat Res 2006;450:82–8.

34. Murakami H, Kawahara N, Tomita K, et al. Biomechanical evaluation of reconstructed lumbosacral spine after total sacrectomy. Biomechanical analysis of anterior versus circumferential spinal reconstruction for various anatomic stages of tumor lesions. J Orthop Sci 2002;7:658–64.

35. Lowery GL, Harms J. Titanium surgical mesh for vertebral defect replacement and intervertebral spacers. In: Thalgott JS, Aebi M, editors. Manual of internal fixation of the spine. Philadelphia: Lippincott-Raven Publishers; 1996.

Cervical and Thoracic Spine Tumor Management: Surgical Indications, Techniques, and Outcomes

Christian Mazel, MD*, Laurent Balabaud, MD, S. Bennis, MD, S. Hansen, MD

KEYWORDS
- Spinal neoplasms • Spinal surgery • Cervical vertebrae
- Thoracic vertebrae • Pancoast syndrome • Vertebral artery

Over the last 30 years, advances in spinal surgery have brought widespread changes in the management of primary and metastasis tumors of the spine. The use of surgery was once controversial and many doubted its effectiveness. Today, attitudes are different. Several recent studies[1,2] have demonstrated that surgery offers significant advantages over other treatments in addressing spinal cord compression, in relieving pain, and in improve quality of life with low rates of complications.[3–5] The aims of spinal surgery are decompression and stabilization. Usually, the surgery has only a palliative role. Sometimes, however, though rarely, surgery is used for curative management in primary and, even more rarely, secondary tumors. Some medical pioneers[6–9] described the first curative resection for primary tumors of the spine by vertebrectomy with complete removal of tumor. In the multidisciplinary therapeutic management of spinal tumors, spinal surgery offers an extensive array of potential uses and benefits.

PATIENT EVALUATIONS AND DIAGNOSTIC ASSESSMENT

The initial evaluation of a patient with a spinal tumor must include a complete history and physical examination, laboratory investigations (with tumors markers), and radiological evaluation. Plain radiograph, CT, and MRI determine the local and systemic extents of the spinal tumor. In cases where the primary site of a spinal metastasis tumor is unknown, the initial evaluation must find the primary tumor. A complete evaluation requires a chest radiograph; a CT scan of the chest, abdomen, and pelvis; a technetium body scan; and, for women, a mammogram. For tumors of the thoracic apex (Pancoast-Tobias syndrome) and posterior mediastinum tumors, the initial evaluation includes chest radiograph, a CT scan of the brain and abdomen, an MRI of the chest, a flexible bronchoscopy, pulmonary function tests, and a technetium body scan.

A biopsy sampling establishes histopatholologic diagnosis. Knowledge of the primary tumor is essential to determine the surgical strategy and to evaluate the tumor's stage. Different techniques may be used, depending on the level and location of the tumor on the vertebral arch. The biopsy is usually percutaneous under CT guidance. At cervical level, an anterolateral approach is used with a fine-needle aspiration. At the thoracic level, a needle biopsy is performed by a large double-tube trocar 3 to 5 mm in diameter. Results can sometimes be inadequate, and a surgical biopsy is necessary via an anterolateral approach in cervical body tumors, a posterior approach in posterior arch locations, and a transpedicular approach for thoracic vertebral body tumors. In rare instances,

Institut Mutualiste Montsouris, 42 Boulevard Jourdan, 75014 Paris, France
* Corresponding author.
E-mail address: cristian.mazel@imm.fr (C. Mazel).

Orthop Clin N Am 40 (2009) 75–92
doi:10.1016/j.ocl.2008.09.008
0030-5898/08/$ – see front matter © 2008 Elsevier Inc. All rights reserved.

an excisional biopsy may be performed if the potential differential diagnosis is limited (osteoma osteoid or osteoblastoma). If spine surgery is subsequently decided upon, the excision of the biopsy wound tract should be performed but is not always possible. In some cases, such as cases in which the primary tumor is known or in cases of recurrent tumors, biopsy can be avoided.

STAGING

After this assessment, it is necessary to stage the tumor on the vertebral arch[10,11] and its extent along and around the spine.[12] General assessment of the patient in metastasis disease is done with the Tokuhashi Staging System.[13] Tomita's Scoring System,[12] the Weinstein-Boriani-Biagini (WBB)[10,11] Staging System, and the Tokuhashi Scoring System[13] are used to assess the patient's prognosis and to determine the best therapeutic option for the patient.

Tomita's Scoring System

Tomita's scoring system[12] provides an anatomic description of the tumoral vertebra and its local extent. This scoring system is a modification of the Enneking system.[14] The vertebral body is divided into five anatomic sites: (1) the vertebral body, (2) the pedicle, (3) the lamina and spinous process, (4) the spinal canal (epidural space), and (5) the paravertebral area. The numbers used to denote the anatomic sites reflect the common sequence of tumor progression. The authors classify most lesions as either intracompartmental lesions (lesions in sites 1, 2, and 3) or extracompartmental lesions (lesions in sites 4, 5, and 6). Multiple or skip lesions are classified as type 7. This scoring system helps surgeons determine whether curative or palliative treatment is the best course. Total en bloc vertebrectomy is recommended for types 2, 3, 4, and 5 lesions, relatively indicated for types 1 and 6 lesions, and contraindicated for type 7 lesions.

Weinstein-Boriani-Biagini Staging System

The WBB Staging System[10,11] is designed first of all to help the surgeon plan the most appropriate tumoral resection. The WBB Staging System is also useful in homogenous data collection in multicenter studies. The vertebra is divided into 12 equal zones radiating off of the spinal canal and numbered clockwise 1 through 12. Moreover, the tumor is classified into one or more of five concentric layers (six in the cervical spine) from the paravertebral extraosseous soft tissue (A) to the dura (E) and the vertebral artery canal (F) for cervical spine.

Tokuhashi Scoring System

The Tokuhashi Scoring System[13] is essential to the preoperative assessment of metastasis spinal tumor prognosis irrespective of treatment modality or local tumor extent. Six parameters are used: (1) the general condition, (2) the number of extraspinal bone metastases, (3) the number of metastases in the vertebral body, (4) metastases to the major internal organs (lungs, liver, kidneys, and brain), (5) the primary site of the cancer, and (6) the severity of spinal cord palsy with Frankel score.[15] Each parameter ranges from 0 to 2 or 5 points, and the total possible score is 15 points. Conservative treatment or palliative procedures are indicated in patients with a total score of 8 or less (predicted survival period <6 months) or those with multiple vertebral metastases, while excisional procedures are performed in patients with a total score of 12 or more (predicted survival period 1 year or more) or those with a total score of 9 to 11 (predicted survival period 6 months or more) and with metastasis in a single vertebra.

TERMINOLOGY

Enneking[14] defined the original terms of surgical management for tumors. Originally described for long bones, these principles are thus not entirely applicable in describing spinal tumors and must be adapted. The term *intralesional* is appropriate for a dissection passing within the tumor mass; *marginal* for a dissection through the pseudocapsule or reactive tissue about the tumor; and *wide* where the tumor is removed with a surrounding cuff of normal tissue. The epidural space and the cord make a "radical" resection impossible without evident neurologic injury. Moreover, it is important to define *piecemeal* as *curettage*, which is an intralesional procedure, and *en bloc* as the removal of a tumor in one piece. Finally, in spinal tumoral surgery, the resection is rarely "wide," and the histologic analysis gives the final result, which can be different from what was planned. Moreover, spinal tumoral surgery must be aggressive to perform the most complete resection to increase the survival period in primary tumor and isolated metastasis.[4,16–20]

The Global Spine Tumour Study Group (GSTSG), an international multicentric group, has proposed a classification of the different types of resections in consideration of the palliative surgical tactic, as opposed to total vertebrectomy;[5] the piecemeal surgical method, as opposed to the en bloc procedure; and the intralesional histopathological margin, as opposed to the wide histopathological margin (**Fig. 1**).

TREATMENT INDICATIONS IN SPINE TUMORS

In the surgical treatment of spine tumors, two opposing strategies prevail: (1) palliative surgery with cord decompression and spine stabilization and (2) curative surgery with en bloc tumor radical resection and stabilization. Curative en bloc resection requires total or partial vertebrectomy. Resection can be piecemeal with tumor opening or en bloc with or without tumor opening. These possibilities have been well described as previously stated by the GSTSG group.[5] Indications depend on the aims of the primary disease treatment.

Palliative Versus Curative Surgery

Palliative surgery, which is indicated in most metastases cases, aims to stabilize the spine and to decompress roots or the cord. In some exceptional cases, total resection of the tumor mass is recommended. Total resection is performed mostly in cases where no medical treatment is accessible (eg, renal cell carcinoma not responding to chemotherapy or radiotherapy, recurrence of

tumor in cases with a previous radiotherapy) and in some other cases where reduction of tumor volume is important (eg, thyroid metastases). Interestingly, resection can decrease local recurrence in patients with short life expectancy. Isolated metastases can be an indication for curative surgery with the aim of curing the patient of cancer. In such cases adjuvant or neoadjuvant efficient therapy is required. All curative en bloc resections should target primary tumors. However, depending on the tumor's location on the spinal ring, such resections are not always feasible. A Pancoast tumor invading the spine is not a metastases, but a primary tumor. A Pancoast tumor will thus respond to usual carcinologic criteria.

INDICATIONS OF TREATMENT IN SPINE METASTASIS
Nonsurgical Treatment Versus Surgery

The medical treatment of spinal metastasis is recommended when (1) local tumor development has produced no related neurologic complications, (2) neither a mechanical complication fracture nor axial destabilization is present, and (3) pain responds to usual treatment.

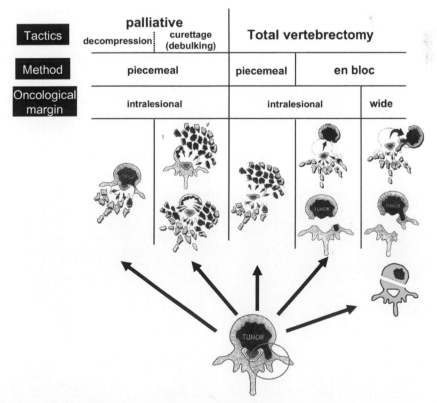

Fig. 1. GSTSG proposed classification for describing the different possible techniques of resection at spine level considering tactics, methods, and postoperation oncology margin.

Vertebroplasty/Kyphoplasty Versus Surgery

Vertebroplasty, developed only few years ago, is taking on an increasingly important role in the treatment of spinal tumors. Usually performed by radiologists, vertebroplasty can be useful in cases where surgery has not yet been indicated or in patients with a poor general status. Vertebroplasty is the injection of polymethylmethacrylate (PMMA) by a percutaneous bilateral pedicle approach. Kyphoplasty is performed by the same approach. However, with kyphoplasty, the PMMA injection is preceded by the insertion of an inflated balloon, which creates a cavity for PMMA and corrects the vertebral height or sagittal alignment. Such procedures can be performed through an open wound or in association with a surgical palliative procedure in multilevel metastasis. These percutaneous procedures are rarely indicated in the cervical spine but more often in the thoracic and lumbar spine (**Fig. 2**). Also, such procedures are employed mostly in cases of osteolytic lesions involving the vertebral body, totally or partially, and the pedicles to a large or small extant. These techniques can also be used in combination with surgical techniques (**Fig. 3**). Some have speculated about the possible carcinologic effects of PMMA as a result of heat from polymerization, but such effects have never been documented.

Surgical Versus Conservative Treatment

The surgical treatment of spinal metastasis is recommended (1) when there are neurologic complications related to local tumor development with local compression or fracture, (2) when there is a mechanical complication with fracture or axial destabilization, (3) when pain does not respond to medical treatment, and (4) in cases of radioresistant tumors (eg, renal cell carcinoma not responding to chemotherapy or radiotherapy; recurrence of tumor in cases of previous radiotherapy).

CERVICAL LEVEL
Indication of Palliative Versus Curative Surgery in Cervical Tumor

In upper cervical tumors, neurologic symptoms are unusual because the neural canal is wide at this level. Neurologic symptoms, when they appear, are most likely due to cord compression from a major instability rather than directly from the tumor. Direct cord compression is thus less likely than occipitocervical instability. If surgery is indicated in such cases, an occipitocervical fixation is necessary. A laminectomy in association with the fixation is rarely required. An anterior decompression is unusual and can be performed by a transoral approach. This rare approach is not discussed in this article. At this level, we can describe two specific anatomic situations where palliative surgery is indicated: (1) when the C2 body is severely damaged, with or without cord compression, and (2) when there is unilateral or bilateral involvement of a C1 lateral mass responsible for a rotatory or axial instability. A wide surgical resection is useful in upper cervical tumors only for treating an exceptional isolated tumor of the posterior arch of C1 or C2.

At the lower cervical spine, the surgical indications are more frequent for several reasons: (1) Tumor localization at this level is more frequent; (2) the neural canal is narrow here, resulting in early neurologic symptoms; and (3) segments are highly mobile, and thus carry a greater risk of instability (**Fig. 4**).

In metastasis tumors, palliative surgery is generally indicated. Surgery can be performed with an

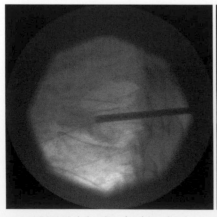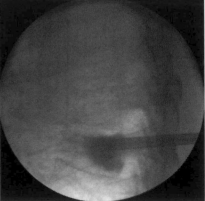

Fig. 2. Percutaneous PMMA injection by bipedicular port is usually recommended in osteolytic lesions without neurologic or mechanical impairment.

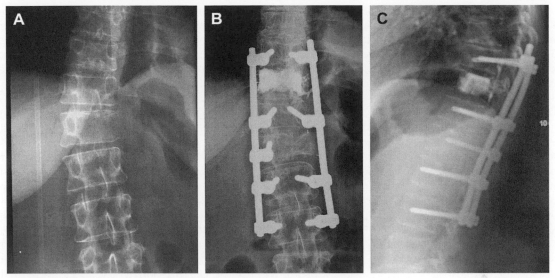

Fig. 3. Combining techniques is an interesting option and PMMA injection perioperation or preoperation can supplement the mechanical characteristics of the construct.

anterior approach, a posterior approach, or a combination of the two. We often prefer a combination of posterior and anterior approaches in a same surgical session. When this surgical procedure is chosen, we usually prefer to begin by the posterior approach, trying to avoid neurologic complications more often observed during resection of the anterior compressive elements. The posterior laminectomy performed in connection with the fixation enables the cord to withstand the potential anterior trauma at the time of the anterior resection.

To ensure the best possible postoperative quality of life, careful consideration must be made to provide good biomechanical characteristics to the three columns during reconstruction. The anterior procedure following the posterior approach accommodates total removal of the remaining anterior vertebral body tumor.

The indications of curative surgery are limited to primary tumors (malignant or apparently benign giant cell and pseudoaneurismal cysts) and, in rare cases, isolated metastasis tumors. The

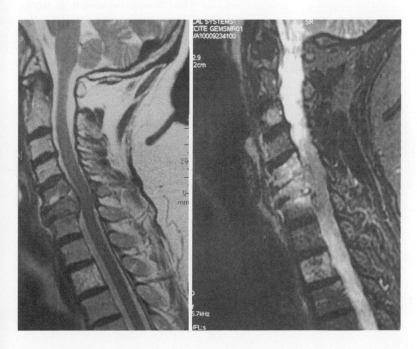

Fig. 4. Lower cervical spine metastases rapidly lead to mechanical and neurologic complications.

involvement of roots and the vertebral artery limits such radical procedures. Cervical roots have a functional value that cannot be sacrificed lightly. The patient must be thoroughly made aware preoperatively about the possible neurologic consequences on the upper limbs of a root section. The problem of the vertebral artery can be solved by unilateral or bilateral vascular bypass. A laterolateral carotidovertebral bypass is also possible, allowing partial or total vertebrectomy. In the partial vertebrectomy, unilateral ligature of the vertebral artery can be performed after arteriography with occlusion test or when the diameter of the involved vertebral artery is no larger that the noninvolved artery.[21] Thus, the preoperative evaluation must include an arteriography of vertebral arteries. Moreover, cervical vertebrectomy is rare and requires a high degree of surgical skill and a multidisciplinary team.

Surgical Technique: Palliative Surgery at Cervical Level

Fixation and laminectomy of the upper cervical spine: occipitocervical fixation

For occipitocervical fixation, the patient is placed in a prone position over a head holder, enabling flexion-extension ranges of motion. A posterior approach is performed over the spinous processes and the occipital bone. The paraspinal muscles are elevated from the spinous processes and the laminae. The approach is extended laterally to the facets of the levels below C2. In C1 and C2 levels, the dissection must be classically limited 1.5 to 2 cm from the midline to avoid injury to the vertebral artery. This dissection is accomplished by making a loop in the form of a horizontal S over the lateral part of C1 posterior arch. For the occipital bone, the approach can be extended 3 to 4 cm laterally from the midline. The posterior longitudinal sinus is in the midline and the fixation is performed laterally to the midline. The thickness of the occiput lateral to the posterior sinus is about 10 to 12 mm with two strong cortexes, which allows a firm implantation of screws. To restore normal curvature of the occipitocervical junction allowing a horizontal view, the device must respect the normal occipitocervical angulation, which is 105° (**Fig. 5**). Usually, we use premolded devices. The first step of this procedure is the cervical fixation. At the cervical level, the fixation is performed with lateral mass screws and rods like those described in the next paragraph (cervicothoracic level), and must go down to C4 or C5. Fixation to the occiput is then achieved with screws that are 13 mm long. In patients with a prolonged life expectancy, an iliac unicortical graft is fixed between the occiput and the C4 or C5 spinous processes. In the case of a tumor involving C1 lateral mass, a transpedicular C2 fixation is a good solution to increase stability. Prevention of neurologic and vascular perioperative injuries can be avoided by precise knowledge of anatomic landmarks. The posterior approach must be extended to the lateral mass of C2, which can be divided into quarters. The vertebral artery adheres directly to the two inferior and the upper lateral quarters. Thus, the upper medial quarter corresponds to the pedicle entrance point. The implantation of the C2 pedicle screw must respect the obliquity of the C2 pedicle, which is 10° to

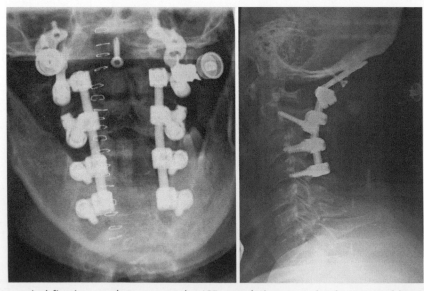

Fig. 5. Occipitocervical fixation needs to respect the 105° angulations to maintain correct vision capacities.

15° upward and inward. After clearing the superior border of the C2, a curved spatula is introduced carefully into the vertebral canal along the medial aspect of the pedicle. From the starting point previously described guided by the spatula and under direct view of the pedicle, the drilling is performed obliquely inward respecting the obliquity of the C2 pedicle. Drilling extends to a depth of 25 to 35 mm, enough to accommodate a screw the same length.

Fixation and laminectomy of the lower cervical spine

For fixation and laminectomy of the lower cervical spine, the patient is placed in a prone position over a head holder, enabling flexion-extension ranges of motion. A posterior approach is performed over the spinous processes. The paraspinal muscles are elevated from the spinous processes and the laminae and the approach is extended laterally to include the lateral mass. The first step is the spinal fixation performed by means of lateral mass screws and rods like those described in the next paragraph (cervicothoracic level). This first step of spine fixation is important for helping to decrease bleeding during the resection of the tumor. Spine fixation also helps in restoring the stability and in correcting the lordosis of the cervical segment before the laminectomy. If a combination of anterior and posterior surgical approaches is planned, the spinal fixation is limited to the adjacent levels of the tumoral vertebrae. In case of a single posterior approach, the quality of the fixation often requires the inclusion of two levels above and below the tumoral vertebrae. The second step of this approach is a bilateral complete laminectomy, which can be extended laterally to the facets and sometimes to the pedicles. Knowledge of the vertebral artery position in front of the roots, helps the surgeon to determine the anterior limits of the resection.

Corporectomy of the lower cervical spine

For a corporectomy of the lower cervical spine, the patient is placed in a supine position. An anterior approach is performed by retracting laterally the carotid sheath and sternocleidomastoid muscle and medially the aerodigestive tractus. After removal of the discs adjacent to the tumoral vertebrae, the resection of the involved vertebral body is achieved and extended posterior to the epidural space. The lateral dissection and resection is related to the tumor extension. One must always be aware of the vertebral artery trajectory. To avoid injury to that artery, a correct preoperative evaluation of its trajectory is essential. A titanium mesh cylinder or an iliac or fibular autograft associated with an anterior plate is inserted to provide a satisfactory primary fixation. In patients with a short life expectancy, we do not use PMMA, but this option can be advocated when the aim is to avoid the detrimental effect of subsequent radiation therapy on an autograft.

Partial and Total Vertebrectomy at Cervical Level

Partial vertebrectomy of the posterior arch

Partial vertebrectomy of the posterior arch is rare and indicated in the primary tumor and in isolated metastasis of the posterior arch (**Fig. 6**). The patient is placed in a prone position over a head holder. A posterior approach is performed with the purpose of achieving a marginal or a wide resection. The paraspinal muscles are dissected from the spinous processes and the laminae at a distance from the tumor. If the tumor is limited to the spinous process and not extended laterally to the articular mass, a laminectomy can be achieved respecting a satisfactory margin to the tumor and the articular mass. After section of the spinous ligament adjacent of the tumoral level, an en bloc resection is performed with a posterior traction on the involved posterior arch. Anteriorly, the careful section of the ligamentum flavum is done with a spatula. Stabilization is not necessary because the articular masses are respected. In case of lateral mass involvement, an en bloc resection is also possible (**Fig. 7**). The first step of the resection is a laminotomy on the nontumoral side at a distance from the tumor. Then on the side of the tumor, the approach is extended laterally over the portion of the articular mass involved with the tumor. Dissection is extended anteriorly to the root and vertebral artery, which are preserved. The pedicular section, which is necessary to free the tumor mass, is performed with a Kerrison or T-saw[22,23] below the root. Posterior traction

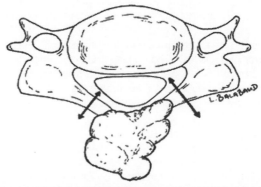

Fig. 6. Partial vertebrectomy in isolated metastasis of the posterior arch. Arrows indicate the directions of the osteotomies. (*Courtesy of* L. Balabaud, MD, Paris, France.)

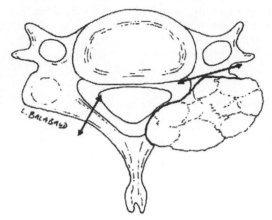

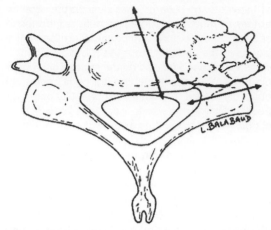

Fig. 7. Partial vertebrectomy in isolated metastasis of the posterior arch extended to the lateral mass. Arrows indicate the directions of osteotomies. (*Courtesy of* L. Balabaud, MD, Paris, France.)

Fig. 8. Partial en bloc vertebrectomy. Arrows indicate the directions of osteotomy. (*Courtesy of* L. Balabaud, MD, Paris, France.)

of the mass and dural adhesion are removed to free the mass. A complementary reconstruction of the articular mass is performed with an iliac crest bone graft and bilateral instrumentation.

Partial en bloc vertebrectomy

For a partial en bloc vertebrectomy, a preoperative arteriography must be performed to decide how best to deal with the vertebral artery: ligature or vascular bypass. The patient is placed in a supine position. An anterior approach is performed by retracting laterally the carotid sheath and sternocleidomastoid muscle and medially the aerodigestive tractus. The dissection is extended laterally to the tumor side while preserving a satisfactory margin to the transverse process, the root, and the vertebral artery. A vascular surgeon performs the vascular bypass or ligature of the vertebral artery at the adjacent levels after liberation of the vertebral artery (**Figs. 8** and **9**). The vertebral body osteotomy is achieved with a motorized drill respecting the preoperative imaging and limited cephally and caudally to the adjacent levels. The pedicular section and the opening of vertebral foramen are done with a Kerrison or T-saw.[22] The tumor piece is removed en bloc and a tricortical iliac autograft is inserted between the adjacent vertebrae. An anterior plate increases the stability and decreases risk of pseudarthrosis.

Total cervical vertebrectomy

Total resection at the cervical level always requires a vertebral arch opening. Even if a bypass or a ligature of both vertebral arteries or a root section and ligature are planned, going around the cord means opening the vertebral arch and illustrates the limits of such surgery.

Surgery is performed in two and sometimes three successive steps with alternating anterior and posterior approaches. Simultaneous approaches have been described, but this access is not always the best for performing a complex and demanding surgery on roots, vertebral artery, and cord. We usually begin with the posterior approach to perform a first resection of the posterior arch extended anteriorly to the plane

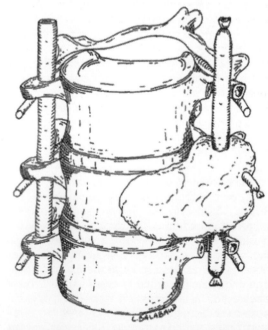

Fig. 9. Partial en bloc vertebrectomy. The dissection is extended laterally to the tumor side, preserving a satisfactory margin to the transverse process, the root, and the vertebral artery. Ligature of vertebral artery is performed at the upper and lower adjacent levels after its dissection. (*Courtesy of* L. Balabaud, MD, Paris, France.)

of the roots, then completed by a strong fixation at least two levels above and two below the resection level. Surgery is then completed by a horizontal anterior skin incision giving a bilateral presternocleidomastoidian access to the spine. Control to the vertebral arteries is usually done under C6 before its access in the vertebral canal. Surgeons can perform ligature or a progressive dissection going from caudal to cranial. Ligature or bypass is performed over the tumor level. In rare cases, a unilateral carotidovertebral anastomosis is performed at the level of C1 vertebral arch. Total resection at cervical level always means tumor opening. Even if a bypass or a ligature of both vertebral arteries is planned and, in the same way, a root section and ligature are called for, going around the cord means opening the vertebral arch and thus limits such surgery.

Anterior vertebral body reconstruction depends on a massive mesh cage or iliac tricortical bone graft. Posterior reconstruction may be necessary to reconstruct the facets and three spinal columns.

CERVICOTHORACIC AND THORACIC LEVEL

Metastases to the cervicothoracic junction are frequent. Posterior mediastinum tumors are also challenging with the necessity to deal with neurogenic as well as Pancoast-Tobias tumors. Cervicothoracic fixation of the unstable spine is mechanically difficult because of the change of cervical lordosis to thoracic kyphosis. Stress and motion are important at the cervical level in contrast to the rigid upper thoracic spine. The anterior approach is also very demanding and needs a good knowledge of surgical anatomy to be able to achieve large anterior corpectomy. Posterior decompression and stabilization is, in our opinion, the gold standard, considering anatomic and biomechanical goals. Long fixations are mandatory. The posterior construct provides the majority of stabilization from a biomechanical point of view.

Indication of Palliative Surgery Versus Curative in Cervicothoracic Tumors

In treating spine tumors, surgeons need to choose between two opposing strategies: (1) palliative surgery with cord decompression and spine stabilization or (2) curative surgery with en bloc radical resection of the tumor and stabilization. Palliative procedures are usually performed through a standard midline posterior approach. Curative en bloc resection requires total or partial vertebrectomy performed through an extended posterior approach combined with an anterior approach, as described by Grunenwald and Mazel.[24,25] In cases of Pancoast tumors, the origin of the tumor is the lung. Often the local extension reaches the junction between the rib and the vertebral body, but the vertebra itself is not invaded. The tumor is only strongly attached to it. In such cases, resection is carcinologic with the vertebra cut giving the only available safe margin (**Fig. 10**). In cases where the tumor arises from the vertebral body itself or when the Pancoast is invading, the adjacent vertebra resection can still be en bloc, as opposed to piecemeal. At least one of the pedicles needs to be assessed safe on preoperative CT and MRI. Skip metastases are still possible and thus the word *carcinologic* as in lower limb surgery cannot be used. In any case, we emphasize the necessity to perform complete en bloc resections as opposed to piecemeal resections.

Palliative Surgery at Cervicothoracic and Thoracic Levels

For palliative surgery at the cervicothoracic and thoracic levels, the approach is a midline access to the spine. Soft tissue elevation is done at both extremities of the wound and progressively reaches the tumor. Resection is not immediately achieved and it is necessary to prepare the fixation before dealing with the resection itself. Facet and pedicle identification is the first step. The key is a unilateral fixation that helps in reducing bleeding. Preoperative embolization of the tumor is necessary in renal cell, thyroid, and prostate metastases. The contralateral fixation is performed at the end of the procedure. Piecemeal resection is always an option and it is usually easier to perform an en bloc resection turning around the tumor mass and cutting at the necessary levels even if, at the end, it is necessary to open the tumor mass to conclude the resection. A posterolateral extension of the dissection is often necessary to turn around the cord. The pedicle and costotransverse joint invaded by the tumor are resected and the access to the posterior part of the vertebral body is possible. A partial vertebral body piecemeal resection can thus be performed. This procedure will free the root from the tumor. However, in some cases, the root will still need to be ligated and cut (**Fig. 11**).

Surgical technique screw implantation characteristics

The fixation devices must accommodate lateral mass screw fixation in the cervical spine and pedicle screw fixation in the thoracic spine.[26] The freedom provided by the screw-rod connection allows the screws to be inserted in the ideal position. Furthermore, variable rod length allows extension of the construct to any necessary length. With regards to screw placement, screws in the cervical spine are placed in the lateral masses at the

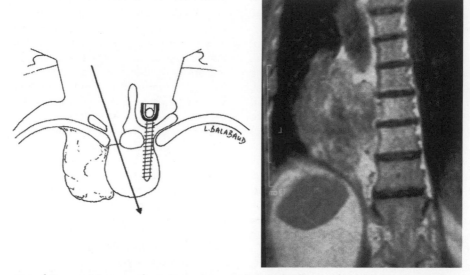

Fig. 10. In cases of Pancoast tumors, the primary tumor origin is the lung. Often the local extension reaches the junction between the rib and the vertebral body, but the vertebra is not itself invaded. In such cases, resection can be carcinologic if the resection osteotomy is done at the level of the vertebral body giving a safe margin. Arrow indicates the level of the osteotomy. (*Courtesy of* L. Balabaud, MD, Paris, France.)

midpoint of the top of the cervical articular mass using the Roy-Camille implantation technique.[27–29] Magërl's positioning can also be proposed.[30] In the thoracic spine, screws are transpedicular, angled 5° to 10° medially and 10° to 20° caudally in T1 and T2. Medial orientation decreases progressively from T3 to T12.

Length of fixation, anterior reconstruction, bone grafting
Long fixation devices and symmetric constructs are recommended. Multiple screw fixation increases the stability of the construct even in weak bone and explain why few such implantations fail. In rare cases, an anterior complementary approach is necessary for complementary bone grafting. In cases of total or partial vertebrectomies, instrumentation must include three levels above and three below the resection. Autologous iliac bone graft can be used in partial resections. Such a graft is screwed to the lateral body of the remaining vertebra. For total vertebrectomies, long-term survival is the challenge and autologous fibula strut graft is the best solution in multilevel

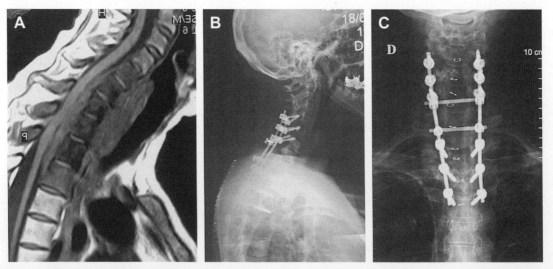

Fig. 11. Multilevel cervicothoracic involvement. Posterior decompression and stabilization are the recommended ways of dealing with such lesions.

cases. Femoral head bank bone is a good alternative in a one-level vertebrectomy, providing immediate stability to the construct (**Fig. 12**).

Technique of En Bloc Tumor Resection at the Thoracic and Cervicothoracic Levels

The strategy for total resection at the thoracic level is similar to that for the cervical level and always means vertebral arch opening. Even if it is determined that a section and ligature of the roots will have few consequences at this level, going around the cord means opening of the vertebral arch and explains the limits of such surgery. En bloc resection at such levels needs a complete soft tissue release to avoid tumor opening and significant bleeding. The esophagus and major vessels are at risk because of their close relation to the spine. The traditional approach is the open thoracotomy. Investigators have described successful surgeries using the coelioscopic approach and transmanubrial accesses, resulting in modifications to surgical procedures.

Anterior soft tissue release

Traditionally, the anterior and posterior sessions are performed the same day but can be performed a day apart without real problem.

The development of the transmanubrial cervicothoracic anterior[24] approach allowed execution of the thoracic steps of the resection without a conventional thoracotomy. With this approach, one elevates an osteomuscular flap from the manubrium, including the entire clavicle and cervical muscles, sparing in particular the sternocleidomastoid muscle and the sternoclavicular joint. Resection of the anterior part of the first rib and, if necessary, the second or even the third ribs allows a formal upper lobectomy through the pulmonary scissura, as well as hilar, carinal, paratracheal, and ipsilateral supraclavicular and superior mediastinal lymph node dissection. The cervical step of the operation allows separation of the tumor from the cervical structures; vascular resection and reconstruction, if needed; division of the external part of the parietal thoracic wall according to the planned resection; and dissection of the anterior vertebral plane free from the posterior mediastinal organs (great vessels, aorta, esophagus). The upper lobe is left attached to the thoracic apex by the tumor involvement, respecting oncologic principles (ie, without violating the tumor margins).

In the case of a medium thoracic posterior mediastinum tumor, a traditional posterolateral thoracotomy is performed, and tumor dissection is achieved as described previously. More and more in our daily practice, we prefer coeliscopic soft tissue elevation. This technique is less aggressive and better tolerated by patients.

Total vertebrectomy

After the first step of anterior soft tissue release, the patient is turned to the prone position in a head holder for the final step. Through a midline

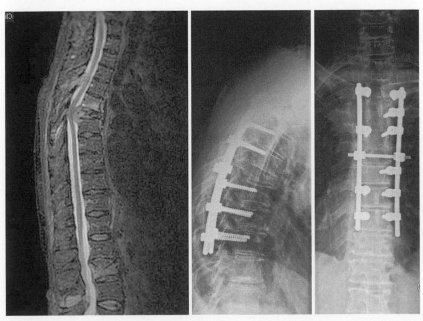

Fig. 12. In multilevel spinal involvement, surgery is indicated at the compressed or unstable level. Other means of treatment are used for other levels.

skin incision, muscle and fibrous tissue are cleared from the spine. Dissection is extended as far as 5 to 6 cm laterally on the ribs adjacent to the tumoral vertebrae. The surgical technique varies at this point according to the type of vertebrectomy necessary for en bloc resection, which is in turn based on vertebral involvement. When the tumor extends to the vertebra itself, the vertebral body, pedicle, or the transverse process, a total vertebrectomy is the only option to obtain complete extralesional resection.

In the case of total vertebrectomy, a bilateral complete laminectomy is performed. It is extended far laterally on the facets, transverse processes, and pedicles on the side opposite the tumor. On the uninvolved side, following dislocation of the costovertebral joints, the ribs at the level of the involved vertebrae and at the adjacent upper and lower levels are transected. At that time, the cord is exposed in the midline with the roots emerging laterally. On the involved side, the transverse processes, as well as the pedicles and ribs, are carefully kept in place. Subcutaneous dissection of the invaded ribs is performed from the midline and allows identification of the distal rib resection zone. The anterior vertebral body plane, previously dissected through the anterior approach is identified. It is now possible to go around the entire vertebral body (**Fig. 13**). Disks adjacent to the resection are carefully identified. Using a unilateral posterior rod and transpedicular screws, spinal fixation on the opposite side is performed before spondylectomy. After division of the roots entering the lateral aspect of the tumor and following ligation

of these roots adjacent to the cord inside the canal, the spondylectomy is performed by Gigli saw from anterior to posterior (**Fig. 14**). After careful division of the posterior longitudinal ligament, which is anterior to the cord, the surgical specimen, including the parietal wall, the pulmonary lobe, the tumor itself, and the vertebral bodies, is pushed forward, rotated around the cord, and extracted laterally en bloc. Contralateral fixation with transpedicular screws completes stabilization of the spine and spinal cord. Vertebral body reconstruction is done using bone graft. Femoral head bank bone gives a good 5-cm height reconstruction. Fibula strut grafts are more efficient in longer reconstructions. A mesh cage filled with autologous cancellous bone is another option (**Fig. 15**). The bone graft is then fixed to the posterior construct with screws avoiding its possible mobilization. Spine stabilization is then completed (**Fig. 16**).

Partial vertebrectomy

A complete resection of the vertebral body is not necessary when the tumor is only attached to the lateral aspects of the spine, without invasion of the vertebral body itself. Such situations are observed in Pancoast-Tobias, where the tumor is only sticking to the lateral side of the vertebral body, and in cases of dumbbell tumors.[24] In

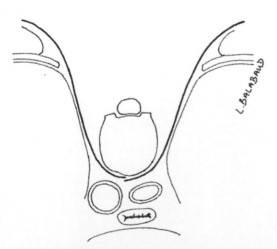

Fig. 13. The anterior soft tissue release enables positioning of a malleable retractor anterior to the vertebral body plane. (*Courtesy of* L. Balabaud, MD, Paris, France.)

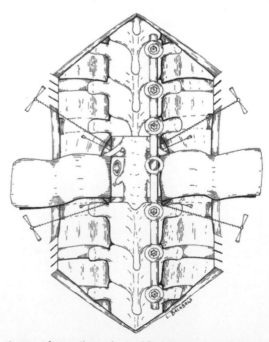

Fig. 14. After unilateral spinal fixation on the side opposite to the tumor and ligature of the roots, the spondylectomy from anterior to posterior is performed with a Gigli saw. (*Courtesy of* L. Balabaud, MD, Paris, France.)

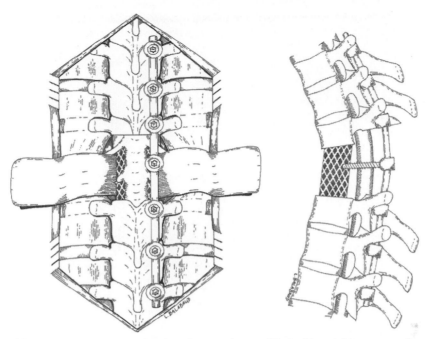

Fig. 15. Vertebral body reconstruction can be done by a mesh cage filled with autologous cancellous bone. (*Courtesy of* L. Balabaud, MD, Paris, France.)

such cases, in which only the foraminal and the costovertebral groove are involved, only a partial or hemivertebrectomy is necessary to achieve an extended and complete resection (**Fig. 17**). This should provide an adequate tumor-free tissue margin, thus respecting principles of oncologic surgery. Bilateral laminectomy and rib control are not necessary.

After the first step of anterior soft tissue release, the patient is turned to the prone position in a head holder for the final step. A midline posterior approach is performed and pedicle identification is performed on the tumor opposite side. The unilateral instrumentation is positioned. The first step of the resection is the ligature and section of the involved roots. For this purpose, a bony furrow is drilled (**Fig. 18**) at the level of the facet joints on the tumor side. Then corresponding roots are identified and divided following the proximal ligature (**Fig. 19**). The vertebral body posterior part is then accessible and the posteroanterior cut is possible. An oblique osteotomy from posterior to anterior is completed on the vertebral body (**Fig. 20**). The osteotomy is completed on the upper and lower parts of spine by transsection of the vertebral isthmus. By this means, a variable portion of the vertebral body or bodies can be resected according to the obliquity of the vertebral

osteotomy. A transpedicular screw device is implanted on the side opposite to the tumor before osteotomy for stabilization as described for complete vertebrectomy. Reconstruction is performed with autologous bone fixed laterally with screws on the remaining vertebral bodies, before inserting a second transpedicular posterior plate or rod. Associated iliac bone grafting can be added on the remaining posterior arch. Patients are immobilized in a plastic jacket until fusion 3 to 6 months postoperatively, depending on the extent of the vertebral resection (**Fig. 21**).

Outcome in Patient Operated for Tumors

Evaluation of the outcome is not always easy and reliable. We refer to individual cases and multicentric series in which we have been involved.

Outcome in en bloc resection of Pancoast-Tobias tumors

We are familiar with 36 cases of Pancoast-Tobias tumors that have been operated on using en bloc resection techniques.[24] Vertebrectomy was complete in 7 cases and partial in the 29 remaining cases.

Follow-up ranged from 6 days to 12.2 years, averaging 46 months. One patient died 1-year postoperation from an unrelated cause. Only 35

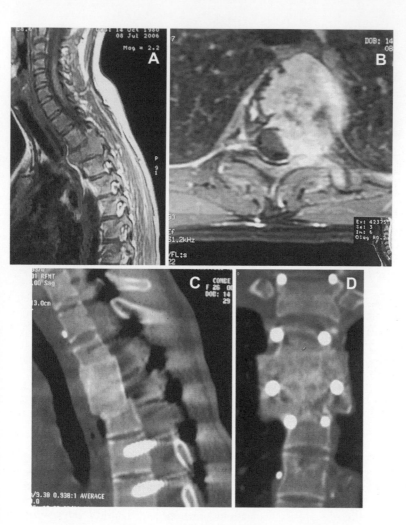

Fig. 16. (*A–D*) Case of total spondylectomy reconstruction is performed with a hallograft (frozen femur head).

patients are available for follow-up analysis. Twenty-one patients (60%) died with average survival duration of 16.7 months (range 8 days to 44 months). The 14 others (40%) are alive an average of 78.26 months postoperatively (range 46 to 144 months). Recently, our oldest patient died 12 years after the initial operation. He had been operated on for lumbar stenosis 1 year prior his death. Although selective preoperative screening of patients is mandatory, and a steep learning curve is necessary to achieve success with this extreme type of surgery, positive results confirm the feasibility of en bloc resection as a possible treatment of tumors usually considered unresectable.

Outcome in malignant dumbbell schwannomas

We have reported[24] on results after radical en bloc resections of three dumbbell-shaped neurogenic tumors. All three were malignant schwannomas. Patients were observed from 8 to 27 months after surgery. All tumors were completely excised, with

histologically controlled extratumoral resection limits. The surgical technique used was the one developed by the authors for extended Pancoast-Tobias resections. The patients had been operated on previously with possible local contamination and the previous surgical wound needed to be excised with the tumor mass. The patients died 8, 12, and 27 months postoperation. This short series of three malignant dumbbell tumors dramatically shows that prognosis is related more to adequacy of the previous resection and to the tumor malignancy than to the surgical technique itself. Indications to such extended surgery are relevant in malignant tumors. No other treatment could have avoided the neurologic incoming deficit and adjuvant therapy has proven ineffective in such cases.

Outcome in metastasis

A group of surgeons from six tertiary centers based in Denmark, France, Germany, Italy, Japan,

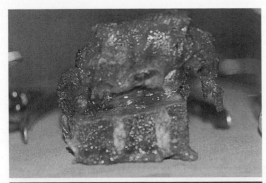

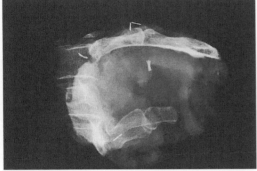

Fig. 17. Partial or hemivertebrectomy is necessary to achieve an extended and complete resection in Pancoast tumor.

classified as either aggressive or palliative. Patients had a histologically confirmed diagnosis of spinal metastasis of epithelial origin and postoperatively oncological specialists performed appropriately indicated adjuvant therapy.

Mean age was 61 years. Seventy-four percent underwent aggressive (excisional en bloc or debulking) surgery; the rest had (minimal) palliative decompression. All patients considered for surgery were included. Ninety-two percent of patients presented with pain, 24% with paraparesis, and 22% with abnormal urinary sphincter (5% were incontinent). Breast, renal, lung, and prostate accounted for three fourths of the cancers and, in 60% of patients, there were widespread spinal metastases (Tomita 6 or 7).

Perioperative mortality (within 30 days of surgery) was 5.8%. Postoperatively for the whole group, 72% had improved pain control, 53% regained or maintained their independent mobility, and 39% regained urinary sphincter function. The median survival for the cohort was 352 days (11.7 months), with those who had aggressive surgery surviving significantly longer than those in the palliative group ($P = .003$). As with survival results, functional improvement outcome was better in those who had aggressive surgery. Surgical treatment was effective in improving quality of life by enabling better pain control, helping patients regain or maintain mobility, and improving sphincter control. Thus, surgical treatment is feasible with acceptably low mortality and morbidity. While not a treatment of the systemic cancer, surgery for many improves the quality of their remaining life.

and the United Kingdom participated a prospective study.[5] This group formed the GSTSG. Included in this study were 223 patients referred by oncologists and physicians over a 2-year period. All patients in this study were treated surgically. Surgery was

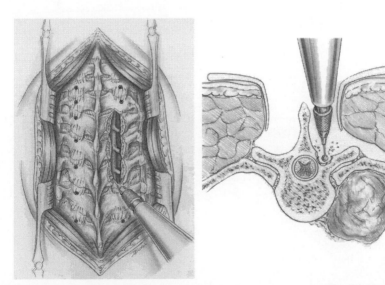

Fig. 18. The first step of a partial vertebrectomy is to drill of a groove to identify the roots. (*From* Mazel C, Hoffman E, Antonietti P, et al. Posterior cervicothoracic instrumentation in spine tumors. Spine 2004;29(11):1246–53; with permission.)

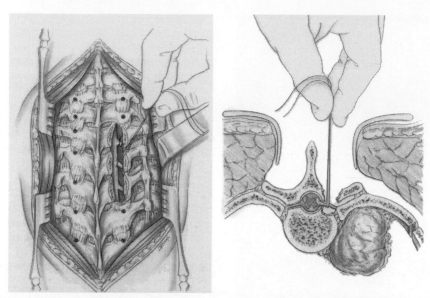

Fig. 19. The second step of a partial vertebrectomy is the ligature of the root inside the drilled groove. (*From* Mazel C, Hoffman E, Antonietti P, et al. Posterior cervicothoracic instrumentation in spine tumors. Spine 2004;29(11):1246–53; with permission.)

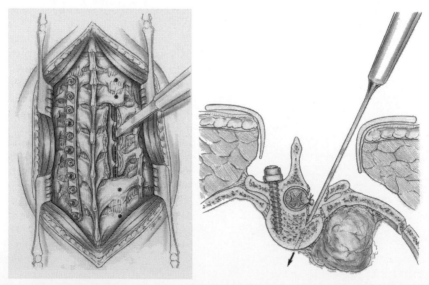

Fig. 20. The third step of a partial vertebrectomy is the osteotomy of the vertebral body and tumor resection. (*From* Mazel C, Hoffman E, Antonietti P, et al. Posterior cervicothoracic instrumentation in spine tumors. Spine 2004;29(11):1246–53; with permission.)

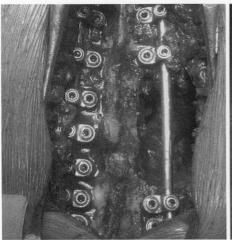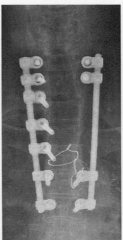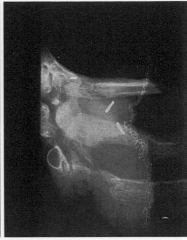

Fig. 21. Operative and postoperative view after partial vertebrectomy at cervicothoracic level. Resections include half of three vertebral bodies, the adjacent ribs, and the pathologic lung segment.

SUMMARY

Resection of spinal tumors at cervical cervicothoracic and thoracic levels is a challenging surgery but favorable, even spectacular, results can be achieved.

Complications and recurrence must be reduced as much as possible, underscoring the need for complete preoperative evaluations, precise surgical techniques, and knowledge based on experience in such resections or surgical procedures.

REFERENCES

1. Klimo P, Thompson CJ, Kestle JRW, et al. A meta-analysis of surgery versus conventional radiotherapy for the treatment of metastatic spinal epidural disease. Neuro-oncol 2005;7:64–76.
2. Patchell RA, Tibbs PA, Regine WF, et al. Direct decompressive surgical resection in the treatment of spinal cord compression caused by metastatic cancer: a randomised trial. Lancet 2005;366:643–8.
3. Falicov A, Fisher CG, Sparkes J, et al. Impact of surgical intervention on quality of life in patients with spinal metastases. Spine 2006;31:2849–56.
4. Fisher CG, Keynan O, Boyd M, et al. The surgical management of primary tumor of the spine: initial results of an ongoing prospective cohort study. Spine 2005;30:1899–908.
5. Ibrahim A, Crockard A, Antonietti P, et al. Does spinal surgery improve the quality of life for those with extradural (spinal) osseous metastases? An international multicenter prospective observational study of 223 patients. J Neurosurg Spine 2008;8:271–8.
6. Lièvre JA, Darcy M, Pradat P, et al. Tumeur à cellules géantes du rachis lombaire, spondylectomie totale en deux temps. Rev Rhum 1968;35:125–30.
7. Roy-Camille R, Saillant G, Bisserié M, et al. Résection vertébrale totale dans la chirurgie tumorale au niveau du rachis dorsale par voie postérieure pure. Rev Chir Orthop 1981;67:421–30.
8. Stener B. Total spondylectomy in chondrosarcoma arising from the seventh thoracic vertebra. J Bone Joint Surg 1971;53B:288–95.
9. Stener B. Complete removal of vertebrae for extirpation of tumors. A 20-year experience. Clin orthop 1989;245:72–82.
10. Boriani S, Weinstein JN, Biagini R. Spine update. Primary bone tumors of the spine. Spine 1997;22:1036–44.
11. Hart RA, Boriani S, Biagini R, et al. A system for surgical and management of spine tumors. Spine 1997; 22:1773–83.
12. Tomita K, Kawahara N, Baba H, et al. Total en bloc spondylectomy: a new surgical technique for primary malignant vertebral tumors. Spine 1997;22:324–33.
13. Tokuhashi Y, Matsuzaki H, Oda H, et al. A revise scoring system for preoperative evaluation of metastatic spine tumor prognosis. Spine 2005;30:2186–91.
14. Enneking WF, Spainer SS, Goodman MA. A system for the surgical staging of musculoskeletal sarcomas. Clin Orthop 1980;153:106–20.
15. Frankel HL, Hancock DO, Hyslop G, et al. The value of postural reduction in the initial management of closed injuries of the spine with paraplegia and tetraplegia. Paraplegia 1969;7:179–92.
16. Boriani S, Biagini R, Delure F, et al. En bloc resections of bone tumors of the thoracolumbar spine: a preliminary report on 29 patients. Spine 1996;21: 1927–31.
17. Boriani S, Chevalley F, Weinstein JN, et al. Chordoma of the spine above the sacrum. Treatment and outcome in 21 cases. Spine 1996;21:1569–77.

18. Sundaresan N, Rothman A, Manhart K, et al. Surgery for solitary metastases of the spine: rationale and results of treatment. Spine 2002;27:1802–6.

19. Tomita K, Kawahara N, Kobayashi T, et al. Surgical strategy for spinal metastases. Spine 2001;26:298–306.

20. Weinstein JN, McLain RF. Primary tumors of the spine. Spine 1987;12:843–51.

21. Hoshino Y, Kurokawa T, Nakamura K, et al. A report on the safety of unilateral artery ligation during cervical spine surgery. Spine 1996;21:1454–7.

22. Tomita K, Kawahara N. The threadwire saw: a new device for cutting bone. J Bone Joint Surg 1996; 78-A:1915–7.

23. Grunenwald D, Mazel C, Girard P, et al. Total vertebrectomy for en bloc resection of lung cancer invading the spine. Ann Thorac Surg 1996;61:723–6.

24. Mazel C, Grunenwald D, Laudrin P, et al. Radical excision in the management of thoracic and cervicothoracic tumors involving the spine: results in a series of 36 cases. Spine 2003;28(8):782–92.

25. Mazel CH, Hoffmann E, Antonietti P, et al. Posterior cervicothoracic instrumentation in spine tumors. Spine 2004;29:1246–53.

26. Roy-Camille R, Mazel CH, Saillant G, et al. Treatment of malignant tumors of the spine with posterior instrumentation. In: Sundaresan N, Schmideck HH, Schiller AL, et al, editors. Tumor of the spine. Philadelphia: WB Saunders; 1990. p. 473–87.

27. Roy-Camille R, Saillant G, Mazel C. Internal fixation of the unstable cervical spine by a posterior osteosynthesis with plates and screws. In: HH Sherk, EJ Dunn, FJ Eismont, et al, editors. The Cervical Spine. 2nd edition. Philadelphia: J.B. Lippincott; 1989. p. 390–403.

28. Roy-Camille R, Saillant G, Mazel C. Treatment of cervical spine injuries by a posterior osteosynthesis with plates and screws. In: Kehr P, Weidner A, editors. Cervical Spine I. Wien: Springer-Verlag; 1987. p. 163–74.

29. Magerl F, Seemann P. Stable posterior fusion of the atlas and axis by transarticular screw fixation. In: Kher P, Weidner A, editors. Cervical Spine I. Wien: Springer-Verlag; 1987. p. 322–7.

30. Mazel C, Topouchian V, Grunenwald D. Effectiveness of radical resections in malignant dumbbell tumors of the thoracic spine: review of five cases. J Spinal Disord Tech 2002;15(6):507–12.

Lumbar Tumor Resections and Management

Todd Alamin, MD[a],*, Robert Mayle, MD[b]

KEYWORDS

- Lumbar tumors • Lumbar tumor resections
- Lumbar metastatses • Lumbar instrumentation
- Tumor kyphoplasty

More than one third of patients with cancer have vertebral metastases found at autopsy.[1] Primary and metastatic tumors to the spinal column can lead to pain, instability, and neurologic deficit. Symptomatic lesions are most prevalent in the thoracic spine (70%), followed by the lumbar spine (20%) and cervical spine (10%).[2] Lesions in larger vertebral bodies are more likely to be asymptomatic given the increased ratio between the diameter of the spinal canal and the traversing nerve roots.

ANATOMY

Several important structural considerations surround the vertebral column. Anterior to the lumbar vertebrae, in the retroperitoneal space, are the aorta, vena cava, iliolumbar vein, crura of the thoracic diaphragm, sympathetic chain, psoas muscles, genitofemoral nerve, and the ureters. Posterior and lateral to the vertebral column is the paraspinal musculature compartment, with several prominent subdivisions (**Fig. 1**). The border of each of these structures is important to be aware of in spinal tumor surgery because the position and extent of the tumor dictates which tissue planes must be resected in excisions with curative intent.

The spinal cord terminates at the conus medullaris, corresponding roughly to the L1 vertebral level in the adult. The nerve roots in the lumbar spine exit below their corresponding pedicle—an important consideration for placement of pedicle screws and when considering surgical approaches to the lumbar spine. The arterial supply to the spinal cord is rich, with dependence on three main arterial sources: the anterior median longitudinal arterial trunk and a pair of posterolateral trunks. In the lumbar spine, there are segmental arteries adjacent to each lumbar vertebra, taking origin from the aorta. The segmental arteries branch to form an anastomotic network at the intervertebral foramen and again in the extradural space of the spinal canal. Venous drainage for the lumbar spine occurs through Batson's plexus. The extradural venous plexus, extravertebral venous plexus, and the veins of the bony structures of the vertebral column form Batson's plexus. Batson's plexus lies on the dorsal surface of the peridural membrane along the entire length of the spinal column, penetrating it at several points to enter the vertebral body.[3] This valveless venous system for the spinal column communicates directly with the venous systems of the head, chest, and abdomen—allowing for spread of metastatic disease.

CLASSIFICATION

The Enneking staging system for classification of long bone tumors has been applied to spinal tumors. This staging system is based on clinical features, imaging (computed tomography [CT] scan, magnetic resonance imaging [MRI], x-rays),

a Stanford University Department of Orthopaedic Surgery, Spinal Surgery Section, Stanford University School of Medicine, 300 Pasteur Drive, Stanford University Hospitals and Clinics, Room R171, Stanford, CA 94305, USA
b Stanford University Department of Orthopaedic Surgery, Stanford University School of Medicine, 300 Pasteur Drive, Stanford University Hospitals and Clinics, Room R171, Stanford, CA 94305, USA
* Corresponding author.
E-mail address: tfalamin@aol.com (T. Alamin).

Orthop Clin N Am 40 (2009) 93–104
doi:10.1016/j.ocl.2008.09.011

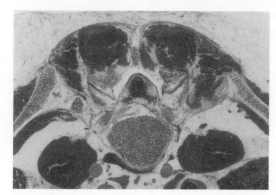

Fig. 1. Axial section. (*Courtesy of* W. Raushning, MD, PhD, Sigtuna, Sweden.)

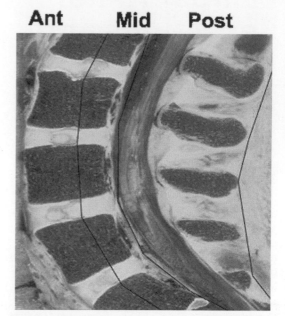

Fig. 2. Sagittal section. (*Courtesy of* W. Raushning, MD, PhD, Sigtuna, Sweden.)

histologic findings based on biopsy, and an isotopic scan.[4] These biological stages were described to classify tumors based on their aggressiveness and systemic extent, which is reflective of how amenable the tumor is to surgical treatment.

Several staging classifications specific to the spine are useful in helping crystallize relevant elements of the anatomic extent of the spinal tumor: the WBB system by Weinstein and modified by Boriani and Biagini divide the vertebrae into 12 radiating zones and into five concentric layers, which help the surgeon plan for en bloc resection via vertebrectomy, sagittal resection, or resection of the posterior arch. The Tomita system classifies tumors according to the site of the tumor, based on the most common sequence of progression: vertebral body (1), pedicle (2), lamina and spinous process (3), spinal canal (epidural space included) (4), and paravertebral area (5), and then subclassifies lesions in these locations as intracompartmental (three subtypes), extracompartmental (three subtypes), or multiple with skip lesions. Recommendations of the appropriateness of spondylectomy made by Tomita are based on this classification.

Denis' three-column theory of the spine can be used to understand the biomechanical significance of lesions of the lumbar spine.[5] The anterior column includes the anterior longitudinal ligament to the anterior portion of the vertebral body. The middle column extends from the posterior vertebral body to the posterior longitudinal ligament. The posterior column includes the posterior bony arch/ligamentous complex. (**Fig. 2**) Given the rich blood supply and sinusoidal vascular distribution, the vertebral body typically is affected first.[6] Involvement of the dorsal elements is rare. When this does occur, facet involvement or destruction may lead to rotational or translational instability at the affected level.[7]

Tumor location within the vertebral body, tumor size, bone mineral density, and cross-sectional area of the intact body correlates with the development and pattern of pathologic fracture. Tumors in the ventral third of the vertebral body, on sagittal imaging cuts, and those located in the central one third of the vertebral body, on axial imaging cuts, are the most destabilizing. Given the intrinsic lordosis of the lumbar spine, lesions located in these areas are subject to compression forces in line with the internal axis of rotation, which can more commonly than in the thoracic spine lead to a burst fracture pattern.[7]

Although primary tumors of the spine have a predilection for the posterior elements, they are rare, comprising less than 10% of all spinal tumors. Metastatic lesions in the spine are far more common and arise from one of four different mechanisms.[8,9] The rich arterial blood supply to the vertebral bodies allows for hematogenous seeding in the bone marrow. Second, Batson's venous plexus permits transmission of metastases with deposition in the epidural space. Batson postulated that an increase in intra-abdominal pressure diverts blood flow into the vertebral venous system, allowing for seeding of metastatic disease (a classic example is that of prostate cancer).[10] Third, spread through cerebral spinal fluid, pathways allow for "drop metastases" to develop in the intradural space. Finally, extension of paraspinal tumors into the epidural space occurs via venous channels through the foramina.

TREATMENT CONSIDERATIONS

Management of primary and metastatic tumors of the lumbar spine can involve single modalities or combinations: chemotherapy, radiation therapy, and/or surgery. The surgeon is an integral part of the decision-making process and should collaborate closely with the oncologist and radiation oncologist in developing a treatment plan.

Chemotherapy is a valuable treatment option for some primary and malignant tumors of the spine, including multiple myeloma, osteosarcoma, and Ewing's sarcoma. Use of chemotherapy has improved 5-year event-free survival rate in patients with osteosarcoma to greater than 70%.[11]

Historically, isolated treatment response with radiation therapy alone has been reported to be 66% to 80%.[11] Of the patients in this series, 50% had improvement in functional status, whereas 33% had stabilization of symptoms. Indications for radiotherapy include radiosensitive tumors, expected survival time less than 3 to 4 months, inability to tolerate surgical intervention, neurologic deficit greater than 24 to 48 hours, and multilevel or diffuse spinal involvement.[2] Conventional radiation therapy delivers 2500 to 4000 cGy to a targeted region over 8 to 10 days. Five centimeter margins (equivalent to the height of two vertebral bodies) are desired. Conventional radiation therapy, however, exposes and irradiates healthy tissue (spinal cord included), which can lead to radiation-induced myelopathy. Radiation to the spinal cord may be reduced by the use of nonconventional radiotherapy. This includes stereotactic radiotherapy and intensity-modulated radiotherapy. By these means, radiation is delivered to the target while decreasing the amount delivered to normal tissue. Benign tumor irradiation should be avoided given the risk of radiation-induced sarcoma. Radiation therapy can aid in alleviation of pain, but cannot reverse destruction of bone. Timing of radiation is an important consideration. Radiation is toxic to fibroblasts, which are responsible for collagen deposition, remodeling, and wound contracture. When performed within 3 weeks after surgery, radiation treatment has been shown to decrease the tensile strength of wounds.[12] Moderately dosed, fractionated radiation given 3 to 6 months before surgery or 7 to 12 days after surgery, however, has been shown to have little affect on wound strength and healing and is unlikely to significantly increase surgical morbidity.[12]

Surgical indications include radioresistant tumors (sarcoma, lung, colon, renal), spinal instability, clinically significant neural compression, intractable pain, or failure of radiation. The patient's life expectancy and ability to tolerate a surgical procedure are crucial elements in the decision-making process. The goal of surgery is to correct instability and prevent any further deformity of the spine with instrumentation, decompression of neural elements to aid in pain relief and potential functional loss (if applicable), and to obtain tissue samples if needed for diagnostic purposes.

When a combination of surgical resection and radiation therapy is used, studies have found that postoperative radiation is more beneficial than preoperative administration.[11] In a comparison between radiation therapy administered preoperatively versus postoperatively, wound healing and ambulatory function were improved if surgical resection was performed first. Seventy-five percent of patients retained ambulatory function compared with 50%. Wound complication rates of 32% were seen in the group that underwent radiation therapy preoperatively.[11]

Embolization of primary or metastatic tumors of the spine can be useful as a means of occluding the vascular supply of the tumor, reducing its size preoperatively, decreasing spinal canal compromise, and improving neurologic function—through reduction of tumor size. When performed before surgical intervention of hypervascular tumors, reduction of intraoperative blood loss can be achieved.[11] Aneurysmal bone cysts, giant cell tumors, renal cell carcinoma, and chordomas are known to respond favorably to embolization.[11]

Use of corticosteroids in the treatment of metastatic disease has resulted in palliation of pain and useful symptomatic remission. Corticosteroids exert their effect through direct action on neoplastic cells, their vascular and soft tissue environment, and alteration of endocrine trophism important to sustained growth.[12] However, they also are immunosuppressive, anti-inflammatory, and catabolic in nature. These characteristics decrease wound healing and potentiate infection. The risk of their use may sometimes outweigh their benefits, especially when used in conjunction with other therapies that affect lymphocyte production and wound healing.

ANESTHETIC/PREOPERATIVE CONSIDERATIONS

Surgical intervention can vary from a straightforward kyphoplasty to an extensive anterior–posterior resection/stabilization. Given this, preoperative workup will vary. Medical comorbidities, the patient's generalized condition, type of tumor, extent of cancer, and the surgical procedure to be performed, including duration and approach, dictate the extent of preoperative workup. Use of nonsteroidal anti-inflammatory medication, common in this population, should be discontinued. Any formal anticoagulation therapy should be discontinued as well, in coordination with the prescribing specialist. Preoperative laboratory investigations should include complete blood count, basic metabolic profile, coagulation panel, and a type and cross. Malnutrition commonly afflicts cancer patients. Evaluation of nutritional status, preoperatively, is essential. Albumin and total lymphocyte count are clinical parameters that help assess the nutritional status of a patient. Both markers are decreased in the malnourished patient and have been associated with postoperative complications including infection, wound healing problems, mortality, and immune suppression. A patient with an albumin level of less than 3.5 g/dL and a total lymphocyte count less than 1500 to 2000 cells/mm,[7] is considered malnourished.[13] Patients that meet these parameters are likely to benefit from nutritional supplementation or replenishment before surgery.

Significant blood loss can occur with resection of lumbar spinal tumors. Invasive blood pressure monitoring (via an arterial line) is typically used in these patients. Patients with known cardiovascular disease should be considered for central venous and pulmonary arterial pressure monitoring. It is critical in these often long procedures to pay close attention to positioning of the patient: their position should be stable, and all potential pressure points should be well padded especially the neck, arms, and eyes. Extremity positioning should be checked carefully to minimize the risk of positional nerve palsies: the most common being brachial plexus and ulnar nerve palsies. Electrophysiologic monitoring, including somatosensory-evoked potentials and motor-evoked potentials, can be useful in cases in which surgical resection of tumor and reconstruction may place neural elements at risk.

Postoperatively, depending on the length and extent of surgery, stay in the intensive care unit may be warranted. Determination of timing of extubation should be based on the complexity and extent of surgery, the patient's existing comorbidities, blood loss or transfusions, and perioperative complications.

Potential perioperative complications include fluid volume deficit, neurologic injury or deficit, infection, dural tear, anemia, urinary retention, ileus, atelectasis or pneumonia, venous thrombosis, and vision loss. Vision loss is a devastating complication with an incidence of 0.028% in spinal surgery, making this 10 times more common than occurrence in any other nonophthalmologic surgery. Risk factors for this condition include direct ocular compression, surgically induced anemia, hypotension, prolonged surgical time, and increased venous pressure.[14,15] In a population-based study of 987 patients with spinal metastasis treated with surgery, the overall complication rate was 39%, in which 27% had one major complication, and 12% had two or more postoperative complications.[16] The rate of postoperative wound infection was 11%, graft and instrumentation complications were seen in 9%, urinary tract infection developed in 21%, and deep-venous thrombosis developed in 6%. Wise and colleagues[17] reported that the complication rate was higher in patients who had a preoperative neurologic deficit. Careful attention to detail in the perioperative period, both from an intraoperative technical standpoint but also encompassing pre- and postoperative care, can help to minimize these risks.

Preoperative Planning

A detailed and well thought-out preoperative plan is critical to achieve an acceptable result in a surgery for spinal tumor. Probably the most important issues to address preoperatively in formulating a surgical plan are the main goals of the surgery. These must be agreed on by the patient, the oncologist, and the surgeon. Is the surgery to be done for palliation of symptoms or with a curative goal? If the surgery is being done for palliative reasons, what is the likely life expectancy of the patient? Does the patient require a stabilization procedure or simply a decompression? How destabilizing will the decompression be? Are there other lesions beyond the symptomatic one that should be addressed, given the patient's life expectancy? What is the preoperative or postoperative plan for chemotherapy or radiation treatment? Clear answers to these questions are of paramount importance because they significantly affect the primary choice of surgery versus nonsurgical treatment, and then the secondary choice of surgical approach and timing.

Most surgeries for spinal tumor are performed for reasons of palliation; therefore, the surgical goals are those of decompressing the spinal canal, stabilizing the involved spinal segment(s), or minimizing the risk of local recurrence. In these more common cases, excision of the vertebral lesion is performed to the degree necessary to both decompress the spinal canal and minimize the risk of local recurrence for the projected lifespan of the patient. This tumor resection typically is performed in an intralesional fashion to minimize the morbidity of the surgery. Stabilization is then performed as necessary based on the assessed degree of instability.

Occasionally, a patient presents with a primary spinal tumor or an isolated metastatic lesion and is a good candidate for an attempted curative surgery. There are several different staging systems, noted above, that are useful for determining if this is a reasonable goal. In the rare cases in which an en bloc resection is necessary for attempted cure, careful consideration needs to be given to balancing the goals of curative resection and minimizing postoperative functional morbidity—this balance is an issue that the patient and his or her family needs to understand and be in agreement with the surgeon preoperatively.

Vertebroplasty/Kyphoplasty

Initially described as a technique for the treatment of vertebral hemangiomas, vertebroplasty has been used as a method for the treatment of both pathologic fractures of the vertebral body, and for prophylactic treatment of large vertebral body lesions. In this procedure, the vertebral body is cannulated percutaneously with a 10-gauge needle for the thoracic and lumbar spines, and a 15-gauge needle for the cervical spine.[18] Cement is injected into the vertebral body during fluoroscopic visualization. A transpedicular approach is used typically in the lower lumbar spine, but in the upper lumbar spine because of the smaller diameter and more sagittally oriented pedicles, an extrapedicular approach is preferred (**Fig. 3**). During vertebroplasty, we use simultaneous biplanar fluoroscopy to ensure good enough visualization to minimize the risk of extravasation of polymethylmethacrylate (PMMA) outside of the vertebral body into the retroperitoneum, the spinal canal, or the paraspinal tissues.

Kyphoplasty is a more recently described method that involves the use of a balloon tamp to both create a void in the vertebral body and to elevate the depressed endplate(s) to reduce the deformity of the vertebral body. Kyphoplasty relies on access to the vertebral body through cannulae that are 4 mm in diameter and can either be placed via a transpedicular route (in the lower lumbar spine) or an extrapedicular route (usually in the upper lumbar spine). Through these cannulae, a biopsy can be obtained of the vertebral body lesion. this biopsy typically is performed before the deployment of the inflatable bone tamps (IBTs). Once, if indicated, a biopsy specimen has been obtained, a passage for the IBTs is created in the vertebral bodies by the use of a drill. The use of a drill is necessary in sclerotic lesions of the vertebral body but often not necessary in lytic lesions of the vertebra. The IBTs are then deployed and inflated progressively in an attempt to reduce the fracture deformity. Preoperative supine hyperextension lateral views can be useful in determining whether fracture reduction will be possible. Improvement in height or a vacuum sign in the vertebral body noted on the supine hyperextension lateral x-ray correlates well in our experience with the ability to effect a significant reduction. If reduction is anticipated, then sequential IBT inflation is performed until the desired reduction is effected or until IBT breakout into the disc space is noted. This inhibits further reduction because expansion of the IBT into the disc will ensue, disrupting the endplate further and increasing the risk of extravasation of cement into the disc space. If reduction is not anticipated, then the IBT is used for a different purpose—creation of a cavity into which PMMA can be inserted at low pressure and from which the PMMA can interdigitate into the rest of the vertebral body. If a reduction is effected, it is critical that the PMMA interdigitate from the superior to the inferior endplates; if this is not the case, the pathologic bone around the PMMA will collapse with subsequent loading.

Kyphoplasty/Vertebroplasty: Open Technique

The vertebroplasty and kyphoplasty procedures may also be done in an open technique to allow simultaneous canal decompression and stabilization of a pathologically fractured anterior column, while directly assessing and protecting the spinal canal to minimize the risk of significant cement extravasation. This technique is useful for pathologic fractures of the vertebral body with significant extension into the vertebral canal when

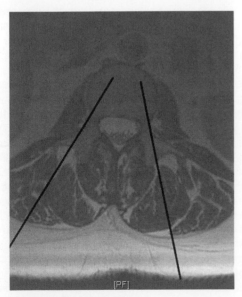

Fig. 3. Extrapedicular route.

a formal complete excision is not indicated and the posterior elements are not insufficient. The lumbar segment is exposed in the standard fashion via a midline posterior approach. The cephalad interlaminar window (eg, L4-5 for an L5 lesion) is exposed if only the superior portion of the pathologic fracture involves extension into the epidural space, which is the more typical situation. If the inferior portion of the pathologic vertebra has burst into the canal, then the more caudal interlaminar window is exposed as well. Laminotomies are performed bilaterally, sparing the posterior midline structures whose integrity is important if no fusion is to be performed. If severe central canal compression is noted, the central ligamentum flavum and the anterior portions of the spinous process and central lamina are resected. The lateral border of the thecal sac is identified, and the thecal sac is retracted medially to expose the underlying burst fragment or epidural tumor mass. Care needs to be taken at this point to ensure that the tissue plane between the tumor mass (if present) and the anterior dura have been developed with a nerve hook, Penfield elevator, or other instrument; this markedly facilitates the canal decompression if performed first. The pathologic bone from the posterior part of the vertebral body is removed piecemeal, creating a space in this position that epidural fragments can be pushed into. The epidural tumor mass (if present) and burst fragment are then impacted into the more anterior portions of the vertebral body with a down-going curette; they then are removed sequentially from the more anterior position into which they have been impacted. Once the canal has been decompressed in this manner, a drill is used to create a path into the anterior portion of the residual vertebral body. This may be performed either unilaterally or bilaterally, depending on the size of the vertebral body. The IBTs then are deployed into the paths that have been created and then inflated sequentially to effect a reduction if possible. As the posterior cortex has been partially resected, PMMA is then inserted into the resultant cavities under low pressure and under direct visualization as the thecal sac is retracted with a nerve root retractor. If cement is noted to encroach upon the canal, it is pushed back toward the anterior portion of the vertebral body with a Woodson elevator. The cement is flushed with irrigant to minimize heating of the thecal sac. This technique cannot be used if significant kyphotic deformity exists and also should not be used if significant portions of the facet joint have been removed with the resultant chance of significant postoperative instability. It may be used in the thoracic spine as well as in the lumbar spine; the stabilizing effect of the rib cage has allowed us to perform this technique with a unilateral pedicular resection in the thoracic spine, obviating retraction of the spinal cord.

Posterior Decompression and Stabilization

This is perhaps the most commonly performed operation in the lumbar spine for spinal tumor; it allows decompression of the spinal canal as well as resections of portions of the involved vertebral body and then posterior stabilization and fusion of the necessary segments. Because of the position and importance of the lumbar nerve roots, an anterior reconstruction after piecemeal excision of the vertebral body is difficult. If this is thought to be necessary, either a transpedicular approach or an anterior and posterior approach is more appropriate.

The issue of bone graft needs to be considered carefully in patients with a lumbar tumor for whom a fusion is planned. It is more difficult to obtain a solid fusion in these patients who often have undergone chemotherapy or irradiation and who may be in a poor nutritional state.[19–21] In such circumstances, use of the most reliable technique to secure a solid fusion is generally accepted to be beneficial if the expected lifespan of the patient is longer than 6 months, but longer-term good results have been obtained with the use of PMMA alone for anterior reconstructions.[22] In considering the options available, imaging studies of the iliac crest are important to rule out the presence of a pathologic lesion at this site; if one was present, then the risk of seeding uninvolved areas by using bone from this location is high.

If the decision to use bone from the iliac crest has been made, then a separate incision is first performed in a longitudinal fashion directly overlying the posterior iliac crest. We perform a corticotomy of the posteromedial wall of the ilium after dissecting the paraspinal musculature off its medial side to not disrupt the gluteal muscles. Cancellous graft then is obtained from between the tables of the ilium and stored for later use. The site is irrigated, a small drain is placed, and then the fascia is re-approximated to the remaining posterior cortex. The skin is closed in the standard fashion before proceeding with the posterior approach to the lumbar spine. When iliac screws are necessary, these are placed first, followed by the harvesting of bone graft, leaving at least a 3-cm section of intact posterolateral cortex between the posterior crest harvest site and the iliac screw site.

A standard midline posterior approach is performed down to the lumbodorsal fascia. If there is involvement of the posterior elements by tumor, the soft tissue dissection of the midline elements is performed first proximally and distally to expose the posterior elements to the tips of the transverse processes to allow for the placement of transpedicular instrumentation at least two levels above and below the level of the tumor. During this portion of the dissection, a soft tissue cuff of normal tissue is left in place around the involved posterior elements to minimize the risk of contamination of the rest of the operative field. Meticulous hemostasis is obtained. Pedicle screws are placed bilaterally at this point in the procedure, before the exposure of the tumor. Once the screws are in good position, it often is best to prebend and then attach the rods to the screws so that the spine may be rendered stable before the decompression. If a reduction in a kyphotic deformity is planned, it is performed at this point to render the canal decompression technically easier.

The posterior elements of the involved level, and typically half of the spinous process and lamina above and below the lesion are resected along with their surrounding soft tissue cuff. The ligamentum flavum is resected along the length of this decompression, and then the lateral border of the thecal sac at the involved level is identified bilaterally. Foraminotomies are performed as needed bilaterally, and then the roots and thecal sac are retracted to expose anterior epidural tumor, if present. This exposure typically necessitates, for an L5 lesion, first retracting the L5 root medially to expose the most cephalad portion of the epidural tumor, and then retracting the L5 root laterally and the rest of the thecal sac medially to expose the more caudal portion of the tumor. A piecemeal partial vertebrectomy can be then performed to remove unstable portions of the pathologically involved vertebral body.

Once an adequate decompression has been performed, careful decortication of the posterolateral gutter is performed, and then this site is packed with iliac crest bone graft and bone graft extender (synthetic or allograft bone). Mobilization is allowed on the first postoperative day, and bracing typically is not necessary.

Because of the extent of bony resection necessary to effect both a complete canal decompression and tumor resection, and the fact that the bone from the decompression (pathologically involved) cannot be used for fusion, it is sometimes difficult to procure enough bone graft from a unilateral iliac crest bone graft harvest.[1] This situation can be managed by either harvesting bone from the contralateral iliac crest as well or by using a bone graft extender. In our institution, we prefer to use synthetic bone graft extender, but understand that there are no good study findings to establish the desired ratio of autograft to extender. There has been recent interest in the use of the commercially available bone morphogenetic proteins (Infuse, Medtronic Spine, LLC, Minneapolis, Minnesota; OP-1, Stryker Spine LLC, Allendale, New Jersey) because of the risk of nonunion in fusions for spinal tumor.[19] There is a theoretic risk of tumor stimulation by the use of these bone morphogenetic proteins, which are part of the transforming growth factor–b superfamily, but this risk has not been documented clinically. This risk seems most concerning in bone-forming tumors such as osteogenic sarcoma; we could find no case reports in the literature of its clinical use in spinal tumor patients.

Posterior Transpedicular Decompression and Anterior Column Reconstruction

The advantage of a transpedicular decompression when compared with a standard posterior decompression is the ability to more effectively visualize the central portion of the spinal canal as well as the more anterior and lateral portions of the vertebral body. This approach allows also for a much gentler anterior column reconstruction by providing better access to the anterior column and improving the ability to retract salient nerve roots, eg, the L3 nerve root for an L3 lesion.

A standard midline posterior approach is performed as above after obtaining sufficient bone graft from the iliac crest. The side of the canal most compressed is chosen for the side of the transpedicular decompression. After transpedicular instrumentation has been placed, a rod is attached to the side contralateral to the planned transpedicular decompression. Slight distraction and reduction of kyphotic deformity, if present, can render the canal decompression less difficult because of the indirect decompression effected by this maneuver. The pars interarticularis above and below the pedicle is resected, and the facet joint overlying the pedicle is resected. The transverse process is freed from the pedicle and facet via an osteotomy at its root. The traversing and exiting nerve roots are then protected carefully, and the pedicle is resected back to its base using a high-speed burr. It is possible to encounter significant epidural bleeding during this portion of the procedure; control of this with bipolar cautery and gelfoam soaked in thrombin is critical.

A small elevator then is used to develop the plane between the lateral wall of the vertebral body and the psoas muscle and exiting nerve root. This elevation may then be continued progressively more anterior, taking care to stay posterior to the aorta and vena cava anteriorly. Once this elevation is complete proximally, it may also be performed distal to the root level— eg, distal to the L3 root for an L3 lesion—to complete exposure of the lateral border of the vertebral body. A blunt Hohmann retractor then is placed in this developed tissue plane and used to retract the lateral and anterior structures to allow direct access to the vertebral body. The thecal sac is protected carefully with a nerve root retractor, and the posterior cortex is impacted anteriorly into the vertebral body and then removed piecemeal, along with the involved portions of the vertebral body. The plane between the thecal sac and epidural tumor mass, if present, is then developed with a nerve hook and Penfield elevator. Once this has been performed, the epidural mass is resected via sequential impaction with a down-going curette into the defect in the vertebral body, followed by piecemeal removal.

It often is necessary to then incise and remove the disc above and below the involved level to allow for an endplate-to-endplate fusion graft. Once this has been performed, the appropriate-size graft is selected: an expandable vertebral body replacement (preferred because of the ability to place it into position in a compact form, and then distract it up to the desired length); structural allo- or autograft; or mesh cage. It then is positioned carefully during retraction of the nerve root with extreme care taken to avoid its direct injury. In the upper lumbar spine (L1, L2), the nerve root may be taken with relatively little morbidity— this typically is not performed in the lower lumbar spine unless the root is invaded directly by tumor. When the anterior graft is in position, the ipsilateral rod is attached, and compression is performed via the pedicle screws bilaterally to load the graft before final locking of the posterior instrumentation.

Anterior Decompression and Stabilization

Anterior decompression and fusion is best used for lesions of a single vertebral body without posterior element involvement, in which all of the compression of the spinal canal is anterior. It is also best performed at the L4 level or above because exposure of the entire L5 body anteriorly is difficult, as is anterior instrumentation across the lumbosacral junction. This approach can be performed in such lesions in conjunction with posterior instrumentation; in this manner it may be extended down to the L5 level. In such cases, the posterior decompression and grafting typically are performed first to both stabilize the vertebral body to be resected and indirectly decompress

the thecal sac via segmental distraction and reduction, making the direct decompression less difficult.

If there is significant compression and displacement of the great vessels anteriorly, then the assistance of a vascular surgeon is obtained for the exposure. For L4 level lesions and above, a left-sided lateral incision is preferred, followed by a retroperitoneal approach. At the L5 level, a midline retroperitoneal approach proceeding between the rectus muscles is preferred, allowing exposure of the vertebral body both in between and lateral to the common iliac vessels. The segmental vessel at the level of the lesion is clipped and transected, along with the vessel at the levels above and below, allowing mobilization of the great vessels across the midline. For an exposure at the L5 level, the middle sacral artery and vein are controlled and transected, along with the ascending iliolumbar vessels.

The disc above and below the lesion is excised back to the posterior longitudinal ligament; this allows the surgeon to determine the location of the posterior aspect of the spinal canal. The pedicle then is osteotomized carefully at its base, anterior to the exiting root at this level. The middle and desired anterior portions of the vertebral body then are resected with large rongeurs back to the posterior cortex. The posterior cortex and ventral epidural mass are then removed via development of the plane anterior to the thecal sac with an elevator and down-going curette followed by impaction into the anterior void and resection. The resection is completed on the contralateral side by resection of the posterior cortex and epidural mass with a Kerrison rongeur to the base of the pedicle.

The distance from endplate to endplate is measured, and an appropriately sized graft is chosen of either structural allo- or autograft, an expandable vertebral body replacement, or a mesh cage packed with graft. PMMA may also be chosen for anterior reconstructions in which the life expectancy of the patient is less than 18 months.[22] If no posterior instrumentation is planned, then an anterior dual rod/dual screw construct or plating is performed. Postoperative bracing typically is used without posterior instrumentation for 3 to 6 postoperative months; the patient is allowed to mobilize on the first postoperative day.

CASE STUDIES

Patient 1 was a 65-year-old woman with a diagnosis of breast cancer 17 years before evaluation and was noted to be metastatic 7 years before evaluation. She had multiple known metastases at the time of evaluation and had a chief complaint of lower thoracic pain radiating along the left T12 rib to the abdominal midline, only relieved by rest, and atraumatic in its onset. She was also undergoing irradiation for a left femoral neck fracture with some left groin pain, but her lower thoracic pain was far more significant. She had been unable to walk for 6 weeks because of her pain, and spent most of her waking hours lying down. There was no bowel or bladder incontinence, and no complaint of weakness or gait imbalance. Her motor examination on the left was limited because of pain, but no long-tract signs were present on examination. MRI scans showed multiple spinal metastases along with a pathologic T12 burst fracture with a left-sided retropulsed fragment at the superior portion of the vertebra, compressing the left T12 nerve root (**Figs. 4, 5**). She had not previously undergone irradiation of her spine, and her oncologist felt that her overall prognosis at this point was poor. After an extensive discussion of the different options for treatment, she elected to proceed with a microdecompression and kyphoplasty, to be followed by postoperative irradiation and continued chemotherapy.

A 3-cm incision was made in the midline directly overlying the T11/T12 interlaminar window, and a left-sided fascial incision was made. Under the operative microscope, the inferior portion of the left T11 lamina and the superior portion of the left T12 lamina were resected. The ligamentum flavum of the interspace was excised, and then the superomedial portion of the pedicle was removed with a high-speed burr. The lateral border of the spinal cord was identified along with the T12 nerve root. The burst fragment was identified and carefully removed, along with unstable portions of the T12 vertebral body anterior to this. The residual T12 body, noted to enhance on preoperative MRI scan, was probed and felt to be structurally capable of

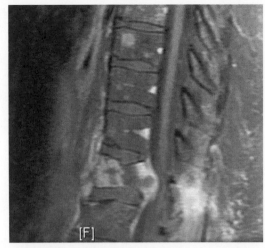
Fig. 5. Contrast sagittal MRI.

containing cement. The working instrumentation for kyphoplasty was placed through the residual left T12 pedicle into the vertebral body, and then a drill was used to penetrate the anterior portion of the T12 body. A 15-mm balloon was placed and sequentially inflated to create a void anteriorly. PMMA was then inserted into this void until it began to extravasate into the surrounding bone. A Woodson elevator was used to prevent contact of the PMMA with the dura and was also used to press any PMMA proceeding posteriorly back into the anterior portion of the body (**Figs. 6, 7**).

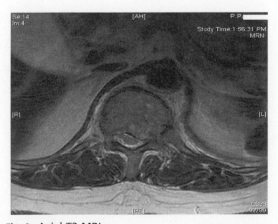
Fig. 4. Axial T2 MRI.

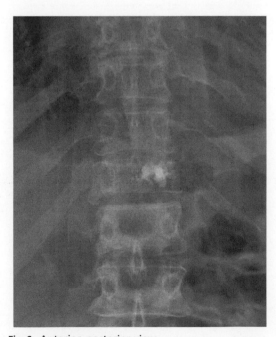
Fig. 6. Anterior–posterior view.

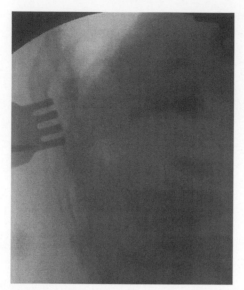

Fig. 7. Lateral view.

Her thoracic and left-sided radiating pain resolved postoperatively, and she began ambulation on postoperative day 1. She began to be limited by her left groin pain, and underwent femoral neck pinning 1 week after surgery. She was treated with radiation to her thoracolumbar junction 2 weeks after surgery and had no recurrence of her thoracic pain before her death 4 months after surgery from complications related to hypercalcemia.

Case 2

Patient 2 is a 40-year-old man who presented with a large, rapidly expansile posterior lumbar mass over a 2-month period. Plain radiographs followed by an MRI scan were obtained eventually by the primary care physician, and the patient was referred on for surgical evaluation with a large multi-loculated mass that appeared to originate in the right L5 transverse process and pedicle, massively extending into the paraspinal musculature and retroperitoneum (**Figs. 8, 9**). After an initial needle biopsy was nondiagnostic, an open biopsy was obtained that showed a high-grade telangiectatic osteosarcoma. He was noted to have severe pain with an upright posture in his lower back radiating to his right thigh and had significant weakness of his quadriceps, hip flexors, and tibialis anterior. A metastatic survey was notable for a concerning lesion in the right proximal femur and in the right posterior iliac crest. No other lesions were noted. Preoperative chemotherapy was planned, followed by wide excision of the primary lesion and concerning area of posterior iliac crest, and biopsy of the proximal femoral lesion.

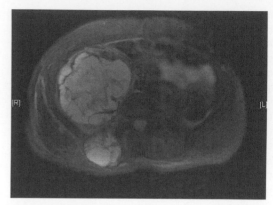

Fig. 8. Axial T2 MRI.

After initial chemotherapy, during which there was, unfortunately, increase in size of the tumor mass, the patient was brought for surgical excision in conjunction with a vascular surgeon and pelvic oncologic surgeon.

He was positioned prone first, and a left-sided longitudinal posterior incision 7 cm lateral to the midline was made first. A paraspinal muscle-splitting approach was performed down onto the transverse processes, facet joints, and sacral ala. Autograft was harvested from the left posterior iliac crest, and then pedicle screws were placed at L3, L4, L5, and S1. A rod was prebent into lordosis and attached to the screws in the standard fashion. Bone graft was packed into the left posterolateral gutter and facet joints, and this incision was closed. A right-sided incision then was made, incorporating the open biopsy incision from the lower thoracic spine to the inferior portion of the sacrum, and a careful dissection superficial to the fascia to the right flank around the paraspinal mass superficial to the fascia, inferiorly to the gluteus fascia, and to the left across the midline was made. An incision was made 1 cm left of the

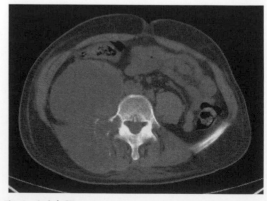

Fig. 9. Axial CT scan.

midline from L3 to the sacrum in the lumbodorsal fascia, and a subperiosteal dissection was performed to elevate the left paraspinal musculature off of the posterior elements. At the L2 level, the fascial incision was continued proximally to the right up to the thoracolumbar junction. The spinous processes of L3, L4, L5, and S1 were osteotomized at their base to prevent violation of the tissue plane around the right paraspinal extension of the tumor. A midline laminectomy was performed, and the L4/5 and L5/S1 discs were incised along their right sides. A sagittal osteotomy was performed through the L5 body in the midline and connected to the disc incision above and below. The right L4 pars interarticularis was resected, and the L5 inferior articular facet was released from the L5/S1 facet joint, freeing the right lateral portion of the vertebral body, pedicle, and transverse process. The right paraspinal muscle insertions then were incised at their insertions onto the 10th, 11th, and 12th ribs, and off of the midline posterior elements proximal to the L3 spinous process. A transverse incision was made in the gluteus muscle down on to the lateral wall of the right ilium; an osteotomy was performed in the ilium to excise the paraspinal muscle origin and the high signal area noted in the posterior superior iliac spine.

An anterior abdominal midline incision then was made with an oblique extension along the femoral canal to the proximal femur at the level of the lesser trochanter. A transperitoneal dissection was performed, and the great vessels were dissected off of the large retroperitoneal tumor. The dissection proceeded down to the insertion of the psoas on to the lesser trochanter. The femoral nerve was entwined extensively in tumor and incised. The iliacus was elevated off of the ilium, and the tumor was dissected off of the floor of the pelvis. The L4 and L5 nerve roots on the right were sacrificed to allow mobilization of the tumor. The L5 sagittal osteotomy performed during the posterior approach was found and completed, as was the mobilization of the L4/5 and L5/S1 disc spaces. The right ilio-psoas was dissected off of the lumbar transverse processes L1-L4 as well as the anterior portions of the posterior T11 and T12 ribs. The osteotomy through the ilium was found and mobilized, and then the tumor was removed in its entirety.

A titanium mesh cage was cut, packed with iliac crest bone graft and bone graft extender, and placed in between the L4 and S1 endplates. The anterior incision was closed, and the posterior incision was opened again. Transpedicular instrumentation was placed into the right L3, L4, and S1 pedicles, and a porcine pericardial flap was

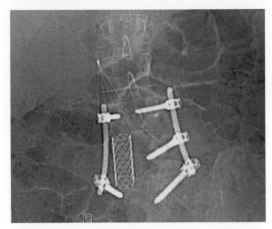

Fig. 10. Anterior–posterior view.

sutured in place to serve as a posterior barrier to the peritoneal contents (**Fig. 10**). His postoperative course was complicated by a symptomatic dural tear that was repaired postoperatively in a subsequent procedure. He began postoperative chemotherapy 3 weeks after surgery. At 6 months from surgery, he has been ambulating with hip-knee-ankle-foot orthosis on the right leg, and there has been no evidence of local recurrence or pulmonary metastasis.

REFERENCES

1. White AP, Kwon BK, Lindskog DM, et al. Metastatic disease of the spine. J Am Acad Orthop Surg 2006;14(11):587–98.
2. Klimo P, Kestle JR, Schmidt MH. Treatment of metastatic spinal epidural disease: a review of the literature. Neurosurg Focus 2003;15:1–9.
3. Wiltse LL, Fonseca AS, Amster J, et al. Relationship of the Dura, Hoffman's ligaments, Batson's Plexus, and a fibrovascular membrane lying on the posterior surface of the vertebral bodies and attaching to the deep layer of the posterior longitudinal ligament. An anatomical, radiologic, and clinical study. Spine 1993;18(8):1030–43.
4. Boriani S, Weinstein JN, Biagini R. Primary bone tumors of the spine. Terminology and surgical staging. Spine 1997;22(9):1036–44.
5. Denis F. Spinal instability as defined by the three-column spine concept in acute spinal trauma. Clin Orthop Relat Res 1984;189:65–76.
6. Harrington KD. Metastatic tumors of the spine: diagnosis and treatment. J Am Acad Orthop Surg 1993; 1(2):76–86.
7. Krishnaney AA, Steinmetz MP, Benzel EC. Biomechanics of metastatic spine cancer. Neurosurg Clin N Am 2004;15(4):375–80.

8. Perrin RG, Laxton AW. Metastatic spine disease: epidemiology, pathophysiology, and evaluation of patients. Neurosurg Clin N Am 2004;15(4):365–73.

9. Quinones-Hinojosa A, Lyon R, Ames CP, et al. Neuromonitoring during surgery for metastatic tumors to the spine: intra-operative interpretation and management strategies. Neurosurg Clin N Am 2004;15: 537–47.

10. Oge HK, Cagavi AF, Benli K. Migration of pacemaker lead into the spinal venous plexus: case report with special reference to Batson's theory of spinal metastasis. Acta Neurochir (Wien) 2001; 143:413–6.

11. Simmons ED, Zheng Y. Vertebral tumors: surgical versus non-surgical treatment. Clin Orthop Relat Res 2006;443:233–47.

12. McPhee IB, Williams RP, Swanson CE. Factors influencing wound healing after surgery for metastatic disease of the spine. Spine 1998;23(6):726–32.

13. Klein JD, Hey LA, Yu CS, et al. Perioperative nutrition and post-operative complications in patients undergoing spinal surgery. Spine 1996;21(22): 2676–82.

14. Petrozza P. Major spine surgery. Anesthesiol Clin North America 2002;20:405–15.

15. Chang SH, Miller NR. The incidence of vision loss due to perioperative ischemic optic neuropathy associated with spine surgery: the Johns Hopkins experience. Spine 2005;30(11):1299–302.

16. Finkelstein JA, Zaveri G, Wai E, et al. A population-based study of surgery for spinal metastases: survival rates and complications. J Bone Joint Surg Br 2003;85(7):1045–50.

17. Wise JJ, Fischgrund JS, Herkowitz HN, et al. Complication, survival rates, and risk factors of surgery for metastatic disease of the spine. Spine 1999; 24(18):1943–51.

18. Gangi A, Guth S, Imbert JP, et al. Percutaneous vertebroplasty: indications, technique, and results. Radiographics 2003;23(2):e10.

19. Narayan P, Haid RW, Subach BR, et al. Effect of spinal disease on successful arthrodesis in lumbar pedicle screw fixation. J Neurosurg 2002;97(Suppl 3):277–80.

20. Fourney DR, Schomer DF, Nader R, et al. Percutaneous vertebroplasty and kyphoplasty for painful vertebral body fractures in cancer patients. J Neurosurg 2003;98(Suppl 1):21–30.

21. Wiekopf M, Ohnsorge JA, Niethard FU. Intravertebral pressure during vertebroplasty and balloon kyphoplasty: an in vitro study. Spine 2008;22(2):178–82.

22. Harrington KD. Anterior decompression and stabilization of the spine as a treatment for vertebral collapse and spinal cord compression from metastatic malignancy. Clin Orthop Relat Res 1988;233:177–97.

Sacral Tumors and Management

Peter Paul Varga, MD[a,*], Istvan Bors, MD[a], Aron Lazary, MD[a,b]

KEYWORDS

• Sacrum • Tumor • Surgery • Stabilization • Outcome

Sacral tumors are rare pathologies, but their management generally generates a complex medical problem. Different types of primary tumors can occur in the sacrum because of its peculiar embryogenic development. The diagnosis is difficult because of the lack of specific symptoms and signs. Sacral tumors usually are diagnosed in advanced stages with extended dimensions involving the sacral nerves and surrounding organs (**Fig. 1**). Surgical treatment is one of the most challenging fields in spine because of the complicated anatomy of the sacral site. In most cases, only radical surgical procedures, such as partial or total sacrectomy, can guarantee optimal local control, but several problems such as bowel, bladder, and sexual dysfunction; infection; massive blood loss; and spino–pelvic instability can be associated with sacral resections. Beyond the primary goal of the surgery (eg, wide resection of the tumor mass), the optimal spino-pelvic reconstruction focused on biomechanical stability and soft-tissue restoration is also indispensable.

Primary benign and malignant tumors of the sacrum are 2% to 4% of all primary bone neoplasms and 1% to 7% of all primary spinal tumors.[1] Most common primary sacral tumors are chordomas, representing 40% of all primary sacral neoplasms.[2] Comprehensive U.S. incidence data are available in the literature. The incidence of sacral chordoma is about 0.02 to 0.03 per 100,000, and it is rare below the age of 40; it is more frequent in males.[3] Chondrosarcoma is the second most frequent primary malignant bone tumor of the sacrum in adults, with an overall incidence of 0.8 per 100,000; however, its sacral location is rarer than 5% of all cases.[4] In contrast, more than 25% of chondrosarcomas are primary pelvic lesions, which can also involve the sacrum. Overall survival depends on the histologic grade and the location of the tumor, because patients with the pelvo–sacral chondrosarcomas generally have poor prognosis.[5,6] Giant cell tumor (GCT) is the most common benign neoplasm of the sacrum, which is a relatively frequent bone tumor, usually occurring in the sacrum within the spine[2,3] Aneurysmal bone cyst (ABC) and Ewing sarcoma are not common but are more often diagnosed at a younger age (in the first two decades).[7] Beyond rare bone-forming tumors, such as osteoblastoma, osteosarcoma, and osteochondroma, other types of neoplasms, such as hemangioma, angiosarcoma, nerve sheath tumors, multiple myeloma, and lymphoma may primarily involve the sacrum.

About half of all sacral tumors are metastases. Lung, breast, prostate, and rectal cancers and sarcomas are the most common origins of spinal metastases affecting more often the thoracic and lumbar spine but also occurring in lumbo–sacral junction and rarely in sacral segments.[8] Invasive rectal carcinomas can directly infiltrate the sacral bone, increasing the complexity of surgical resection.

Table 1 shows the distribution of the sacral tumors operated on in the Hungarian National Center for Spinal Disorders in a 10-year period.

CLINICAL SIGN AND SYMPTOMS

Sacral neoplasms generally grow insidiously, causing ambiguous symptoms in the early stages; thus, patients often have a long nonspecific

Conflict of interest: Authors have nothing to declare. Neither the manuscript nor any part of it has been published or is being considered for publication elsewhere.
[a] National Center for Spinal Disorders, Buda Health Center, Királyhágó u. 1-3, Budapest, Hungary, H-1126
[b] 1st Department of Internal Medicine, Semmelweis University, Budapest, Hungary
* Corresponding author.
E-mail address: vpp@bhc.hu (P.P. Varga).

Orthop Clin N Am 40 (2009) 105–123
doi:10.1016/j.ocl.2008.09.010

disease course as well as false diagnoses and treatment procedures. Most of the patients initially report low back or buttock pain for months or years, but a painless visible sacral mass can also be the first sign of the disease. Low back or sacral pain at night may be a warning symptom, but sacral tumors often are (under)diagnosed at this stage as nonspecific low back pain or disc herniation because of the lack of an available diagnostic process, frequently resulting in a delayed diagnosis. Neurologic symptoms may be present with or without pain. Some patients may present with numbness, paresthesias, sphincter dysfunction, or muscle weakness. Others have decreased reflexes, perianal hypoesthesia, and moderate lower extremity weakness that can only be diagnosed via detailed neurologic examination. Subclinical levels of bowel and bladder dysfunction can also be found in detailed medical histories. The cauda equina syndrome refers to the specific and serious constellation of sensory, motor, and vegetative symptoms occurring when the cauda equina is compressed by a tumor mass supporting emergent therapeutic interventions.[9] A large presacral mass often causes constipation because of rectal compression, whereas a smaller tumor may be palpable on digital rectal examination in the early stages. General signs of neoplastic diseases, such as weight loss, blood abnormalities, or weakness are typical of metastatic lesions rather than primary sacral tumors.

IMAGING

Because of the nonspecific symptoms and their insidious development, sacral tumors usually are discovered with advanced imaging studies. Plain radiography is often the first imaging modality performed; however, this often remains inefficient because of the difficulty in evaluating the sacrum on x-ray films. The absence of the sacral foramina and the sacroiliac joint, as well as the posterior iliac wing, can be considered radiographic signs of a lytic lesion of the sacral ala.[10] More accurate visualization of the region may be obtained by using computerized tomography (CT) and magnetic resonance imaging (MRI). In most cases, because of the different characteristics of the two methods, both should be used for the correct imaging of the disease. Some types of sacral tumors have specific CT or MRI signs (**Table 2**), but the imaging process is appropriate for estimating the anatomic situation and the dimensions of the tumor rather than for definitive diagnosis. CT scans show well the osseous relations as well as intratumoral calcification (see **Fig. 1**B and **Fig. 2**C). Hypervascularity also appears on CT scans as enhancement. Rectal or venous contrast can be administered to visualize the involvement of pelvic structures. Possibility of three-dimensional reconstruction is a great advantage of the CT scan (**Fig. 3**). MRI may be used to visualize the relationship between the tumor and the bone and soft tissues. The combination of T1- and T2-weighted imaging is suitable

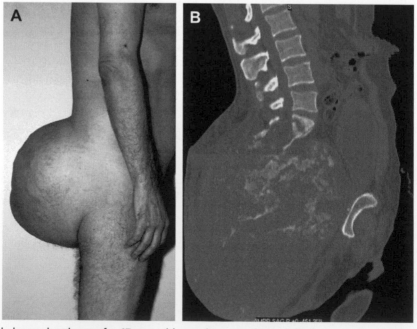

Fig. 1. Extremely large chordoma of a 47-year-old man (no neurologic deficit).

Table 1
Distribution of the sacral tumors operated on in the Hungarian National Center for Spinal Disorders between 1997 and 2007 according to the WHO histologic classification (N=122)

Histology	Number (%)[a]
Bone-forming tumors	
Osteoid osteoma	3 (4)
Osteoblastoma	2 (2)
Osteosarcoma	2 (2)
Cartilage-forming tumors	
Osteochondroma	2 (3)
Chondrosarcoma	10 (13)
Giant cell tumor	2 (2)
Hemopoietic tumors	
Myeloma	6 (8)
Lymphoma	2 (2)
Primitive neuroectodermal tumor	
Ewing sarcoma	7 (9)
Vascular tumors	
Angiosarcoma	1 (1)
Connective tissue tumors	
Desmoplastic fibroma	1 (1)
Fibrosarcoma	1 (1)
Neurogenic tumors	6 (8)
Notochordal tumors	
Chordoma	35 (44)
Total number of primary tumors	**80**
Metastatic tumors	35
Tumorlike conditions	
Aneurysmal bone cyst	2
Langerhans Cell Histiocytosis	1
Fibrous dysplasia	3
Echinococcus cyst	1
TOTAL	**122**

[a] Rate among primary neoplasms (n=80) without metastases and tumorlike conditions.

for evaluating nerve root, muscle, and visceral structure involvement. When performing diffusion-weighted MRI scans, sacral metastases can be differentiated clearly from insufficient fractures of the sacrum.[11] Bone scan is used to determine whether the lesion is monostotic or polyostotic and for searching for bone metastasis (**Fig. 4**A). Chordomas can be identified with positron emission tomography (PET). This could also be feasible for monitoring nonsurgical treatments of the tumor;[12] however, it has not yet been accepted as part of everyday clinical practice. Regarding the site and extent of the tumor, one of the most important questions to be answered is the extent of involvement of the sacral (or lumbar) segments

and the sacroiliac joint, because they influence the surgical strategy and may definitely determine the surgical outcome. The CT and MRI scans are necessary tools in the diagnostic process of a sacral mass and very helpful in the preoperative planning as well as in the postoperative follow-up phase (**Fig. 5**A).

BIOPSY AND HISTOLOGY

Obtaining a sample of the tumor tissue is essential for setting up the final diagnosis of the sacral mass. The biopsy procedure must be planned based on previous imaging studies and any additional tests before the invasive process. For

Table 2
Type of common sacral tumors with imaging properties

Tumor Type	Typical Imaging Findings
Benign sacral tumors	
Giant Cell Tumor	Low to intermediate signal intensity on T2-weighted MRI, thin cortical rim (CT)
Aneurysmal bone cyst	Fluid-fluid levels on T2-weighted MRI and CT
Osteoblastoma	Expanded lesion with multiple small calcifications and peripheral sclerotic rim (CT)
Nerve sheath tumors (neurofibroma, schwannoma)	"Target" sign on T2-weighted MRI with a low signal center surrounded by high signal mass (occasionally)
Hemangioma	High signal intensity on T1- and intermediate on T2-weighted MRI
Malignant sacral tumors	
Chondroma	Intratumoral calcification (CT), very high intensity on T2-weighted MRI (enhances after Gadolinium administration)
Myeloma	Multiple round "punched-out" lytic lesions or a large, expanded lytic lesion (plasmacytoma)
Ewing sarcoma	Highly destructive lesion involving a large soft-tissue mass
Osteosarcoma	Mixed lytic/sclerotic pattern on radiograph (Paget disease)
Chondrosarcoma	High signal intensity on T2-weighted MRI with lobular configuration

example, in very rare cases, echinococcosis can appear as a sacral tumorlike mass, and a biopsy might cause anaphylaxis and disease dissemination. A retrospective study of Özerdemoglu and colleagues[13] reported the advantage of open biopsy compared with percutaneous needle procedures. The study showed the effective accuracy of open biopsies to be 81%, and that of conventional percutaneous samplings were only 12%. Although the necessity for a second biopsy was also significantly lower in open biopsies, the accuracy and safety of the percutaneous approach may be increased using CT fluoroscopy guidance.[14,15] Taking into consideration that the sacral region is generally well accessible for surgical sampling, and the disadvantages of the percutaneous procedures, open biopsy would be the recommended method for obtaining a histologic diagnosis (see **Fig. 3**D).

The histologic classification and diagnosis of primary sacral tumors is based on the World Health Organization (WHO) Tumor Classification Systems. Experimental studies suggest that for certain types of sacral tumors, further immunohistologic and molecular studies could be useful in evaluating the biological nature of the tumor.[16,17] In chordomas, such genetic abnormalities as structural chromosomal abnormalities,[18] microsatellite instability,[19] and polyclonality[20] were also described, but these results were not validated

and have not had any therapeutic consequences. Histologic examination can clarify the diagnosis in cases of rare sacral tumorlike conditions, such as osteomyelitis[21] and tuberculosis[22] as well as determine the origin of sacral metastases.[23]

THERAPEUTIC CONSIDERATIONS OF SACRAL TUMORS
Metastatic Lesions

Treatment of sacral metastatic lesions can be different from the therapeutic approach of primary tumors. Radiotherapy may be chosen as initial therapy for sacral metastases in patients without spinal instability or acute plegia in which significant pain reduction and neurologic improvement are attainable.[24,25] Surgical treatment of sacral metastases is done for palliative reasons. Percutaneous osteoplasty with polymethyl methacrylate (PMMA) can be used successfully for palliative management of osteolytic sacral metastases.[26] Pain relief and neurologic improvement can be achieved through the biological and mechanical effect of injected PMMA. Decaying neurologic functions and increasing local and radicular pain are indications of surgical decompression with or without sacrectomy as well as internal stabilization.[27] Pain while walking occurs in cases of metastases infiltrating the sacroiliac joint and is

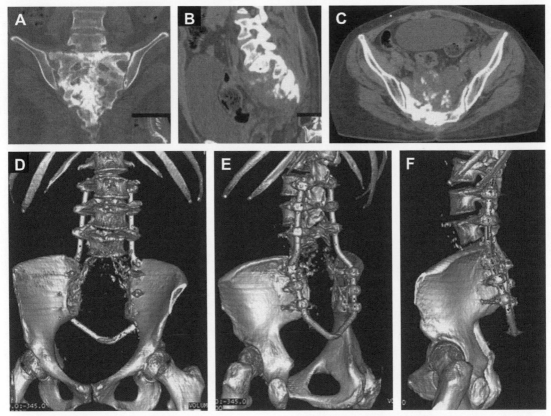

Fig. 2. (*A–C*)Imaging of chondrosarcoma (grade II) on preoperative CT scans in a 54-year-old woman. (*D–F*)Imme-diate postoperative pictures of lumbo–pelvic stabilization with closed loop technique after en bloc hemicorpor-ectomy including total sacrectomy and L5 spondylectomy as seen on three-dimensional CT reconstruction (Morselized bone graft could be observed in a bilateral gelatin sponge scaffold between the L4 vertebral body and the ilium.)

a notable symptom necessitating surgical inter-vention. Patchell and colleagues[28] published the advance of combined therapy (decompressive surgery followed by radiotherapy) compared with radiotherapy alone for spinal metastases regard-ing the ability to walk.

Primary Sacral Tumors

In cases of primary sacral neoplasms, goals of the therapeutic process are to be curative. The complex management is based on the complete removal of the tumor tissue in conjunction with adequate rehabilitation process and long-term follow-up. Local control can be achieved via proper surgical intervention in a majority of sacral tumors; however, conventional oncologic therapeutic methods, such as radiotherapy and chemotherapy, should be performed as neoadju-vant or adjuvant treatment in certain histologic types.

RADIOTHERAPY

Benign primary sacral tumors have high local con-trol rates with radiotherapy; however, it should be performed circumspectly for these lesions and only in assorted inoperable cases because of the risk of malignant transformation.[29] For low-grade malignant tumors, radiotherapy is a possible adju-vant option especially for further management of subtotally resected lesions,[30] local recurrences,[31] and inoperable cases.[32] Carbon-ion radiother-apy,[33] as well as high-dose proton/photon ther-apy,[34] was reported to have better results compared with conventional radiotherapy be-cause of increased effective doses and the lower incidence of side effects. Radiation can also be combined with percutaneous therapy. Nakajo and colleagues[35] reported on percutaneous etha-nol injection therapy combined with irradiation for successful management of recurrent sacral chor-doma. Intensity-modulated radiation therapy and stereotactic radiosurgery (SRS) allow spatially

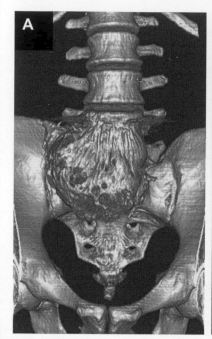
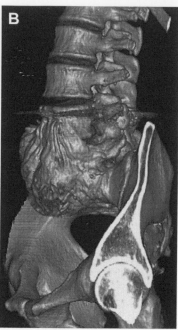

Fig. 3. Aggressive osteoblastoma affecting L5–S3 segments in a 23-year-old man.

well-positioned treatment delivery and high-dose hypofractionation, minimizing side effects such as radiation-induced injuries of the lumbo–sacral plexus, skin reaction, and visceral lesions. Cyber-Knife is a frameless, image-guided SRS system combined with a linear accelerator successfully applicable for sacral neoplasms.[36,37] In addition, use of radiosensitizing agents (razoxane) with interesting results has also been reported.[38] Radiotherapy is an important therapeutic tool for high-grade malignant sacral sarcomas. Osteosarcomas are relatively radiation resistant, but recently developed techniques can also improve the rates of local control for subtotally resected cases.[39] For patients with sacral Ewing sarcoma, definitive radiotherapy must be relied on for local control when wide surgical excision is not feasible.[40] Whole-lung radiotherapy may be of some benefit for patients whose metastatic Ewing sarcoma is confined to the lung.[41]

CHEMOTHERAPY

Most sacral tumors are benign aggressive lesions or low-grade malignancies. Therefore, chemotherapy does not play a crucial part in the treatment of these diseases; however, there is new published evidence regarding this therapeutic option. Recurrence of aggressive GCTs of the jaw was significantly reduced because of adjuvant alpha interferon therapy in the prospective study of Kaban and colleagues[42] Adjuvant chemotherapy

was also used successfully for visceral metastasis of GCTs.[43] Regarding chordomas, some case reports were found citing partial tumor response to chemical agents.[44,45] Lately, new types of anticancer drugs have been considered potential options based on the molecular studies of the biological properties of the chordomas. Imatinib mesylate is an inhibitor of some tyrosine kinases, and one of their targets, the platelet-derived growth factor receptor-b, is highly expressed and activated in chordoma samples, suggesting a potential target for imatinib on low-grade malignancies with poor response to conventional chemotherapy. Casali and colleagues[46] first published the oncologic effectiveness of imatinib on chordoma and also reported that additional low-dose cisplatin could restore tumor sensitivity after imatinib resistance.[47] The positive effect of imatinib on progression-free survival was also supported in a multicenter phase II study[48] Another molecular pathway activated in chordomas was targeted by Hof and colleagues[49] who administered cetuximab and gefitinib—drugs interfering with the epidermal growth factor signal transduction—with a good response in a patient with local recurrence and pulmonary metastases. Chemotherapy has a significant role in the management of high-grade primary malignant sacral tumors (Ewing and osteosarcoma) based on the results of chemotherapy applied for sarcomas of other skeletal sites. Relapse-free survival is increased significantly with combined adjuvant chemotherapy in the case of

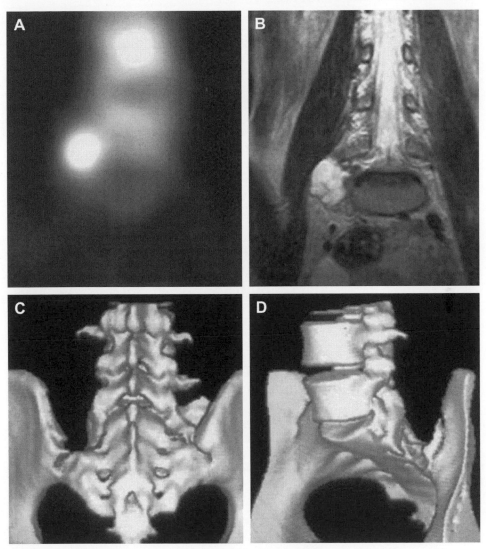

Fig. 4. Bone scan (*A*) and preoperative MRI (*B*) of a grade I chondrosarcoma in S1 of a 27-year-old woman. Three-dimensional CT reconstruction (*C, D*) 7 years after en bloc partial lateral sacrectomy.

osteosarcoma,[50] and several trials have reported the biological response of the primary tumor and metastases for various drugs.[51,52] Combined adjuvant chemotherapy increased the 5-year survival rate to 70% to 80% in Ewing sarcomas.[53,54] In sacral Ewing sarcomas, adjuvant chemotherapy is reported to be crucial regarding disease-free survival.[55] Chondrosarcomas are typically resistant to chemotherapy.

EMBOLIZATION

Various agents, such as Gelfoam (Pfizer Inc., New York), polyvinyl alcohol, and coils are available for percutaneous embolization, which is a valuable technique for primary treatment of certain sacral tumors and also can be used as a neoadjuvant or adjuvant option. Embolization of certain cases of ABC and GCTs can result in pain relief, tumor ossification, and arrested tumor growth. After this procedure, recurrence rate of these tumors could also be low. According to some authors' experiences, these tumors can be treated by repeated embolization with favorable long-term results.[56,57] As a preoperative application, selective arterial embolization plays an important role reducing intraoperative blood loss in cases of hypervascular primary malignant lesions and metastatic tumors.[58] In the

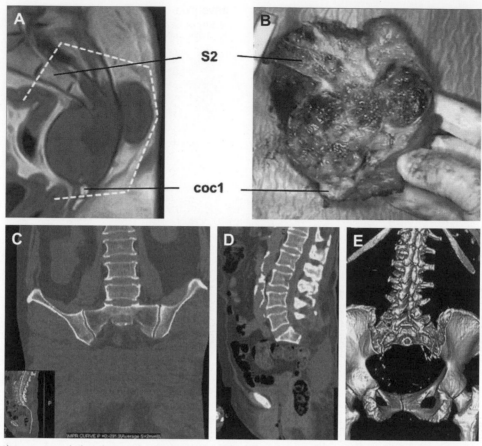

Fig. 5. (*A*) Large sacral chordoma of a 76-year-old woman on preoperative median sagittal MRI (Dashed line indicates the preoperative planning of wide surgical margins of the high sacrectomy). (*B*) Surgical en bloc specimen. (*C–E*) CT reconstructions at 30 months' follow-up shows tumor-free surgical margins and healed soft tissue reconstruction.

latter, embolization is also used for palliative treatment of advanced metastatic stage and for surgically nonresectable tumors. Tumor size, pain, and neurologic symptoms can be influenced with this technique.[59]

INDICATIONS AND TECHNIQUES OF SURGICAL INTERVENTIONS

The surgeon should decide on the appropriate surgical technique based on the knowledge of the histologic characteristics of the sacral tumors. The only exception may be osteoid osteoma, in which the radiologic appearance (especially on CT) (**Fig. 6**) already provides enough data for decision making (eg, resection of the core of the tumor).

Benign lesions (eg, ABC), could be resected intralesionally in a piecemeal fashion, but some of these lesions (such as aggressive osteoblastomas, see

Fig. 3) show high recurrence rates if inadequately resected.

En bloc resection with wide surgical margins is the optimal technique in the majority of the tumors of the sacrum. Because of the special anatomic and biomechanical position of the sacral bone, the resection itself could result in severe lumbopelvic disturbances in load transmission from the lumbar spine to the pelvic girdle. The transverse axis of rotation passes through the second sacral segment, thus, together with the first segment, they are the key components of physiologic stability and load transmission.[60] The strong ligamentous structures connecting the sacrum and coccygeum to the ischial tuberosity (sacrotuberous ligaments) and the ilium (posterior sacroiliac and sacrospinous ligaments bilaterally), play an important role in the sacro–pelvic balance and serve as a solid base for the muscle actions of the pelvic roof and the wider gluteal function as

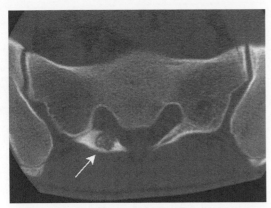

Fig. 6. Osteoid osteoma in S2 (*white arrow*) is treatable with resection alone.

well as the perianal muscle complex. The sacral canal and foramina contain the terminal part of the dural sac and sacral nerve roots, and, across them, a rich venous network (Batson) extends from the cranial-central section to the cavity of the lumbar spinal canal. Ventrally to the sacral bone, the very rich network of small veins and the autonomic nerve system require special surgical considerations and techniques as do the retroperitoneal large vascular structures (iliac artery and vein). Also, the lower sacral segments and the coccyx are in a very close topographic relationship to the rectum.

These anatomic characteristics make en bloc sacral resections a very demanding and challenging procedure. The size of malignant tumors (eg, chordoma and chondrosarcoma) can be enormous (see **Fig. 1**). However, these tumors generally respect the nerve sheets and do not penetrate through them, instead, they completely surround the sacral nerves during the growing stages, making it practically impossible to dissect them from the nerves. Ventrally, the tumors also respect the presacral connective tissue layers, seldom infiltrate the rectum, but could involve the large retroperitoneal vessels (most frequently), the left common iliac vein. These are the main reasons why the surgical margins of the sacral tumors are not only a technical challenge for the surgeon but also a very severe ethical–moral issue to be covered in the preoperative discussion with the patients regarding the proper surgical intervention, its advantages and disadvantages, and its effects on the quality of life after the surgery.

It is widely accepted in the literature[6,16,61,62] that the risk of local recurrence of primary malignant sacral tumors depends primarily on the feasibility of performing an en bloc resection with wide surgical margins as the initial procedure. Because of the magnitude of the en bloc technique in the

prevention of the local tumor recurrence and the patient's survival, the role of the preoperative surgical planning cannot be overestimated. The essential component of the planning process is the careful investigation of the extent of the bony (lateral–lateral and cranio–caudal) involvement of the sacral segments; the localization of the extraosseous components; the cranial end of the soft tumor penetration into the sacral canal (indicating the level of the nerve root resection); the lateral extension of the tumor into the gluteal muscles (including piriformis muscle); the relationship between the tumor and the retroperitoneal organs (vessels and rectum); and the posterior muscle boundaries, the fascia, subcutaneous, and cutaneous layers.

Various levels of sacral resections are described in detail in the fundamental article of Fourney and colleagues[61] They categorized sacral resections into two groups: those used for midline tumors and those used for eccentric lesions. The midline group was then divided into subgroups according to the level of nerve root sacrifice: the low subgroup contained those that sacrifice S4; the midsacral subgroup included those that sacrifice at least the unilateral S3 (**Fig. 7**); and the high subgroup contained those whose sacrifice involves at least the unilateral S2 (see **Fig. 5**). When the plane of the resection is higher, total sacrectomy is performed. When the tumor spreads beyond the sacrum to the lumbar spine, the extended resection called "hemicorporectomy" (translumbar amputation) is done (see **Figs. 2** and **8**). The lateral group of sacral resections includes en bloc resections of eccentrically located tumors involving the sacroiliac joint. In our clinical practice, we use their terminology and follow the surgical principles summarized in this very well structured article (**Table 3**).

As a result of the preoperative surgical planning, the surgeon should decide on the surgical approach. Anterior, posterior, and combined approaches are widely used and described in the literature depending on the tumor anatomy and the clinical experience of the surgeon. It seems there is a wider consensus regarding the use of the combined anterior–posterior approach when the tumor involves the retroperitoneal organs or in the cases of hemicorporectomy, total sacrectomy, or selected cases of high sacral amputations.[61,63–65] The goal of the anterior approach is to ligate the main tumor vessels and to expose the anterior aspect of the tumor to help identify the proper plane of the resection at the anterior cortex of the involved bony structures. Some investigators prefer using the rectus abdominis myocutaneous flap for the cavity on the site of the resected

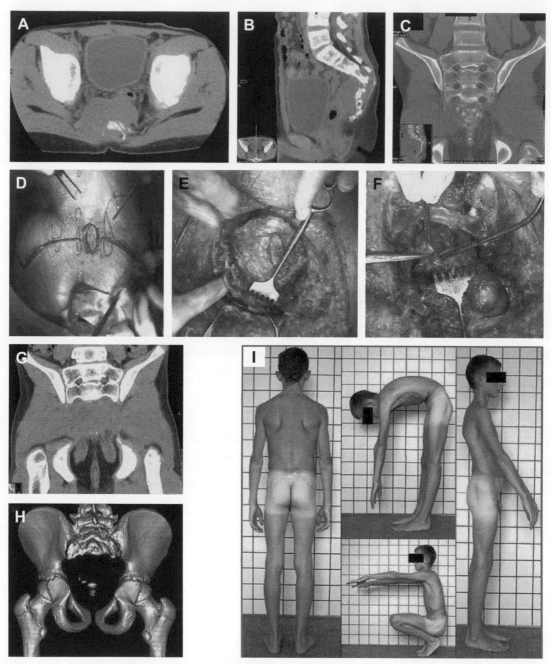

Fig. 7. (*A–C*) Sacral fibrosarcoma in a 13-year-old boy with rectal contact on preoperative CT scans. Intraoperative images show skin incision with isolated scar of the previous open biopsy (*D*), specimen of middle en bloc sacrectomy (*E*), specimen turned caudally and biopsy sampling of the affected rectal wall (surgical margin) (*F*). Twenty-four months' follow-up (sacral osseous margin and rotatory gluteal flaps are well visible) without local recurrence (*G–H*). Functional outcome (*I*).

sacral tumor. This flap is prepared and created as a last step of the anterior approach before wound closure.[64–66] Simultaneous antero–posterior approaches are also described.[67]

In the authors' experience, the single posterior approach works well in the majority of high, middle, or low sacral resections. The size and shape

of the skin incision depends on the size and location of the tumor. If the tumor has no posterior extraosseous extension, we sharply dissect the dorso–lumbar fascia and the caudal portion of the erector muscle in one flap, lifting it from the sacrum and turning it cranially, exposing the posterior aspect of the sacrum (**Fig. 9**D). We then

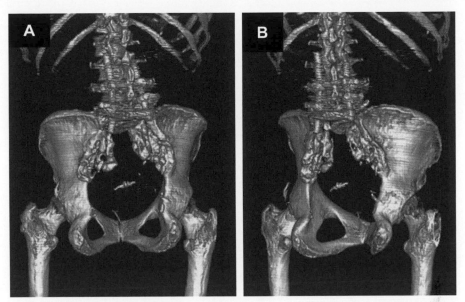

Fig. 8. Hemicorporectomy (en bloc total sacrectomy and L5 spondylectomy) because of sacral chordoma (47-year-old woman) stabilized by modified Luque-Galveston technique at 3 years' follow-up, as seen on the three-dimensional CT reconstruction (*A–B*). Strong bony bridge developed bilaterally between the L4 vertebral body and the ilium.

continue the dissection bilaterally, transecting the gluteal muscles carefully and keeping the proper oncologic margin from the tumor. In the last few years, we have routinely resected the piriformis muscle bilaterally because of our belief that this is a frequent site of local tumor recurrence (**Table 4**). We then approach the caudal end of the planned resection: the os coccygeum, or, if they are involved, the coccygeal muscles and the anococcygeal ligament. Then, from the caudal direction, by blunt dissection, we separate the specimen from the rectum and continue the blunt dissection on the ventral surface of the sacrum (or the tumor) up to the preoperatively measured cranial plane of the sacral resection. After placing a soft cloth to protect the presacral anatomic structures, following proper sacral laminectomy, the sacral nerve roots carefully selected for sacrifice are identified. The thecal sac is then closed and a sacral osteotomy is performed. After this step, the entire specimen becomes free and can be dorsally removed en bloc (see **Fig. 5**). During the procedure, we try to carefully protect the remaining sacral nerve roots as well as the vascular

Table 3 Types of sacrectomy in the National Center for Spinal Disorders, Budapest (*N*=122)	
Sacrectomy Type	**Number**
Hemicorporectomy	4
Total sacrectomy	13
High partial sacrectomy	8
Midsacral partial sacrectomy	25
Low sacral sacrectomy	21
Eccentric sacrectomy	
With total sacroiliac resection	4
With partial sacroiliac resection	29
Without sacroiliac involvement	18
TOTAL	122

Data from Fourney DR, Rhines LD, Hentschel SJ, et al. En bloc resection of primary sacral tumors: classification of surgical approaches and outcome. J Neurosurg Spine 2005;3(2):111–22.

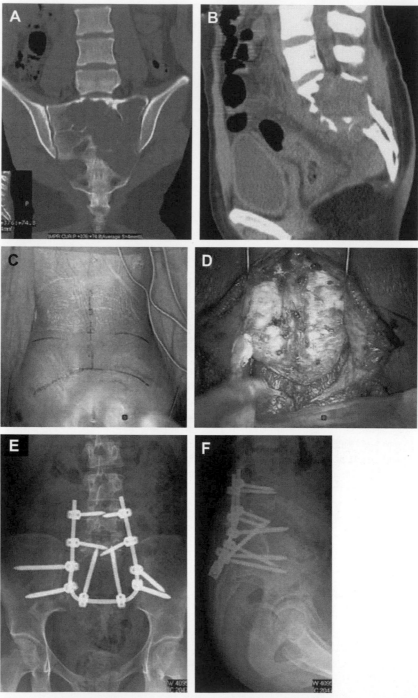

Fig. 9. Sacral schwannoma in a 25-year-old woman with pathologic fracture resulting in unilateral sacroiliac instability. Preoperative coronal (*A*) and sagittal (*B*) CT reconstruction. Intraoperative set-up with planned incisions (*C*). Extension of the routinely used sacral musculo–fascial flap before lifting from the posterior aspect of the sacrum (*D*). Postoperative X-rays (*E, F*) of the lumbo–pelvic stabilization (Closed loop technique with double median screws between the rod and the L5 vertebral body acting against the flexion–extension loading forces) after high sacral amputation (the right side of S3-5 segments and the coccyx were kept).

Table 4
Recurrence of chordoma after "en bloc" sacral resection

ID	Type of Resection	Bone Resection Level	Bilateral Piriformis Muscle Resection	Surgical Margins	Time of Local Recurrence (mo)	Site of Local Recurrence
1	Low	S3/4	None	Wide	28	Gluteal
2	Low	S3/4	None	Contaminated	16	Piriformis
3	Low	S3/4	Yes	Wide	42	Sacral Bone
4	Low	S3/4	None	Marginal	48	Sacral Bone
5	Low	S3/4	None	Marginal	22	Piriformis
6	Middle	S2/3	Yes	Wide	15	Gluteal
7	Middle	S2/3	Yes	Wide	16	Gluteal
8	Middle	S2/3	Yes	Wide	29	Sacral Bone
9	High	S1/2	Yes	Wide	52	Gluteal
10	High	S1/2	Yes	Marginal	10	Widespread
11	High	S1/2	Yes	Marginal	12	Widespread
12	Total	L5/S1	Yes	Wide	36	Gluteal

structures. Bone wax is applied immediately to the free bony surfaces, and even the small bleeding muscle parts are carefully electrocauterized for hemostasis.

After tumor resection, the large sacrectomy defects should be closed. Several techniques can be used for soft tissue reconstruction. Rectus abdominis myocutaneous flap,[64] "turnover," and "sliding" types of gluteus maximus adipomuscular flaps[68] were used successfully to prevent the creation of large cavities, rectal prolapse, and walking disturbances. Abhinav and colleagues[69] implanted allogen acellular collagen-graft (Permacol, Tissue Sciences Lab Inc., Andover (MA)) for the repair of the large pelvic floor defect without any complication.

If, as a result of the sacral resection, spino-pelvic instability is created, bony reconstruction is necessary. The indications for spino-pelvic stabilization described by Gunterberg and colleagues[60] (total sacrectomy or high partial sacrectomy with more than 50% sacroiliac joint resection each side) is widely accepted.[70] However, we do not stabilize when the first sacral segment and its iliac connection are maintained bilaterally, because in our experience we have never met with fatigue fracture of the remaining sacrum, as Gutenberg observed (Fig. 10). We recommend and routinely use lumbo-pelvic stabilization after total sacrectomy and unilateral sacroiliac joint resection (see Fig. 9). The modified Galveston-technique and further modifications (combinations of transpedicular lumbar screws, crosslinks and bicortical–iliac screws) are well accepted and widely published in the literature.[71–74] Recent biomechanical studies found that instrumentation failure and loosening can be caused by the excessive stress concentrated at the iliac bone and the spinal rods in these configurations.[75] In our clinical experience, this has been the preferred method for several years (see Fig. 8); however, during the last few years, as a modification, the "Closed Loop

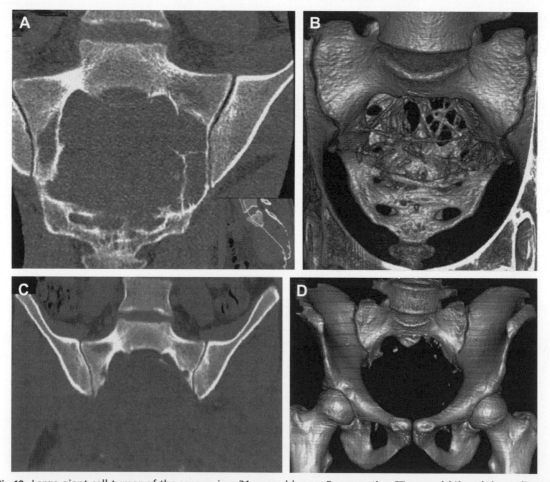

Fig. 10. Large giant cell tumor of the sacrum in a 21-year-old man. Preoperative CT coronal (*A*) and three-dimensional reconstruction (*B*) show the extension of the osteolytic lesion. Coronal (*C*) and three-dimensional (*D*) CT reconstruction 36 months after partial high (piecemeal) sacrectomy.

Technique (CLT)" became the routine method for lumbo-pelvic stabilization (see **Figs. 2** and **9**). The advantage of this method is the use of a single, properly contoured U-shaped rod improving rotational stability and providing better anchoring to the iliac bone by two or three pairs of bicortical–iliac screws, and, with the possibility of using lumbar vertebral support screws (see **Fig. 9**E–F), improved stability of the lumbo-pelvic junction in flexion–extension and rotation could be obtained.

Various techniques of bony fusion are in use, such as structured bone grafts (fibula, tibia) and morselized auto- or allografts. The authors prefer the morselized autograft, which can be obtained from the bilaterally resected iliac crests and sometimes mixed with allografts from our bone bank. Morselized bone graft incorporates well within a year when placed in the proper position for physiologic loading (see **Fig. 8**).

The advantage of the proper soft tissue and bony spino-pelvic stabilization is the possibility of improved and accelerated rehabilitation of the patient. Our patients begin walking a few days after surgery and the careful exercising of the lumbo-pelvic muscles is also commenced (except for the patients with total sacrectomies in which the neurologic deficit prevents the early ambulation). The advantage of the early mobilization helps in the prevention of pneumonia, decubitus ulcers, thromboembolism, and other common complications after major spinal or pelvic surgeries.

Sacral tumor resections are major surgeries. The operating time of partial sacrectomies is between 3 and 8 hours, whereas total resections often require more than 10 hours, depending on the experience of the surgical team and the characteristics of the individual case. Intraoperative bleeding could be enormous. Tomita and colleagues[73] reported total sacrectomies (one chordoma, two GCTs) with 11 L of blood loss. Gokaslan and colleagues[72] reviewed the total sacrectomy literature and noted 6.5 to 40 L of blood loss for single-staged total sacrectomies and 10 to 80 L for two-stage procedures. In the authors' experience, the highest blood loss occurred in a 23-year-old man with GCT, in whom an intralesional total sacrectomy was performed with lumbo-pelvic stabilization, realizing 11.6 L of blood loss. In the authors' institution, the average blood loss of low sacrectomies is 780 mL and of middle sacrectomies is 1170 mL.

COMPLICATIONS

Because of the very complex surgical technique, extended operating time, and intraoperative bleeding, several complications may occur during the surgery or in the immediate postoperative period.[62,63,65,76] Death during the surgery or in the early postoperative period is reported.[65] Unplanned nerve root injuries, rectal perforations, and large vessel injuries are also major intraoperative complications. In the early postoperative period, deep or superficial wound infection may develop, which may require additional surgical interventions (debridement or irrigation). Cerebrospinal fluid fistulas are also reported. Transient bladder or bowel incontinence may occur. Urogenital infections are quite frequent. After lumbo–pelvic stabilization, the risk of hardware failure also has to be considered.

OUTCOME
Rehabilitation After Sacrectomy

Very little data are available in the literature regarding the rehabilitation of patients operated with sacral tumors, and yet, quality of life and long-term outcome strongly depend on the adequate physical and psychologic rehabilitation processes.[77] Rehabilitation may be restorative in cases of curative surgeries, whereas supportive care may be required if only palliative therapy is done. Because common impairments may result after total sacrectomy and prolonged bed rest, special air fluidized beds may be helpful in preventing skin breakdown and in promoting wound healing as well. Rehabilitation must be initiated immediately after the surgery with motor and sensory evaluation of the lower extremity and the degree of bowel and bladder control. Patients should be informed about the definitive neurologic losses and should receive psychologic support if needed. Patients with no neurologic deficits have to undergo early ambulation and trunk–muscle exercise programs. The final goal of the intensive postoperative physical therapy is to increase patient independence and safety with transfers and other abilities. Patients generally return home with the ability to walk with or without the use of a rolling walker. The intensity of the physical therapy is individualized, and involvement of occupational therapists as well as psychologists is almost always necessary to achieve a good overall functional outcome.

Functional Outcome

Functional outcome of sacral tumors is influenced highly by the level of neurologic deficit, which basically determines the quality of the patient's life. Bowel and bladder functions seem to remain quite normal when both S3 roots or the unilateral S1-S5 roots are spared (see **Fig. 7**I).[76,78] When the S2 nerves are also bilaterally resected, major bowel and bladder problems develop in almost all cases. Loss of lower sacral nerves can result in perineal hypoesthesia, whereas resection of all sacral roots cause complete saddle anesthesia and sexual dysfunction. Regarding motor disability, sacrifice of S1 nerves may lead to lower extremity muscle weakness; however, patients with intact L5 nerves, generally are able to walk without external support. Life quality is also strongly influenced by the biomechanical outcome of the sacral surgery. Although the use of self-related disability questionnaires is not reported frequently regarding the management of sacral tumors, the authors strongly suggest the use of the Short Form-36 (SF-36) or the Musculoskeletal Tumor Society Score (MSTS) questionnaires for monitoring the functional outcome during the long-term postoperative period. Depression and other psychologic conditions often develop in patients with severe functional losses after sacrectomies. These patients require long-term adequate psychosocial support as well.

Oncologic Outcome

Primary sacral tumors are predominantly benign aggressive lesions or low-grade malignancies with relatively high risk of local recurrences. Data from the literature show local recurrence rates of 17% to 35% in patients operated with chordoma, the most common primary sacral tumor.[79–82] Local control and long-term survival can be achieved only via complex management and close follow-up. The risk of local and distant recurrences of surgically treated sacral tumors is associated with the histologic type of the tumor and the extent of the resection. En bloc resections with wide surgical margins is the optimum surgical procedure and result in longer disease-free survival in all comparative studies.[6,16,61,62] The authors' clinical experience supports these observations (see **Table 4**). Adjuvant therapy can positively modify the oncologic outcome in the cases of intralesional surgeries and local recurrences. Bergh and colleagues[16] performed a comprehensive study regarding the prognostic factors in chordoma after 30 sacral and nine spinal chordoma patients. They concluded that, regarding local recurrences of their patients, the initial invasive diagnostic and surgical procedures performed elsewhere outside their tumor center are also significant negative prognostic factors. Risk of tumor-related death was significantly associated with local recurrences (21-fold) and metastasis (451-fold) in this study. Other observations confirmed these associations.[61] Sarcomatous transformation and metastases of the locally aggressive sacral GCTs are not uncommon.[83] En bloc resection of these tumors are often complicated but can result in long disease-free survival.[61] A high histologic grade, inadequate surgical margins, and management at institutions not specialized in tumor care in patients with chondrosarcomas and Ewing-sarcomas were shown to be associated with a worse prognosis.[6,55]

SUMMARY

The majority of primary tumors of sacrum are locally aggressive benign or low-grade malignant neoplasms with nonspecific early signs or symptoms. The insidiously growing tumor mass is usually diagnosed in the very late stages when it has reached extensive dimensions, and the involvement of surrounding organs result in a challenging problem in management. The evaluation and complex treatment of these rare tumors require a multidisciplinary approach, optimally at institutions with comprehensive care and experience. En bloc resection with wide surgical margins is essential for long-term local oncologic control, although it is technically quite difficult because of anatomic relationships and the large tumor size. There is a wide consensus regarding the use of standard surgical techniques of the resection and soft tissue reconstruction. Because of the very complex biomechanics of the lumbo–pelvic junction, currently there is no generally accepted and used stabilization technique of the instabilities created by the surgical resections of large sacral tumors. The recently published solutions are promising, making possible the early rehabilitation of the patients. The success of the complex treatment depends on the strict follow-up and each patient's cooperation.

Just a few centers in the world have enough wide experience and perform a large number of sacral tumor surgeries. Therefore, an international cooperation and registry should be organized through which centers with a special interest in these cases could work together according to mutually established protocols.[84]

REFERENCES

1. Feldenzer JA, McGauley JL, McGillicuddy JE. Sacral and presacral tumors: problems in diagnosis and management. Neurosurgery 1989;25(6): 884–91.
2. Disler DG, Miklic D. Imaging findings in tumors of the sacrum. AJR Am J Roentgenol 1999;173(6): 1699–706.
3. McMaster ML, Goldstein AM, Bromley CM, et al. Chordoma: incidence and survival patterns in the

United States, 1973–1995. Cancer Causes Control 2001;12(1):1–11.

4. Pritchard DJ, Lunke RJ, Taylor WF, et al. Chondrosarcoma: a clinicopathologic and statistical analysis. Cancer 1980;45(1):149–57.

5. York JE, Berk RH, Fuller GN, et al. Chondrosarcoma of the spine: 1954 to 1997. J Neurosurg 1999; 90(1 Suppl):73–8.

6. Bergh P, Gunterberg B, Meis-Kindblom JM, et al. Prognostic factors and outcome of pelvic, sacral, and spinal chondrosarcomas: a center-based study of 69 cases. Cancer 2001;91(7):1201–12.

7. Murphey MD, Andrews CL, Flemming DJ, et al. From the archives of the AFIP. Primary tumors of the spine: radiologic pathologic correlation. Radiographics 1996;16(5):1131–58.

8. Vrionis FD, Small J. Surgical management of metastatic spinal neoplasms. Neurosurg Focus 2003;15(5):1–8.

9. Bagley CA, Gokaslan ZL. Cauda equina syndrome caused by primary and metastatic neoplasms. Neurosurg Focus 2004;16(6):11–8.

10. Manaster BJ, Graham T. Imaging of sacral tumors. Neurosurg Focus 2003;15(2):1–8.

11. Byun WM, Jang HW, Kim SW, et al. Diffusion-weighted magnetic resonance imaging of sacral insufficiency fractures: comparison with metastases of the sacrum. Spine 2007;32(26):E820–4.

12. Zhang H, Yoshikawa K, Tamura K, et al. Carbon-11-methionine positron emission tomography imaging of chordoma. Skeletal Radiol 2004;33(9):524–30.

13. Ozerdemoglu RA, Thompson RC Jr, Transfeldt EE, et al. Diagnostic value of open and needle biopsies in tumors of the sacrum. Spine 2003;28(9):909–15.

14. Heyer CM, Al-Hadari A, Mueller KM, et al. Effectiveness of CT-Guided percutaneous biopsies of the spine an analysis of 202 examinations. Acad Radiol 2008;15(7):901–11.

15. Varga PP, Hoffer Z, Bors I. Computer-assisted percutaneous transiliac approach to tumorous malformation of the sacrum. Comput Aided Surg 2001; 6(4):212–6.

16. Bergh P, Kindblom LG, Gunterberg B, et al. Prognostic factors in chordoma of the sacrum and mobile spine: a study of 39 patients. Cancer 2000;88(9):2122–34.

17. Lee FY, Mankin HJ, Fondren G, et al. Chondrosarcoma of bone: an assessment of outcome. J Bone Joint Surg Am 1999;81(3):326–38.

18. Butler MG, Dahir GA, Hedges LK, et al. Cytogenetic, telomere, and telomerase studies in five surgically managed lumbosacral chordomas. Cancer Genet Cytogenet 1995;85(1):51–7.

19. Klingler L, Shooks J, Fiedler PN, et al. Microsatellite instability in sacral chordoma. J Surg Oncol 2000; 73(2):100–3.

20. Klingler L, Trammell R, Allan DG, et al. Clonality studies in sacral chordoma. Cancer Genet Cytogenet 2006;171(1):68–71.

21. Nasir N, Aquilina K, Ryder DQ, et al. Garre's chronic diffuse sclerosing osteomyelitis of the sacrum: a rare condition mimicking malignancy. Br J Neurosurg 2006;20(6):415–9.

22. Kumar A, Varshney MK, Trikha V. Unusual presentation of isolated sacral tuberculosis. Joint Bone Spine 2006;73(6):751–2.

23. Destombe C, Botton E, Le Gal G, et al. Investigations for bone metastasis from an unknown primary. Joint Bone Spine 2007;74(1):85–9.

24. Maranzano E, Trippa F, Chirico L, et al. Management of metastatic spinal cord compression. Tumori 2003; 89(5):469–75.

25. Loblaw DA, Laperriere NJ. Emergency treatment of malignant extradural spinal cord compression: an evidence-based guideline. J Clin Oncol 1998; 16(4):1613–24.

26. Masala S, Konda D, Massari F, et al. Sacroplasty and iliac osteoplasty under combined CT and fluoroscopic guidance. Spine 2006;31(18):E667–9.

27. Fujibayashi S, Neo M, Nakamura T. Palliative dual iliac screw fixation for lumbosacral metastasis. Technical note. J Neurosurg Spine 2007;7(1):99–102.

28. Patchell RA, Tibbs PA, Regine WF, et al. Direct decompressive surgical resection in the treatment of spinal cord compression caused by metastatic cancer: a randomised trial. Lancet 2005;366(9486):643–8.

29. Feigenberg SJ, Marcus RB Jr, Zlotecki RA, et al. Radiation therapy for giant cell tumors of bone. Clin Orthop Relat Res 2003;(411):207–16.

30. York JE, Kaczaraj A, Abi-Said D, et al. Sacral chordoma: 40-year experience at a major cancer center. Neurosurgery 1999;44(1):74–9 [discussion: 9–0].

31. Raque GH Jr, Vitaz TW, Shields CB. Treatment of neoplastic diseases of the sacrum. J Surg Oncol 2001;76(4):301–7.

32. Schwartz LH, Okunieff PG, Rosenberg A, et al. Radiation therapy in the treatment of difficult giant cell tumors. Int J Radiat Oncol Biol Phys 1989;17(5):1085–8.

33. Imai R, Kamada T, Tsuji H, et al. Carbon ion radiotherapy for unresectable sacral chordomas. Clin Cancer Res 2004;10(17):5741–6.

34. Park L, Delaney TF, Liebsch NJ, et al. Sacral chordomas: impact of high-dose proton/photon-beam radiation therapy combined with or without surgery for primary versus recurrent tumor. Int J Radiat Oncol Biol Phys 2006;65(5):1514–21.

35. Nakajo M, Ohkubo K, Fukukura Y, et al. Treatment of recurrent chordomas by percutaneous ethanol injection therapy and radiation therapy. Acta Radiol 2006; 47(3):297–300.

36. Gibbs IC, Kamnerdsupaphon P, Ryu MR, et al. Image-guided robotic radiosurgery for spinal metastases. Radiother Oncol 2007;82(2):185–90.

37. Gibbs IC. Spinal and paraspinal lesions: the role of stereotactic body radiotherapy. Front Radiat Ther Oncol 2007;40:407–14.

38. Rhomberg W, Bohler FK, Novak H, et al. A small prospective study of chordomas treated with radiotherapy and razoxane. Strahlenther Onkol 2003;179(4): 249–53.

39. DeLaney TF, Park L, Goldberg SI, et al. Radiotherapy for local control of osteosarcoma. Int J Radiat Oncol Biol Phys 2005;61(2):492–8.

40. Skubitz KM, D'Adamo DR. Sarcoma. Mayo Clin Proc 2007;82(11):1409–32.

41. Paulussen M, Ahrens S, Craft AW, et al. Ewing's tumors with primary lung metastases: survival analysis of 114 (European Intergroup) Cooperative Ewing's Sarcoma Studies patients. J Clin Oncol 1998;16(9):3044–52.

42. Kaban LB, Troulis MJ, Ebb D, et al. Antiangiogenic therapy with interferon alpha for giant cell lesions of the jaws. J Oral Maxillofac Surg 2002;60(10): 1103–11 [discussion: 11–3].

43. Dominkus M, Ruggieri P, Bertoni F, et al. Histologically verified lung metastases in benign giant cell tumours–14 cases from a single institution. Int Orthop 2006;30(6):499–504.

44. Fleming GF, Heimann PS, Stephens JK, et al. Dedifferentiated chordoma. Response to aggressive chemotherapy in two cases. Cancer 1993;72(3):714–8.

45. Schonegger K, Gelpi E, Prayer D, et al. Recurrent and metastatic clivus chordoma: systemic palliative therapy retards disease progression. Anticancer Drugs 2005;16(10):1139–43.

46. Casali PG, Messina A, Stacchiotti S, et al. Imatinib mesylate in chordoma. Cancer 2004;101(9):2086–97.

47. Casali PG, Stacchiotti S, Grosso F. Adding cisplatin (CDDP) to imatinib (IM) re-establishes tumor response following secondary resistance to IM in advanced chordoma [abstract]. J Clin Oncol 2007; 25(Suppl 18):10038.

48. Stacchioni S, Ferrari S, Ferraresi V. Imatinib mesylate in advanced chordoma: a multicenter phase II study [abstract]. J Clin Oncol 2007;25(Suppl 18):10003.

49. Hof H, Welzel T, Debus J. Effectiveness of cetuximab/gefitinib in the therapy of a sacral chordoma. Onkologie 2006;29(12):572–4.

50. Link MP, Goorin AM, Miser AW, et al. The effect of adjuvant chemotherapy on relapse-free survival in patients with osteosarcoma of the extremity. N Engl J Med 1986;314(25):1600–6.

51. Bacci G, Longhi A, Cesari M, et al. Influence of local recurrence on survival in patients with extremity osteosarcoma treated with neoadjuvant chemotherapy: the experience of a single institution with 44 patients. Cancer 2006;106(12):2701–6.

52. Chou AJ, Merola PR, Wexler LH, et al. Treatment of osteosarcoma at first recurrence after contemporary therapy: the Memorial Sloan-Kettering Cancer Center experience. Cancer 2005;104(10):2214–21.

53. Grier HE, Krailo MD, Tarbell NJ, et al. Addition of ifosfamide and etoposide to standard chemotherapy for Ewing's sarcoma and primitive neuroectodermal tumor of bone. N Engl J Med 2003;348(8):694–701.

54. Ferrari S, Mercuri M, Rosito P, et al. Ifosfamide and actinomycin-D, added in the induction phase to vincristine, cyclophosphamide and doxorubicin, improve histologic response and prognosis in patients with non metastatic Ewing's sarcoma of the extremity. J Chemother 1998;10(6):484–91.

55. Hoffmann C, Ahrens S, Dunst J, et al. Pelvic Ewing sarcoma: a retrospective analysis of 241 cases. Cancer 1999;85(4):869–77.

56. Hosalkar HS, Jones KJ, King JJ, et al. Serial arterial embolization for large sacral giant-cell tumors: mid-to long-term results. Spine 2007;32(10):1107–15.

57. Konya A, Szendroi M. Aneurysmal bone cysts treated by superselective embolization. Skeletal Radiol 1992;21(3):167–72.

58. Gottfried ON, Schmidt MH, Stevens EA. Embolization of sacral tumors. Neurosurg Focus 2003;15(2):E4.

59. Chiras J, Adem C, Vallee JN, et al. Selective intra-arterial chemoembolization of pelvic and spine bone metastases. Eur Radiol 2004;14(10):1774–80.

60. Gunterberg B, Romanus B, Stener B. Pelvic strength after major amputation of the sacrum. An experimental study. Acta Orthop Scand 1976;47(6): 635–42.

61. Fourney DR, Rhines LD, Hentschel SJ, et al. En bloc resection of primary sacral tumors: classification of surgical approaches and outcome. J Neurosurg Spine 2005;3(2):111–22.

62. Hulen CA, Temple HT, Fox WP, et al. Oncologic and functional outcome following sacrectomy for sacral chordoma. J Bone Joint Surg [Am] 2006;88(7): 1532–9.

63. Sar C, Eralp L. Surgical treatment of primary tumors of the sacrum. Arch Orthop Trauma Surg 2002; 122(3):148–55.

64. Zhang HY, Thongtrangan I, Balabhadra RS, et al. Surgical techniques for total sacrectomy and spinopelvic reconstruction. Neurosurg Focus 2003;15(2):1–10.

65. Zileli M, Hoscoskun C, Brastianos P, et al. Surgical treatment of primary sacral tumors: complications associated with sacrectomy. Neurosurg Focus 2003;15(5):1–8.

66. Stener B, Gunterberg B. High amputation of the sacrum for extirpation of tumors. Principles and technique. Spine 1978;3(4):351–66.

67. Localio SA, Eng K, Ranson JH. Abdominosacral approach for retrorectal tumors. Ann Surg 1980;191(5): 555–60.

68. Furukawa H, Yamamoto Y, Igawa HH, et al. Gluteus maximus adipomuscular turnover or sliding flap in the surgical treatment of extensive sacral chordomas. Plast Reconstr Surg 2000;105(3):1013–6.

69. Abhinav K, Shaaban M, Raymond T, et al. Primary reconstruction of pelvic floor defects following

sacrectomy using Permacoltrade mark graft. Eur J Surg Oncol 2008; [epub ahead of print].

70. Hugate RR Jr, Dickey ID, Phimolsarnti R, et al. Mechanical effects of partial sacrectomy: when is reconstruction necessary? Clin Orthop Relat Res 2006;450:82–8.

71. Allen BL Jr, Ferguson RL. The Galveston technique for L rod instrumentation of the scoliotic spine. Spine 1982;7(3):276–84.

72. Gokaslan ZL, Romsdahl MM, Kroll SS, et al. Total sacrectomy and Galveston L-rod reconstruction for malignant neoplasms. Technical note. J Neurosurg 1997;87(5):781–7.

73. Tomita K, Tsuchiya H. Total sacrectomy and reconstruction for huge sacral tumors. Spine 1990; 15(11):1223–7.

74. Jackson RJ, Gokaslan ZL. Spinal-pelvic fixation in patients with lumbosacral neoplasms. J Neurosurg 2000;92(1 Suppl):61–70.

75. Murakami H, Kawahara N, Tomita K, et al. Biomechanical evaluation of reconstructed lumbosacral spine after total sacrectomy. J Orthop Sci 2002; 7(6):658–64.

76. Guo Y, Palmer JL, Shen L, et al. Bowel and bladder continence, wound healing, and functional outcomes in patients who underwent sacrectomy. J Neurosurg Spine 2005;3(2):106–10.

77. Bauer KA, Ghazinouri R. Rehabilitation after total sacrectomy. Rehabilitation Oncology 2005. Available at: http://findarticles.com/p/articles/mi_qa3946/is_200501/ai_n15348089.

78. Todd LT Jr, Yaszemski MJ, Currier BL, et al. Bowel and bladder function after major sacral resection. Clin Orthop Relat Res 2002;(397):36–9.

79. McPherson CM, Suki D, McCutcheon IE, et al. Metastatic disease from spinal chordoma: a 10-year experience. J Neurosurg Spine 2006;5(4):277–80.

80. Osaka S, Kodoh O, Sugita H, et al. Clinical significance of a wide excision policy for sacrococcygeal chordoma. J Cancer Res Clin Oncol 2006;132(4):213–8.

81. Ishii K, Chiba K, Watanabe M, et al. Local recurrence after S2-3 sacrectomy in sacral chordoma. Report of four cases. J Neurosurg 2002;97(1 Suppl):98–101.

82. Jeanrot C, Vinh TS, Anract P, et al [Sacral chordoma: retrospective review of 11 surgically treated cases]. Rev Chir Orthop Reparatrice Appar Mot 2000;86(7): 684–93.

83. Bertoni F, Bacchini P, Staals EL. Malignancy in giant cell tumor of bone. Cancer 2003;97(10):2520–9.

84. Borlani S, Weinstein JN. Oncologic classification of vertebral neoplasms. In: Dickman CA, Fehlings MG, Gokaslan ZL, editors. Spinal cord and spinal column tumors. New York: Thieme Medical Publishers, Inc.; 2006. p. 37.

Complications of En Bloc Resections in the Spine

Stefano Bandiera, MD[a,b,*], Stefano Boriani, MD[a,b],
Rakesh Donthineni, MD, MBA[c,d], L. Amendola, MD[a,b],
Michele Cappuccio, MD[a,b], Alessandro Gasbarrini, MD[a,b]

KEYWORDS

- Spine • Tumor • En Bloc excision • Vertebrectomy
- Complication • Revision • Radiation

En bloc resections[1] are procedures aimed at surgically removing the tumor in a single piece, intact and fully encased by a continuous shell of healthy tissue (margin). These operations also can be performed in the spine.[2–7] If the goal is to achieve a negative margin when resecting the tumor, the process may necessitate resection of functionally relevant anatomic structures (eg, pleura, dura, muscles, nerve roots, nerves, vessels). Intentional transgression of the oncologic principles can be considered, weighing the advantage in term of reducing morbidity and better functional results for the higher risk of recurrence.[5] To perform en bloc resections, multiple approaches or widely enlarged posterior approach must be planned. The surgeon also should be aware of the morbidity of en bloc resections, because it can be caused by multiple extensive approaches or prolonged surgery.[8]

Perioperative adjuvants such as radiation therapy and chemotherapy lead to better oncologic outcomes in some tumor types but also exaggerate the risk of local complications.[9–11] Spine tumor surgeries in children, especially if associated with radiation therapy, also can lead to late deformities with or without hardware failure. Complications can be divided into major and minor, as described by McDonnell and colleagues.[12] Any complication that seemed to substantially alter an otherwise full

and expected course of recovery was considered a major complication. Complications also can be classified into intraoperative, early postoperative, and late postoperative: early (occurring within 30 days of surgery) and late (occurring more than 30 days after surgery). The center of treatment, surgical approach, association with radiation, and risk of local recurrences also were reviewed.

CLASSIFICATION AND DATA

We reviewed our database for complications from en bloc resections. From 1990 to 2007, 1035 consecutive patients with spine tumors were diagnosed and treated at the same institution. En bloc excisions were performed on 134 by the senior author (S.B.) and his team. All the data concerning clinical, histologic, and radiologic figures were included in a specifically built database since the beginning of the study. Complications and related relevant details, such as their relationship to surgical procedures, adjuvant therapies, and previous surgeries, were thoroughly reviewed.

TERMINOLOGY FOR RESECTIONS
Intralesional Excision

Intralesional excision is defined as piecemeal removal of the tumor. It is further organized into

No grants, equipment or other such items were received by any of the authors for the preparation or publication of this article.
[a] Rizzoli Institute, Bologna, Italy
[b] Department of Orthopaedics and Traumatology – Spine Surgery, Ospedale Maggiore 'C. A. Pizzardi', Largo Nigrisoli 1 – 40100 Bologna, Italy
[c] Spine and Orthopaedic Oncology, 5700 Telegraph Avenue, Suite 100, Oakland, CA 94609, USA
[d] Department of Orthopaedics, University of California Davis, Suite 3800, Y Street, Sacramento, CA, 95817, USA
* Corresponding author. Department of Orthopaedics and Traumatology – Spine Surgery, Largo Nigrisoli 2 – 40100 Bologna, Italy.
E-mail address: cocchi1@fastwebnet.it (S. Bandiera).

Orthop Clin N Am 40 (2009) 125–131
doi:10.1016/j.ocl.2008.10.002

these subcategories:[1,13] (1) intracapsular: tumor removal is incomplete because gross or histologic remnants inside the tumor capsule can be expected; and (2) extracapsular: tumor removal includes the whole tumor mass and the peripheral tissue (3–5 mm or more of healthy peripheral tissue).

En Bloc Resection

En bloc resection is complex surgery that aims to remove en bloc the whole tumor mass, including a cuff of healthy tissue encasing the tumor. The pathologist's evaluation of the thickness of the resected extracapsular tissue allows further subclassification of en bloc resections: (1) intralesional: the tumor is violated by planned or unplanned transgression to save the relevant important neurovascular structures, which causes tumor spillage; (2) marginal: a thin layer remains on the tumor (through the reactive zone); (3) wide: a thick layer of peripheral healthy tissue, a dense fibrous cover (eg, fascia), or an anatomic barrier not yet infiltrated (eg, pleura) fully covers the tumor.

The average age of the study group was of 44 years (range: 3–82 years), and the average follow-up time was 64 months (latest clinical follow-up or until death: range 0–180 months). Seventy-two percent had follow-up more than or equal to 24 months. Ninety of the cases involved primary tumors (31 benign and 59 malignant), and the remaining 44 cases involved metastases. The distribution of the tumors was 73 in the lumbar, 57 in the thoracic, and 4 in the cervical spine. Forty-seven procedures were performed by posterior approach alone; 87 included anterior and posterior approaches under the same anesthesia. All of the procedures were performed in one session.

With respect to margins, as reported by the pathologist on the final specimen, "wide" margin was achieved in 88 cases, "marginal" was achieved in 27 patients, and "intralesional" was achieved in 19 cases. Complications after en bloc excision were observed in 48 patients. Thirty-two of these patients (67%) suffered one complication, and the rest suffered two or more (**Table 1**).

SEVERITY
Major

Using the McDonnell classification,[12] 43 major complications were identified in 27 patients (**Table 1**). The most relevant complications were one intraoperative death caused by injury to the vena cava and two late dissections of the aorta wall (**Fig. 1**), one of which was fatal. In the postoperative course, three patients developed myocardial infarctions (no late sequelae), one developed

pulmonary embolism (leading to death), and two developed renal transitory failures related to intraoperative hemodynamic imbalance. Six deep infections (5.4%) required surgical debridement and long-term multiple antibiotic treatment. An iatrogenic injury of the left ureter was recognized during surgery and repaired. Temporary postoperative paraplegia was precipitated by a large hematoma; this patient fully recovered but 8 months later developed paraplegia again because of the previously mentioned aortic wall dissection and died from complications. Another peculiar incident involved an ex vacuo cerebral hematoma (**Fig. 2A**) caused by depletion of cerebrospinal fluid (an unidentified dural tear). Ten patients (7%) required revision of the posterior instrumentation. Overall, three patients died from complications.

Minor

Twenty-nine minor complications were observed in 28 patients. Nine patients had dural tears, which were successfully repaired. Injuries to the iliac vein and the vertebral artery in separate patients were repaired and had no sequelae. In 3 patients, malposition of the hardware resulted in asymptomatic deformity. One patient complained of retrograde ejaculation. Two cases of acute renal failure were treated with medical therapy.

TEMPORAL DISTRIBUTION
Intraoperative Complications

Six major and 14 minor complications were recorded, including vascular injuries and dural tears. One patient died because of injury to the vena cava. Most minor complications, such as small vascular tears and dural tears, were often identified at the time of surgery and were repaired with good outcomes.

Early Postoperative Complications

Seventeen major complications and 10 minor complications were observed in 21 patients. Among the major occurrences were a fatal pulmonary embolism and a postoperative paraplegia caused by a massive hematoma and hemothorax. Deep venous thrombosis, pneumothorax, and tracheal lesions during intubation were also encountered.

Late Postoperative Complications

Eighteen major and 7 minor complications were recorded in 22 patients. The most severe cases were two aortic dissections, which occurred at 3 and 8 months after the surgery (one caused a death and the other was treated successfully

Table 1
List of observed complications

Complications	Major	#	Minor	#
Pulmonary	Embolism	1		
	Pneumothorax	3	Pneumothorax	2
	Respiratory failure requiring tracheostomy	1	Respiratory failure	1
	Tracheal decubitus	1		
Operative wound	Infection requiring surgical debridement	6	Superficial wound necrosis	3
Operative	Hardware failure requiring surgical revision	10	Asymptomatic hardware failure	3
			Kypho-scoliosis caused by hardware malposition	3
Neurologic	Paraplegia	2	Dura tear	9
	cerebrospinal fluid depletion	1	Retrograde ejaculation	1
	Ex vacuo cerebral hematoma	1		
Cardiac	Myocardial infarction	3	Paroxysmal tachycardia	1
Death		3		0
Genitourinary	Ureteral injury	1	Transitory renal incompetence	2
Vascular	Aorta wall dissection	2	Cervical vertebral artery lesion	1
	Vena cava injury	2	Iliac vein injury	1
	Massive hemorrage	1	Hematoma	1
	Deep hematoma	1		
Gastrointestinal	Laparocele requiring surgery	1	Asymptomatic laparocele	1
Hematologic	Deep venous thrombosis	3		
TOTAL		43		29

Number of cases.

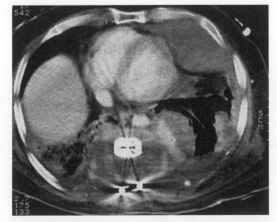

Fig. 1. Dissection of the aortic wall occurred 3 months after double approach en bloc resection of a recurrent osteosarcoma of T12. The patient had a partial excision and internal fixation 6 months previously. Release of the specimen from the aorta was performed by thoracoscopy and was particularly demanding because of the thick fibrous scar.

with open surgery). The other cases involved deep infections, hardware failure or loosening, deformities, laparoceles, and retrograde ejaculation. Overall, three patients died from complications: one died intraoperatively (injury to the cava), one died postoperatively (pulmonary embolism), and one died 6 months after the operation (aortic wall dissection). Intraoperative complications are related to manipulations of the vital structures. The risk of injury increases in patients who already have undergone operation or previously received radiation (fibrous scar, tissue fragility). Manipulation of the spinal cord, especially in the thoracic spine, should be handled carefully.[14] Two patients in this series were paraplegic at the time of recovery from anesthesia, although they had gradual improvement (Frankel A to D) after rehabilitation. Thoracic root transection causes minimal postoperative problems but allows an easier approach to the tumor mass, which reduces traction on the cord.

Dural tears are more likely encountered when operating through the scar of a previous surgery. Immediate suturing with a muscular coverage

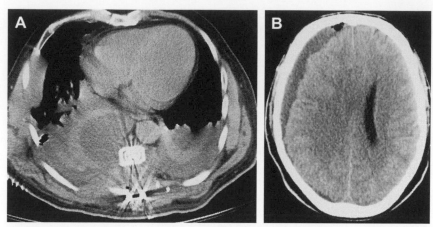

Fig. 2. (*A*) Huge collection of cerebrospinal fluid after non–water-proof suture during double approach en bloc resection. The dura injury occurred during the posterior approach (first step) and resulted in a persistent cerebrospinal fluid leak. (*B*) Epidural brain ex vacuo hematoma as a consequence of the cerebrospinal fluid depletion.

generally leads to prompt satisfactory healing. When waterproof sutures cannot be performed, cerebrospinal fluid depletion can produce further complications (see **Fig. 2**B). Postoperative hematomas form whenever a large void is present after tumor resection can cause paraplegia or lead to early deep infections.[9]

Hemodynamic stability is the major intraoperative concern of anesthesiologists during en bloc resections—similar to any long duration surgeries.[8] This also can affect early postoperative course: myocardial infarction after a quick decrease of intraoperative hemoglobin rate complicated three procedures, and a course of paroxysmal tachycardia was observed, but fortunately the patients recovered in a few months. A postoperative pulmonary embolism was fatal in one patient. Renal failure can also occur because of excessive hemorrhage or poor hemodynamic stability. Late complications also can be related to intraoperative work, such as dissections of the aortic walls in patients previously irradiated (see **Fig. 1**) and in patients in whom a difficult dissection frees the aorta from the tumor. In such cases, an aortic bypass should be included in surgical planning to prevent intraoperative injuries and late dissections.

CENTER OF TREATMENT

Thirty-five patients (26%) were referred from another institution after unsuccessful treatment. A series of patients who had five primary benign tumors (out of 31), 20 malignant tumors (out of 59), and 10 metastases (out of 44) were admitted to our department because of recurrence or progression of their disease. We grouped them in the

previously treated category for analysis. Conversely, the patients who presented to our institution because of initial symptoms and then were diagnosed and treated were grouped in the new presentation category. Of the 35 patients in the previously treated group, 17 (48.5%) had at least one complication (23 major and 12 minor). Among the 99 cases in the new presentation group, 31% suffered 20 major and 17 minor complications. Higher rate of complications were observed in the group of patients who were referred from another center after an open biopsy or previous treatment and then developed a recurrence. In particular, the risk of a major complication was observed in 72% of the previously treated group versus 20% in the new presentation group.

SURGICAL APPROACH

Combined anterior and posterior approaches under the same anesthesia[6,7] were performed in 87 patients, whereas the en bloc resection was achieved by single posterior approach in 47 cases.[2–7] Within the anterior approaches, patients had cervical prevascular approach (1), thoracotomies (20), extrapleural thoracoabdominal (36), lumbar retroperitoneal (28), and transperitoneal (2). Of note is that only 4 patients out of 47 who had a single posterior approach (8.5%) had at least one complication (including deep infection, profuse bleeding, and hardware failures). Conversely, 44 of the 87 (50.5%) patients who had a double approach had at least one complication. A massive hemorrhage caused by injury of the vertebral artery occurred during a prevascular neck approach. En bloc resection via a single posterior approach has fewer associated risks than a double approach.[2–4,6,7] This lessened risk probably can be explained by the fact that a double approach is often chosen when the tumors are large, which requires more extensive dissection and increases the risk for complications. The morbidity of an anterior approach was comparable to that described by Faciszeski.[15]

RADIATION THERAPY

Fifty-one patients received radiation therapy before or after surgery. Fifteen of those patients (29%) had nine complications, including five deep infections that required surgical treatment and one superficial infection that was managed with antibiotics. In two cases treated with anterior resection, late dissection of aorta occurred after adjuvant radiation therapy. Cases of instability caused by postradiation bone necrosis and failure of the posterior hardware that required revision also were encountered. Contrary to what is expected, the rate of complications in the group of patients treated with radiation was not higher in our study. Twenty-nine percent of the radiated group had at least one complication compared with 40% in the nonradiated group. Five of the six infections occurred in the group that underwent radiation therapy, however. It is possible to conclude that radiation-related complications are not more frequent but are more serious and occasionally can be life-threatening.

LOCAL RECURRENCES

The main purpose of an en bloc resection is the local control of disease and prevention of systemic effects. As such, it allows acceptance of a higher level of morbidity. The risk of local recurrence is directly related to the margin of resection.[1] Epidural extension of tumor increases the risk of local recurrence.[1,16–18] Even major neurologic sacrifices could be included in the decision-making process, considering the fact that a future local recurrence places neurologic function at risk, increases the challenge to the treatment strategy, and has a poorer prognosis. After our surgical management, 22 local recurrences (16%) were noted after an average of 37 months (7–126 months); 14 required further surgeries. Nine patients died because of disease, 8 of whom died from primary malignant tumors.

In the previously treated group, 14 local recurrences (40%) occurred. Twelve local recurrences were observed in the primary malignant tumors series. Of the 99 patients in the new presentation group, there were 8 local recurrences (8%). Although the oncologic margins of the en bloc

resection were defined as wide, in three cases, a recurrence was observed after 10, 20, and 88 months. The most relevant finding is the comparison between the incidence of local recurrence in patients initially treated elsewhere (previously treated) and patients treated at our center from initial disease presentation—40% versus 8%. This finding demonstrates that prognosis is closely related to the first treatment and that failing to understand or observe the principles of oncologic surgery can lead to serious consequences.[19]

Hardware Failures

En bloc resection includes not only bone resection but also surrounding soft tissue constraints, which lead to significant instability; therefore, a stable circumferential reconstruction is required.[20] To enable a stable fusion and good long-term outcome, autogenous graft or bone substitute or both should be used.[21,22] Chemotherapy and radiation therapy may delay achievement of fusion.[23] The reconstructive technique proposed includes posterior pedicle screws and titanium rods construct, connected with a carbon-fiber modular anterior column reconstruction filled with autogenous graft or bone substitutes.[21,22] This system failed in 10 patients (7%) because of a short posterior fixation and subsequent imbalance in the column. These events were not related to radiation therapy in our series. No failure of the anterior construct was observed.

DISCUSSION

To identify risk factors, reduce the rate of complications, and improve outcome, we have reviewed a homogeneous series of 134 en bloc resections, which is a highly demanding surgical procedure. It is commonly accepted that morbidity of surgical procedures for spine tumors is related to the altered anatomy secondary to the tumor growth, fibrosis caused by preoperative radiation therapy or previous surgery, and severe bleeding caused by the tumor mass. Intraoperative manipulation of the vascular structures can be a source of bleeding and may even be fatal. The unusual surgical techniques required to achieve en bloc resection are expected to increase the rate of complications, because extratumoral resection includes violation of anatomic barriers and manipulation or sacrifice of vascular and nervous structures. Although bleeding from a tumor mass is not expected in extralesional surgery, bleeding from epidural veins can provoke hemodynamic imbalance if not appropriately replaced. After surgery of such long duration, postoperative complications may include early problems related to wound dehiscence or infections. Late complications may include mechanical failures such as breakage or loosening of the complex circumferential reconstructions. Local recurrences may represent the failure of the oncologic planning.

A correct analysis of all the incidences is difficult because most of the occurrences are multifactorial and may lead to other adverse effects (eg, hematoma after en bloc resection in the thoracic spine may lead to a hemopneumothorax caused by the resection of the barrier for oncologic purposes, causing paraplegia).

SUMMARY

Oncologic criteria should guide the decision-making process for bone tumors of the spine.[1,13] When en bloc resection is the procedure of choice, surgical planning should include possible sacrifices of important neurovascular structures leading to altered function to accomplish the oncologic requirements. Preparation also should include awareness and discussion with patients about the potential morbidity of these procedures. The major risk factors identified after reviewing the reported series are manipulation of the vital structures (including the great vessels) after previous surgery or radiation, incomplete intraoperative management of the hemodynamics, double combined approach, and inadequate posterior fixation.

Overall, the incidence of complications and recurrences is significantly higher in revision surgery, and the first treatment determines of the final outcome. Global treatment, from biopsy to resection, should be performed at the same center. Radiation therapy does not increase the rate of complications (based on our study) but is associated with more severe ones. En bloc resections should be performed by specifically dedicated teams, including trained surgeons and anesthesiologists.

REFERENCES

1. Enneking WF. Muscoloskeletal tumor surgery. New York: Churchill Livingstone; 1983. p. 69–122.
2. Stener B. Complete removal of vertebrae for extirpation of tumors. Clin Orthop 1989;245:72–82.
3. Roy-Camille R, Mazel CH, Saillant G, et al. Treatment of malignant tumors of the spine with posterior instrumentation. In: Sundaresan N, Schmidek HH, Schiller AL, et al, editors. Tumors of the spine: diagnosis and clinical management. Philadelphia: WB Saunders; 1990. p. 473–92.
4. Tomita K, Kawahara N, Baba H, et al. Total en bloc spondylectomy: a new surgical technique for primary malignant vertebral tumors. Spine 1997;22: 324–33.
5. Fisher CG, Keynan O, Boyd MC, et al. The surgical management of primary tumors of the spine. Spine 2005;30:1899–908.
6. Boriani S. Subtotal and total vertebrectomy for tumours. In: Surgical techniques in orthopedics and traumatology. Paris: Editions Scientifiques et Medicales, Elsevier; 2000. p. 55-070-A.
7. Boriani S, Biagini R, De Iure F, et al. En bloc resection of bone tumors of the thoracolumbar spine: a preliminary report on 29 patients. Spine 1996;21: 1927–31.
8. Di Fiore M, Lari S, Boriani S, et al. Major vertebral surgery: intra- and postoperative anaesthesia-related problems. Chir Organi Mov 1998;LXXXIII:65–72.
9. McPhee IB, Williams RP, Swanson CE. Factors influencing wound healing after surgery for metastatic disease of the spine. Spine 1998;23:726–33.
10. Pascal-Moussellard H, Broc G, Pointillart V, et al. Complications of vertebral metastasis surgery. Eur Spine J 1998;7:438–44.
11. Wise JJ, Fishgrund JS, Herkowitz HN, et al. Complication, survival rates and risk factors of surgery for metastatic disease of the spine. Spine 1999;24:1943–51.
12. McDonnell MF, Glassman SD, Dimar JR, et al. Perioperative complications of anterior procedures of the spine. J Bone Joint Surg Am 1996;78: 839–47.
13. Boriani S, Weinstein JN. Differential diagnosis and surgical treatment of primary benign and malignant neoplasm. In: Frymoyer JW, editor. The adult spine: principles and practice. 2nd edition. Philadelphia: Lippincott-Raven; 1996.
14. Miller DJ, Lang FF, Walsh GL, et al. Coaxial double-lumen methyl methacrylate reconstruction in the anterior cervical and upper thoracic spine. J Neurosurg 2000;92:181–90.
15. Faciszewski T, Winter RB, Lonstein JE, et al. The surgical and medical perioperative complications of anterior spinal fusion surgery in the thoracic and lumbar spine in adults: a review of 1223 procedures. Spine 1995;20:1592–9.
16. Biagini R, Casadei R, Boriani S, et al. En bloc vertebrectomy and dural resection for chordoma: a case report. Spine 2003;28:E368–72.
17. Hart RA, Boriani S, Biagini R, et al. A system for surgical staging and management of spine tumors: a clinical outcome study of giant cell tumors of the spine. Spine 1997;22:1773–83.
18. Sundaresan N, DiGiacinto GV, Krol G, et al. Complete spondylectomy for malignant tumors. In: Sundaresan N, Schmidek HH, Schiller AL, et al, editors. Tumors of the spine: diagnosis and clinical management. Philadelphia: WB Saunders; 1990. p. 438–45.
19. Mankin HJ, Mankin CJ, Simon MA. The hazards of the biopsy, revisited: members of the Musculoskeletal Tumor Society. J Bone Joint Surg Am 1996;78:656–63.

20. Fourney DR, Abi-said D, Lang FF, et al. Use of pedicle screw fixation in the management of malignant spinal disease: experience in 100 consecutive procedures. J Neurosurg 2001;94:25–37.

21. Boriani S, Biagini R, De Iure F, et al. Reconstruction surgery in the treatment of vertebral tumors. Chir Organi Mov 1998;83:53–64.

22. Boriani S, Biagini R, Bandiera S, et al. The reconstruction of the anterior column of the thoracic and lumbar spine with the carbon fiber stackable cage system. Orthopedics 2002;25:37–42.

23. Otsuka NY, Hey L, Hall JE. Post-laminectomy and post-irradiation kyphosis in children and adolescents. Clin Orthop 1998;354:189–94.

Radiation for Spinal Metastatic Tumors

Patrick S. Swift, MD

KEYWORDS

- Stereotactic • Radiosurgery • SBRT • SRS
- Spinal • Vertebral • Radiotherapy

IRRADIATION FOR SPINAL METASTATIC TUMORS

In autopsy studies, metastases are found in the vertebral bodies of 5% to 30% patients who have malignant disease.[1–4] At autopsy, vertebral metastases have been found in as many as 90% of patients who had prostate cancer 74% of patients who had breast cancer, 45 % of patients who had lung cancer, 29% of patients who had lymphoma, and 25% of patients who had gastrointestinal malignancies.[5] Up to 20% of these spinal metastases are symptomatic, with associated severe pain, limitation of motion, increasing requirements for pain medication, decreasing quality of life, and potentially decreased duration of life secondary to complications arising from symptoms. Epidural spinal cord compression ultimately occurs in 5% to 15% of patients who have cancer, further degrading the overall quality of life and shortening the duration of life.[1–3,6,7] Pain is present in 83% to 95% of these cases, and two thirds of patients who have cord compression are nonambulatory at presentation.[5,8] Sensory deficits are associated with the compression in 40% to 90% of patients.[5]

Standard methods for dealing with these symptomatic occurrences include the delivery of radiation (alone or in conjunction with chemotherapy), radionuclide therapy, hormonal therapy, bisphosphonate therapy, and surgical decompression (with or without adjunctive irradiation). The magnitude of the problem is increasing as patients with more common malignancies (breast, prostate and lung cancer) survive for longer lengths of time because of the development of new and more effective treatment strategies. The need to prevent or manage the complications arising from spinal involvement is becoming a greater challenge to the clinician, because the short-term duration of control of areas of vertebral involvement is inadequate. At the same time, longer survival posttherapy allows more time for complications resulting from overly aggressive approaches to become manifest. New approaches involving the delivery of much larger doses of radiation in single fraction (stereotactic radiosurgery, SRS), hypofractionated regimens (stereotactic body radiotherapy, SRT or SBRT), or the use of particle therapy (protons) are showing increasing efficacy and duration of control in long-term survivors.

The selection of an appropriate therapeutic intervention depends on a number of factors: histology, extent of disease, existing comorbidities, age of the patient, prior treatment modalities, predicted life expectancy, and availability of resources. Some form of irradiation usually is recommended when the vertebral lesions cause significant pain[9] or neurologic symptoms resulting from nerve root or cord compression[5] or, increasingly, in patients who have oligometastases and a diagnosis with a prolonged life expectancy, such as prostate or breast cancer.[10–16]

Standard External Beam Therapy

For patients who have widely metastatic disease and a relatively short life expectancy, palliation of symptoms is the main reason for considering radiation therapy for spinal metastases. The timing and delivery of the radiation must take into account the past use of and future plans for systemic therapies, because the combined administration of extensive fields of large-dose-per-fraction radiation and certain types of chemotherapies and biologic modifiers may increase the risk of severe toxicity to an already debilitated patient.

Radiation Oncology, Alta Bates Comprehensive Cancer Center, 2001 Dwight Way, Berkeley, CA 94704, USA
E-mail address: pswift@aptiumoncology.com

Orthop Clin N Am 40 (2009) 133–144
doi:10.1016/j.ocl.2008.09.001

orthopedic.theclinics.com

Not all sites of vertebral involvement require radiation intervention. Sites that are actively causing pain, sites of vertebral collapse, and certainly sites with neurologic consequences resulting from spinal cord, cauda, or nerve root compression should be addressed in a timely fashion. It often is difficult to decide exactly how much of the spine to treat in patients who have diffuse involvement of the spinal column demonstrated on bone scans or MRI. Areas that are small and asymptomatic, unless immediately adjacent to the more significant sites that require treatment, may be spared to minimize the impact on marrow capacity for future systemic therapies. These asymptomatic sites should be addressed with the use of bisphosphonates,[17–21] with chemotherapy, or with future irradiation should they become symptomatic.

A prospective, randomized study of 123 patients who had new-onset cord compression (ie, major symptoms present for <48 hours) found initial surgical decompression followed by postoperative irradiation to be superior to irradiation alone in terms of ambulatory rates, maintenance of continence, motor strength, and reduction in long-term opioid and steroid requirements.[6] Patients who had a life expectancy of more than 3 months, duration of paraplegia for less than 48 hours, a single area of radiologically documented spinal cord displacement, and no prior history of spinal cord compression were assigned randomly to either immediate surgical decompression followed within 14 days by irradiation or to irradiation alone to a dose of 30 Gy. Patients who had very radiosensitive tumors (lymphomas, myelomas, germ cell tumors), and those who had brain metastases were excluded from the study. The posttreatment ambulatory rates were 84% for surgery versus 57% for irradiation alone ($P < .001$). The median length of time that patients maintained the ability to walk was 122 days after surgical decompression versus only 13 days after irradiation alone. Of the patients who were able to walk at entry into the study, 94% of those treated with the combined approach continued to be ambulatory, compared with 74% of those treated with irradiation alone. Of those unable to walk at entry into the study, 62% in the surgical decompression group regained the ability after surgery, versus 19% in the irradiation group. These results clearly show a benefit of immediate surgical decompression followed by irradiation in those patients who met the eligibility criteria.

Not all patients who have cord compression necessarily require surgical intervention, however. Based on a multivariate analysis performed on a cohort of 2096 patients who were irradiated for spinal cord compression without surgery from 1992 to 2007, Rades and colleagues[1] proposed a scoring system with the potential to predict the ambulatory rates after irradiation alone using five prognostic factors: histology, the interval between initial diagnosis of malignancy and development of cord compression (<15 months or >15 months), the presence of visceral metastases, pretreatment motor function (ambulatory versus nonambulatory), and the duration of motor deficits before irradiation (1–7 days, 8–14 days, or >14 days). As in Patchell's study, this scoring system identified a subset of patients who had excellent postradiotherapy ambulatory rates who might not require surgical decompression. These patients met all the following criteria: favorable histology (myeloma/lymphoma, breast, prostate), more than 15 months between diagnosis and the development of cord compression, ambulatory before radiotherapy, and slower development of motor deficits (>14 days). Postradiotherapy ambulatory rates of 99% were seen in 750 of 760 patients who met these criteria and underwent irradiation alone.

Irradiation without surgery often is appropriate for patients without evidence of structural instability or epidural cord compression, especially for patients who have radiosensitive histologies (lymphoma, myeloma, germ cell tumors, prostate cancer, or breast cancer). The area treated traditionally has been the involved vertebra(e) plus one additional body above and below the target area. Bone scans or MRIs are helpful in defining the field sizes. The radiation beam delivery approach is determined by the level of the spine involved, the presence nearby of radiosensitive organs such as the kidneys, upper esophagus, and lungs, and any areas of prior irradiation that might overlap with the current area. Simple opposed anterior and posterior fields often are the best choice for the minimizing radiation exposure of nearby organs in thoracolumbar and sacral lesions. Posterior wedge pairs for lumbar lesions may reduce the bowel toxicity (diarrhea, nausea) while respecting the radiation tolerance of the kidneys and liver. Special care is taken with cervical lesions to minimize the risk of severe esophageal irritation; opposed lateral fields are used to minimize esophageal exposure. This precaution is especially important in patients being treated with concurrent systemic therapy, such as taxanes, that may increase the risk of radiation esophagitis dramatically.

The dose fractionation schedule used in these palliative cases has been the focus of a large number of prospective, randomized trials. A recent meta-analysis of 16 major trials worldwide comparing multiple fractionation schemes for palliation of pain secondary to bone metastases failed to show any one regimen to be superior to any other.[9,22–24] A short course of a single 800-cGy fraction is as effective as 400 cGy × 5 or 300 cGy × 10 in providing pain relief. The response rates with these single or multifraction regimens were not found to be statistically different: complete response rates were 23% to 24%, and partial response rates were 58% to 59%. In patients who had vertebral metastases, 4.1% to 5.7% went on to develop subsequent cord compression. In the nine randomized trials that reported this end point, the incidence of re-treatment was greater in patients who received short-course (single-fraction) treatments than in patients treated with higher-dose, more protracted courses (20% versus 8%, $P < .00001$), but this difference may reflect an increased willingness to re-treat an area that previously had been treated with a single fraction. There also was a trend toward increased incidence of pathologic fracture after single-dose treatment, although pathologic fracture was not a primary end point of any of these trials. The overall response rates in these trials were less than desired (an average of 72% of patients experienced some pain relief), however, and the duration of pain relief was only in the range of 11 to 24 weeks. In three of these trials,[22,25–27] reanalysis of results using strict definitions of "response," based on the International Bone Metastases Consensus Working Party criteria, found lower rates of overall response (46%–72%) and complete response (14%–25%). The Dutch Bone Metastasis Trial found that with both single-dose and protracted regimens the median time to progression of symptoms was only 20 to 24 weeks,[28] indicating that the doses used in the palliative setting are insufficient for patients surviving beyond 1 year. In a separate large, multicenter, retrospective study of five different irradiation treatment schedules for patients who had malignant spinal cord compression (no surgery), there was no difference in the post-treatment effect on motor function or ambulatory status favoring one regimen over another (25%–38% of patients improved with treatment).[3] Bone remineralization and in-field local control, however, favored longer fractionation schedules in patients surviving beyond 6 months.

For the debilitated patient who has a relatively short life expectancy (<6 months) and few therapeutic options, it is more humane to treat with a single large fraction of 800 cGy (to minimize the number of trips, often by ambulance, to the treatment facility). For a patient functioning at a higher level, with a life expectancy longer than 6 months, it is more appropriate to select a more protracted course of 300 cGy × 10 to lower the potential need for reirradiation, to increase the chance of remineralization, and to reduce the risk of pathologic fracture. Initiating bisphosphonate therapy should be considered, because multiple trials have shown a reduction in skeletal events and progression in the bones of patients who have breast/prostate/lung cancer and other solid tumors as well as myeloma with bisphosphonate therapy.[17,19,21] Bisphosphonate therapy will limit the need for radiation intervention further. For patients who have a life expectancy of several years, such as the patient newly diagnosed with metastatic breast or prostate cancer, neither of the standard radiation fraction approaches is very satisfying, because of late failures, and a more aggressive approach should be considered to assure maximum duration of control at the treated site.

Stereotactic Radiosurgery and Stereotactic Body Radiotherapy

The development of advanced approaches for the delivery of a single (SRS) or a few (SBRT) very large doses of radiation to a very tightly conformed target immediately adjacent to critical normal tissue structures has provided a possible means of increasing the chance of local control of tumors that have spread to the spinal column. Building on experience developed in years of treatment of intracranial lesions with SRS,[29] in which an external three-dimensional reference frame attached rigidly to the skull allows the delivery of a single, highly focused collection of beams of radiation to a target deep within the cranium, SBRT is a technology that attempts to deliver similarly focused treatment to targets outside the cranium. Lesions within the spine are logical targets for such hypofractionated approaches, as long as intra- and interfraction motion of the target can be accounted for by highly precise set-up.

The proximity of the sensitive spinal cord (an "organ at risk") to the target lesion is in the order of millimeters. The delivery of large doses of radiation risks injuring this serially operating organ, potentially leading to myelopathy, an unacceptable side effect. A steep and reliable dose gradient between the target and the cord must be achieved, and the clinician must be assured that the desired dose is being delivered to the exact location of the intended target. At the doses being delivered, movement of the cord into the high-dose target volume could have disastrous results, and movement of the lesion outside of the target volume will result in local failure. The challenges to be overcome by this technology are many, and a multitude of questions must be answered. What is the precise definition of the target to be treated (grossly identifiable disease only or areas at risk of subclinical spread)? What is the tolerance of any fractional portion of the spinal cord to single large doses of radiation? What is the optimal way to account for motion of the patient and internal target during a relatively long treatment period? What degree of error in set-up of the patient is acceptable to ensure coverage of the target and avoidance of the cord? What dose is necessary to increase the chance of local control but not cause delayed major side effects? Which patients are appropriately selected to receive this costly therapy?

Stereotactic body radiotherapy systems

Building on the processes used extensively for intracranial SRS (externalized three-dimensional reference systems affixed to the skull), early programs used external fixation devices screwed into the spinous processes and attached to external reference frames.[30] This cumbersome and costly approach was replaced by the development of extensive body frames that were fixed to immobilization devices that cradle the body in a relatively stable position without the need for deep surgical instrumentation.[31,32] Later, radiopaque fiducial markers were implanted within the spinous processes of patients as internal landmarks that could be visualized easily by kilovoltage (kV) imaging; these surrogates for the location of the intended target allowed the target location to be verified at the time of dose delivery. This technique, however, still required a surgical procedure that was costly and had the risk of marker migration. As imaging technology has improved, the ability to identify the target itself directly (with kV or MV CT imaging) or nearby bony landmarks (via kV imaging) has reduced the need for such invasive procedures.[32,33]

Several different systems are commercially available for the delivery of stereotactic spinal treatment (Table 1). Each includes the radiation treatment machine with a precise beam-collimating ability, an immobilization method that takes into account inter- and intrafractional movement, a sophisticated image guidance system, and a precise and reliable treatment planning system.

The CyberKnife (Accuray, Inc.) system uses a compact, relatively light-weight 6-MV linear accelerator attached to a robotic manipulator that is maneuverable around six axes.[34] Real-time imaging of the target and internal bony anatomic landmarks is achieved by two kV imaging devices set at 90° to one another, programmed to image the patient repeatedly at set intervals during the treatment process. These images are registered rapidly to the images obtained at the time of planning. Any discrepancies in patient localization compared with the initial set-up can be identified, accounted for, and corrected by compensation of the robotic manipulator in a real-time setting.

The Novalis Shaped Beam Surgery unit (BrainLab, Inc.) includes a dedicated 6-MV linear accelerator with beams defined by a micro-multileaf collimator, opposing pairs of tungsten leaves that are adjusted to control the gaps through which the beam passes toward the target.[35] An infrared system, the ExacTrac, uses skin markers to allow rapid initial set-up and monitoring to detect any change in the patient's position during the treatment delivery. Two kV imagers mounted orthogonally in the floor project obliquely in all three translational axes onto imagers. The images obtained are registered to the planning images (again, looking at bony landmarks and/or implanted fiducials), and any error in translational axes (x-, y-, or z-axis) or error around the rotational

Table 1
Representative commercial stereotactic body radiotherapy systems

System	Position Verification	Treatment Delivery
CyberKnife	Real-time orthogonal kV images	Lightweight 6-MV linear accelerator mounted on robotic arm
BrainLab	Orthogonal kV imaging and infrared surface markers	6-MV linear accelerator with micro-multileaf collimators, IMRT
Varian Trilogy	On-board kV cone-beam CT ± infrared surface markers	6-MV linear accelerator with micro-multileaf collimators, IMRT
Elekta	On-board kV cone-beam CT	6-MV linear accelerator with micro multileaf collimators, IMRT
TomoTherapy HI-ART	Integrated MV CT	Helical IMRT with binary multileaf collimator

Abbreviation: IMRT, intensity-modulated radiation therapy.

axes (pitch, roll, or yaw) can be detected. With the use of a specialized tabletop with six ranges of motion, patient positioning can be corrected in all six degrees of freedom before treatment delivery.

Both the Trilogy system (Varian Medical Systems) and Elekta Synergy S (Elekta, Inc.) have an integrated kV cone-beam CT apparatus built into the gantry of the linear accelerator that allows both orthogonal kV and MV images as well as acquisition of CT images with the patient in the treatment position.[16,32] The CT in treatment position is registered with the CT used for planning to determine the corrections needed along the translational and rotational axes. This approach allows identification of the true target rather than surrogate markers or bony landmarks.

TomoTherapy Hi-ART (TomoTherapy, Inc.) is a CT-based delivery system that uses pretreatment CT scanning to identify the true target and correct patient positioning immediately before treatment.[36] Dose delivery via a helical 360° pattern is achieved by continuous movement of both the gantry and table during the treatment. An intensity-modulated fan beam is mounted on a slip-ring gantry.

In implementing any of these systems, quality assurance programs are essential to determine the degree of spatial accuracy that can be achieved. Extensive work has been published on the analyses of errors caused by the specific characteristics of each system, the image registration programs used, the set-up verification procedures, and the estimation of patient motion.[11,15,16,32,33,35–44]

Stereotactic planning process

Patient selection has varied in the clinical studies of stereotactic approaches to spinal lesions reported to date, but some generalizations can be made (**Box 1**). Patients fall into two major categories: those who have newly identified spinal column metastases, and those who have recurrent disease after prior irradiation. Patients in the former group have a solitary or at most a very limited number of metastases (oligometastatic), a high performance status, a life expectancy in excess of 6 months, and histology not deemed to be exquisitely radiosensitive (thereby excluding myeloma, lymphoma, or leukemia, which can be handled adequately with standard radiation approaches). Patients in the latter group generally are quite symptomatic and are considered to be a poor risk for additional surgery or at high risk of failure even after such surgery. Patients generally considered ineligible for SRS or SBRT are those who have a significant (>25%) canal compromise and significant cord compression or who have

Box 1
Patient selection criteria for SRS/SBRT
Recurrent disease after prior irradiation
Not a good surgical candidate or patient refuses surgery
Significant neurologic/pain symptoms
Newly identified vertebral lesions
Solitary or oligometastatic lesions
Verifiable distance between cord and lesion (preferably >5 mm)
Life expectancy greater than 6 months
Good overall performance status
Systemic disease controlled, stable
Not eligible
Structural instability of spine
Cord compression
More than 25% canal compromise
Radiosensitive histology (myeloma, lymphoma)
Unable to rest comfortably for duration of treatment

spinal instability, two groups that are handled best initially with a surgical decompressive approach, potentially with stabilization instrumentation followed by delayed radiotherapy. Patients must be able to tolerate the treatment position (treatment may last longer than an hour in some circumstances), and there must be some measurable distance (preferably >5 mm) between the cord itself and the target volume to allow dose fall-off from the target to the cord. Because of concerns about the uncertainty of true cord tolerance, concurrent chemotherapy or other biologic agents such as monoclonal antibodies, antiangiogenesis agents, or tyrosine kinase or epidermal growth factor receptor (EGFR) inhibitors, which may have a significant radiosensitizing effect, generally have been avoided. When these agents can be safely restarted after irradiation is not clear but is an important area for discussion.

After patient selection, the first step in the treatment process is patient immobilization and imaging. The safe and successful delivery of the large doses of radiation being prescribed to a target that sits next to the spinal cord requires that the patient's position be stable, reproducible through the planning and delivery process, and comfortable, and that patient motion is extremely limited in all directions. The patient is placed in a vacuum-bag cradle that allows comfortable general alignment of the patient. For cervical lesions, an

Aquaplast mask may be created that allows stabilization of the head. An external stereotactic body frame system may be attached to the immobilization device, although this precaution is less critical in systems that allow direct visualization of the target. Body motion may be restricted further through the use of a clear plastic cover sheet with a vacuum action that constrains voluntary motion of the trunk during the procedures (BodyFix, Medical Intelligence, Inc.) (**Fig. 1**). Patients who are physically and/or psychologically incapable of resting comfortably within these immobilizers for prolonged periods of time may not be good candidates for the treatment. Analgesics are used as necessary to maintain the patient's pain at an acceptable level. Once the immobilization has been accomplished, a treatment-planning CT scan of the region of interest is performed, and the patient is released.

The CT generally is fused with an MRI (**Figs. 2 and 3**) of the spine using software designed for that purpose. The MRI has a superior ability to define the contours of the spinal cord and cauda equina. A CT myelogram may be useful also. The accuracy of the image fusion is critical to the success of the planning process but introduces a potential source of error into the system (eg, through differences in patient deformation during the two separate imaging procedures or variation in spinal geometry).[32,33,42]

The clinicians (radiation oncologists, neurosurgeons, and orthopedic surgeons) next contour the organs at risk, such as the cord, cauda, nerve roots, esophagus, kidneys, and heart, and define the tumor volumes based on the International Commission on Radiation Units and Measurement Report 50 guidelines.[42] The cord and cauda are termed "avoidance structures" in the planning process, and the treatment-planning software is instructed to minimize the dose to these

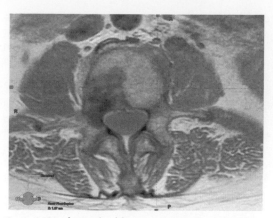

Fig. 2. MRI of vertebral lesion suitable for SRS/SBRT.

structures. A small margin (1–3 mm) may be added around the spinal cord to reduce the risk to the cord conservatively. The gross target volume (GTV) is defined as the identifiable extent of disease as seen on the MRI or CT. The clinical target volume (CTV) is defined as the GTV plus any region thought to be at considerable risk for spread of the disease and therefore requiring full treatment doses (such as the remainder of the vertebral body, the pedicles, or posterior processes). This critically important process is handled differently at various reporting centers[42] and will require further refinement as clinical experience accrues. It ideally is a process that involves the input of the neurosurgeon or orthopedic surgeon as well as the radiation oncologist. Some choose to treat only the GTV, not attempting to deliver full treatment to the entire vertebral body. Others believe that pedicles and possibly spinous processes require treatment as well, resulting in a very different CTV with a potentially higher dose delivery to the nearby cord. Given the ability to vary the dosing across small volumes, a third approach is to attempt to give the highest dose to the GTV and a lesser dose to the remainder of the CTV, a concept known as "dose painting."[29] An example would be treating the GTV to a dose of 16 to 18 Gy and the remainder of the vertebral body (the CTV) to a lesser but still significant dose. The final planning target volume (PTV) may be limited to the absolute GTV with no margin, or it may include the CTV with some minimal expansion to take into account the treatment delivery system and set-up accuracy. Target definition and dose decisions are bound together inextricably but are not yet standardized.[10,12,15,16,40,42] If larger CTVs are selected, then doses must be constrained to safeguard the spinal cord. If larger doses are desired, then potential underdosing of clinical areas of potential spread may occur.

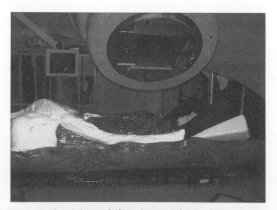

Fig. 1. Patient immobilization with BodyFix system (Medical Intelligence).

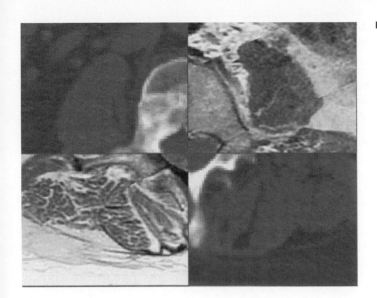

Fig. 3. CT/MRI registration.

Spinal cord radiation tolerance

Many years of experience have shown that fractionated courses of radiation to total doses of 45 to 50 Gy at 1.8 to 2.0 Gy per fraction are well tolerated by the human spinal cord.[42,45] Although case reports have described individual cases of myelopathy at these doses, such instances are rare. An extensive data analysis by Schultheiss[45] found that the incidence of myelopathy after a dose of 45 Gy is 0.03% and at 50 Gy is only 0.2%. These numbers, however, must be viewed cautiously, because many new and potentially radiosensitizing agents, such as the taxanes, kinase inhibitors, and antiangiogenic agents, may lower the tolerance dose of tissues including spinal cord, both when they are delivered concurrently with radiation and when they are used in the postirradiation period, instigating a potentially dangerous recall phenomenon.[11,45,46]

The delivery of large individual doses to a target (the vertebral body and pedicles) that is in extremely close proximity to an organ (the cord and cauda) where injury to even a small portion of tissue can have devastating consequences evokes important questions about the actual tolerance of small volumes of the cord to irradiation. With current technological approaches, a steep dose gradient of radiation is achieved, making the dosage within several millimeters of the cord difficult to define. The fact that this radiation is delivered to patients who often have limited life expectancies further muddies the water, because many patients would not be expected to live long enough to develop late toxicity such as myelitis or nerve root injury.

Initially, limits were set at 8 Gy to 10 Gy for the cord dose that would be accepted in planning treatments for spinal lesions. This limit was based on data about the tolerance of optic nerves obtained from earlier studies in cranial stereotactic radiosurgery.[13] In a report on 177 patients in whom 230 lesions in the spine were treated with single doses of radiation ranging from 8 to 18 Gy, Ryu and colleagues[46] reported on the partial volume tolerance of the human spinal cord, focusing on 86 patients who survived longer than 1 year. None of these patients had received previous irradiation to the region. The average dose delivered to 10% of the spinal cord tissue within the fields treated was 9.2 +/−2.3 Gy. Patients treated to target doses greater than 16 Gy had substantially higher doses of radiation delivered to the cord (9.8 +/−1.5 Gy to the 10% cord volume). At these doses, there were only two late cases of cord injury, one of which was shown to be secondary to disease progression higher in the cord. Based on these data, the authors concluded that the cord tolerance (in a previously untreated cord with no concurrent chemotherapy) is at least 10 Gy to 10% of the cord volume at that level. Additional years of follow-up are essential, however, to determine if late vascular occlusion of the cord vessels may occur in long-term survivors as a result of these doses.

Yamada and colleagues[16] reported on 93 patients in whom 103 lesions were treated with single doses of 18 to 24 Gy, with dose constraints of 12 to 14 Gy as the maximal dose allowed any point in the spinal cord. None of the patients had received prior irradiation to the area. The target volume was the entire vertebral body. The median time to death was 10 months, but the 45-month actuarial survival was 39%. At these doses, no patient developed myelopathy or radiculopathy at a median follow-up time of 15 months. Gibbs and colleagues[11] reported on the Stanford experience with 74 patients who had 102 lesions with a mean follow-up of only 9 months, 50 of whom had received prior irradiation to the area of interest. The spinal cord maximum dose was set at the biologic equivalent of a single dose of 10 Gy (not including the prior radiation dose), with target doses of 16 to 25 Gy delivered in one to five fractions. Three patients developed treatment-related severe myelopathy in the thoracic spine: two of these cases had received prior irradiation courses to the region, and two were treated with antiangiogenic therapy or epidermal growth factor inhibitors within 2 months of the appearance of myelopathy. Gerszten and colleague[34] reported on 500 cases treated to a median target dose of 19 Gy, 344 of whom had prior irradiation. At a median follow-up of 21 months, no cases of myelopathy were reported. More data and longer follow-up are essential to help define the true limits of cord tolerance to the large doses of radiation being delivered in stereotactic cases.

For single-fraction SRS of spinal lesions, doses of 8 Gy to 24 Gy have been prescribed.[10,12,15,32,36,38,40,47,48] For multifractionated SBRT, dosing schedules of 9, 8, or 6 Gy × 3 and of 6 or 4 Gy × 5 have been reported. The decision to fractionate may be based in part on the proximity of the tumor to the spinal cord volume, as well as on the size of the lesion and its location within the vertebra and whether there has been prior irradiation. The smaller the distance between the lesion and the cord, the greater is the tendency to fractionate the course, although institutional preference may dictate the schedule used. Whether a single larger dose is superior to several smaller doses spread out over a week remains an unanswered question, one that a prospective, randomized study may be needed to answer.

Inverse planning systems are used to create a treatment delivery plan based on these dose constraints to the cord (and other nearby organs such as kidneys or esophagus) and the target dose (**Figs. 4** and **5**). Each of the previously mentioned systems has its own solution to this problem,[42,49] either through the use of multiple non-coplanar beams (with or without intensity modulation)[10,11,13,16,29,39,40,47,50–54] or continuous helical delivery.[13,36,55]

The precise delivery of the planned dose to the defined target requires that the patient positioning

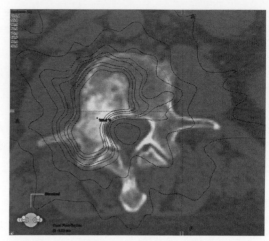

Fig. 4. Axial isodose distribution displaying a steep dose gradient between tumor and spinal cord. The PTV in this case is the MR-identified lesion only.

be exact within six degrees of freedom: the translational planes (x-, y-, and z-planes) and the rotational planes (pitch, roll, and yaw). Slight errors in any of these dimensions can result in the cord moving into the high-dose region of the plan and in the loss of the advantage of the steep dose gradient. The precision of positioning differs from system to system and must be defined clearly before initiating any such program. In an elegant discussion of 540 simulations of translational and rotational errors in set-up, Guckenberger and colleagues[41] introduced stepwise errors in all six directions ranging from 0.5 mm up to 10 mm. Translational errors in the superior–inferior translational direction had only minimal impact on cord dose. Left–right or anterior–posterior translations of 7 and 5 mm, however, resulted in as much as

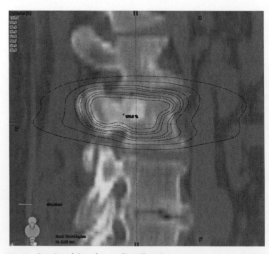

Fig. 5. Sagittal isodose distribution.

a median difference in the dose to the cord of 48% and 34%, respectively. Rotational errors generally resulted in less variance, but, depending on the location of the tumor, a 5° rotation could result in a 25% difference in dose to the cord. These differences clearly demonstrate the critical importance of initial patient positioning and the need to reduce the intrafractional motion of the patient. The patient's position must be verified carefully to assure that it is exactly the same position used for the planning process, preferably within 1 mm in each of the translational axes.[29,37,39,41,43,54]

After the patient's position has been verified, treatment commences. The treatment time can vary from 20 to 90 minutes, so ensuring patient comfort is essential. The patient is monitored closely during the treatment to assure that the position is maintained. At least one of the systems uses an on-going kV-imaging approach intermittently during the treatment and automatic registration of these films to the planning films with analysis of deviations to allow for compensatory moves in the isocentric treatment delivery to account for any patient movement.[10,13,39,40,47,50,54] In the other systems, observed patient movements may require interrupting the treatment fraction and reverifying correct positioning. Overall, the treatments themselves are very well tolerated and only rarely are associated with acute side effects.

Stereotactic radiosurgery/stereotactic body radiotherapy clinical results

Gerszten and colleagues[34] reported on 500 treatment sessions using the CyberKnife system in 393 patients undergoing SRS for spinal metastases at the University of Pittsburgh. This series included a wide variety of histologies, and 344 of the treatments were in locations where radiation (usually 3 Gy × 10 or 2.5 Gy × 14) had been delivered previously. Patients who had significant spinal instability or neurologic findings secondary to cord compression were not eligible for treatment. Fiducial seeds (four to six per case) were implanted into the pedicles adjacent to the lesion, except in cervical spinal lesions. The PTV was the GTV with no margin added. A dose in the range of 12.5 to 25 Gy (mean, 20 Gy) was delivered to the 80% isodose line (ie, there was a 20% inhomogeneity of dose within the GTV). The maximum dose to the spinal cord at any point ranged up to 13.5 Gy; the mean was 10 Gy.[56–58] No instances of radiation-induced spinal injury were seen. Long-term pain improvement (as defined by a 10-point visual pain scoring system) was reported in 86% of all patients at a median follow-up of 21 months, and long-term radiographic improvement was seen in 88%. Differences in radiographic control were noted by histology, with melanoma at 75%, renal cell at 87%, and breast and lung at 100%. No cases of failure were noted in immediately adjacent vertebral bodies.

Yamada and colleagues[16] reported on the SRS experience at Memorial Sloan Kettering in 103 lesions in 93 patients, none of whom had prior surgical resection or irradiation of the involved region. Patients who had spinal instability or cord compression were not eligible for this study. An infrared optical system was used to monitor patient movement during the procedure, and patient position was verified initially by comparing orthogonal films registered to the planning CT-derived digitally reconstructed radiographs. After 2004, a cone-beam CT integrated into the linear accelerator allowed direct CT visualization of the lesion at time of treatment.[29] Intensity-modulated treatment using a combination of multiple non-coplanar fields was used to deliver doses of 18 to 24 Gy to the entire involved vertebral body expanded by 2 mm. The PTV, however, was never allowed to overlap the cord, which was constrained to a dose of 12 to 14 Gy. At a median follow-up time of 15 months, actuarial local control as documented by serial MRI scans was 90%, with a 45-month actuarial survival of 36%. No cases of radiation injury to the spine or cauda were seen, although one case of a tracheoesophageal fistula occurred at the treatment level while the patient was receiving doxorubicin, raising the possible specter of a radiation recall phenomenon.

Ryu and colleagues[15] reported on the experience at Henry Ford Hospital of SRS for 61 lesions in 49 previously unirradiated patients, using the BrainLab system. Twelve of the patients underwent initial decompressive surgery before the SRS. Doses of 10 to 16 Gy at the 90% isodose line were delivered to the entire vertebral body and paraspinal soft tissue component plus 2-mm margins, limiting the cord dose below 10 Gy. Using a 10-point pain scale, 46% of patients experienced complete pain relief by 8 weeks, 19% had partial relief, and 16% had stable pain. Median duration of pain relief was 13.6 months, with a trend toward greater pain relief at doses above 14 Gy. With a 1-year overall survival rate of 74%, no cases of cord injury were seen.

In a separate report by Ryu and colleagues[46] of 230 lesions treated in 177 patients using the BrainLab system, none of whom had prior irradiation, doses of 8 to 18 Gy were delivered as single fractions to a target volume that included the vertebral body and pedicles with no margin.[46] The cord constraint was 10 Gy maximum to 10%

of the adjacent cord. To accomplish this cord constraint, the target dose often required restriction. The 1- and 2-year overall survival rates were 49% and 39%. The maximum cord dose in the cohort that lived longer than 1 year was 12.2 Gy. Two patients in this cohort developed neurologic deterioration, one because of progressive disease at the site and one, who also was treated with subsequent carboplatin, docetaxel, herceptin, and fulvestrant, because of radiation. The latter patient showed symptomatic improvement with the use of dexamethasone.

Gibbs[10] reported on the Stanford experience with the CyberKnife (initially with implanted fiducials but later using the Xsight kV imaging system) in 102 spinal lesions in 74 patients, 50 of whom had received prior irradiation at or near the SRS field. Patients were treated with from one to five fractions to a dose of 16 to 25 Gy (dose per fraction, 7–20 Gy to a wide range of isodose lines, 61%–89%) to the target volume. The cord limit was set at 10 Gy from the stereotactic treatment alone. At a mean follow-up of 9 months, 52 of 62 initially symptomatic patients reported improvement or disappearance of symptoms. Three cases of severe myelopathy were reported. Two of these patients had received prior irradiation to the region (prior doses of 25.2 and 40 Gy, respectively), and two had received antiangiogenic therapy or anti-EGFR therapy within 2 months of the myelopathy.

Chang and colleagues[38] performed a phase I/II study of SBRT for 74 isolated spinal metastases in 63 patients, using a CT-on-rails system in which the patient was positioned before treatment in a body stabilization unit with an external stereotactic reference frame. A CT scan was performed in the treatment position for verification. Based on the CT, the positioning was adjusted, and the tabletop subsequently was swung into position with the linear accelerator for treatment. This protocol consisted of either 3 × 9 Gy or 5 × 6 Gy, and the spinal cord dose was maintained below 10 Gy (a substantially lower equivalent dose than 10-Gy single-dose restraint of the SRS studies mentioned earlier). Patients were eligible if they had prior irradiation (maximum 45 Gy) to the region or if they had prior surgical decompression, but not if the vertebral body was considered unstable. At a median follow-up of 21 months, the actuarial 1-year local control was 84%. The predominant patterns of failure were within the epidural space (in the high-dose gradient region abutting the spine) and within the pedicles and posterior elements of the bone that were not routinely targeted. No cases of grade 3 or grade 4 neurologic toxicity were seen.

SUMMARY

A number of critical questions remain to be answered with regards to SRS and SBRT for spinal lesions. The process requires the close cooperation among a multidisciplinary team that includes the radiation oncologist, neurosurgeon, orthopedic surgeon, and medical oncologist. What is the ideal target of therapy, and what dose and fractionation schemes will maximize results? What is the true long-term dose tolerance of the spinal cord to large individual fraction sizes? How may tolerance be modified by the use of new systemic targeted agents? How can the cost of this procedure be reduced through new technological developments?

The ultimate goal in radiotherapeutic management of spinal metastases is durable improvement of quality of life for the affected individual. SRS or SBRT for spinal lesions achieves higher percentages of pain relief and longer duration of local control than standard fractionation schemes in carefully selected patients who have long life expectancies. The requirement for maximal precision in set-up verification and delivery is paramount but is costly and time-consuming. Not all patients require such complex measures, and adequate palliation certainly is possible with much simpler means for patients who have shorter life expectancies.

REFERENCES

1. Rades D, Dunst J, Schild SE. The first score predicting overall survival in patients with metastatic spinal cord compression. Cancer 2008;112(1):157–61.

2. Rades D, Fehlauer F, Veninga T, et al. Functional outcome and survival after radiotherapy of metastatic spinal cord compression in patients with cancer of unknown primary. Int J Radiat Oncol Biol Phys 2007;67(2):532–7.

3. Rades D, Stalpers LJ, Veninga T, et al. Evaluation of five radiation schedules and prognostic factors for metastatic spinal cord compression. J Clin Oncol 2005;23(15):3366–75.

4. Sundaresan N, Boriani S, Rothman A, et al. Tumors of the osseous spine. J Neurooncol 2004;69(1–3): 273–90.

5. Prasad D, Schiff D. Malignant spinal-cord compression. Lancet Oncol 2005;6(1):15–24.

6. Patchell RA, Tibbs PA, Regine WF, et al. Direct decompressive surgical resection in the treatment of spinal cord compression caused by metastatic cancer: a randomised trial. Lancet 2005;366(9486): 643–8.

7. Rades D, Karstens JH, Hoskin PJ, et al. Escalation of radiation dose beyond 30 Gy in 10 fractions for

metastatic spinal cord compression. Int J Radiat Oncol Biol Phys 2007;67(2):525–31.

8. Maranzano E, Trippa F, Chirico L, et al. Management of metastatic spinal cord compression. Tumori 2003; 89(5):469–75.

9. Sze WM, Shelley M, Held I, et al. Palliation of metastatic bone pain: single fraction versus multifraction radiotherapy—a systematic review of the randomised trials. Cochrane Database Syst Rev 2004;(2): CD004721.

10. Gibbs IC. Spinal and paraspinal lesions: the role of stereotactic body radiotherapy. Front Radiat Ther Oncol 2007;40:407–14.

11. Gibbs IC, Kamnerdsupaphon P, Ryu MR, et al. Image-guided robotic radiosurgery for spinal metastases. Radiother Oncol 2007;82(2):185–90.

12. Rock JP, Ryu S, Yin FF. Novalis radiosurgery for metastatic spine tumors. Neurosurg Clin N Am 2004; 15(4):503–9.

13. Rock JP, Ryu S, Yin FF, et al. The evolving role of stereotactic radiosurgery and stereotactic radiation therapy for patients with spine tumors. J Neurooncol 2004;69(1–3):319–34.

14. Ryu S, Fang Yin F, Rock J, et al. Image-guided and intensity-modulated radiosurgery for patients with spinal metastasis. Cancer 2003;97(8):2013–8.

15. Ryu S, Jin R, Jin JY, et al. Pain control by image-guided radiosurgery for solitary spinal metastasis. J Pain Symptom Manage 2008;35(3):292–8.

16. Yamada Y, Bilsky MH, Lovelock DM, et al. High-dose, single-fraction image-guided intensity-modulated radiotherapy for metastatic spinal lesions. Int J Radiat Oncol Biol Phys 2008;71(2):484–90.

17. Aapro M, Abrahamsson PA, Body JJ, et al. Guidance on the use of bisphosphonates in solid tumours: recommendations of an international expert panel. Ann Oncol 2008;19(3):420–32.

18. Berenson JR. Zoledronic acid in cancer patients with bone metastases: results of phase I and II trials. Semin Oncol 2001;28(2 Suppl 6):25–34.

19. Berenson JR. Recommendations for zoledronic acid treatment of patients with bone metastases. Oncologist 2005;10(1):52–62.

20. Hillegonds DJ, Franklin S, Shelton DK, et al. The management of painful bone metastases with an emphasis on radionuclide therapy. J Natl Med Assoc 2007;99(7):785–94.

21. Ross JR, Saunders Y, Edmonds PM, et al. Systematic review of role of bisphosphonates on skeletal morbidity in metastatic cancer. BMJ 2003; 327(7413):469.

22. Chow E, Harris K, Fan G, et al. Palliative radiotherapy trials for bone metastases: a systematic review. J Clin Oncol 2007;25(11):1423–36.

23. Wu J, Bezjak A, Chow E, et al. A consensus development approach to define national research priorities in bone metastases: proceedings from NCIC CTG workshop. Clin Oncol (R Coll Radiol) 2003; 15(8):496–9.

24. Wu JS, Wong R, Johnston M, et al. Meta-analysis of dose-fractionation radiotherapy trials for the palliation of painful bone metastases. Int J Radiat Oncol Biol Phys 2003;55(3):594–605.

25. Chow E, Hoskin PJ, Wu J, et al. A phase III international randomised trial comparing single with multiple fractions for re-irradiation of painful bone metastases: National Cancer Institute of Canada Clinical Trials Group (NCIC CTG) Sc 20. Clin Oncol (R Coll Radiol) 2006;18(2):125–8.

26. Hartsell WF, Scott CB, Bruner DW, et al. Randomized trial of short- versus long-course radiotherapy for palliation of painful bone metastases. J Natl Cancer Inst 2005;97(11):798–804.

27. van der Linden YM, Steenland E, van Houwelingen HC, et al. Patients with a favourable prognosis are equally palliated with single and multiple fraction radiotherapy: results on survival in the Dutch bone metastasis study. Radiother Oncol 2006;78(3):245–53.

28. Steenland E, Leer JW, van Houwelingen H, et al. The effect of a single fraction compared to multiple fractions on painful bone metastases: a global analysis of the Dutch bone metastasis study. Radiother Oncol 1999;52(2):101–9.

29. Yamada Y, Lovelock DM, Bilsky MH. A review of image-guided intensity-modulated radiotherapy for spinal tumors. Neurosurgery 2007;61(2):226–35 [discussion: 235].

30. Hamilton AJ, Lulu BA, Fosmire H, et al. Preliminary clinical experience with linear accelerator-based spinal stereotactic radiosurgery. Neurosurgery 1995;36(2):311–9.

31. Lax I, Blomgren H, Naslund I, et al. Stereotactic radiotherapy of malignancies in the abdomen. methodological aspects. Acta Oncol 1994;33(6):677–83.

32. Chang BK, Timmerman RD. Stereotactic body radiation therapy: a comprehensive review. Am J Clin Oncol 2007;30(6):637–44.

33. Galvin JM, Bednarz G. Quality assurance procedures for stereotactic body radiation therapy. Int J Radiat Oncol Biol Phys 2008;71(Suppl 1):S122–5.

34. Gerszten PC, Burton SA, Ozhasoglu C, et al. Radiosurgery for spinal metastases: clinical experience in 500 cases from a single institution. Spine 2007; 32(2):193–9.

35. Jin JY, Ryu S, Rock J, et al. Evaluation of residual patient position variation for spinal radiosurgery using the Novalis image guided system. Med Phys 2008;35(3):1087–93.

36. Kim B, Soisson ET, Duma C, et al. Image-guided helical tomotherapy for treatment of spine tumors. Clin Neurol Neurosurg 2008;110(4):357–62.

37. Chang EL, Shiu AS, Lii MF, et al. Phase I clinical evaluation of near-simultaneous computed

tomographic image-guided stereotactic body radiotherapy for spinal metastases. Int J Radiat Oncol Biol Phys 2004;59(5):1288–94.

38. Chang EL, Shiu AS, Mendel E, et al. Phase I/II study of stereotactic body radiotherapy for spinal metastasis and its pattern of failure. J Neurosurg Spine 2007;7(2):151–60.

39. Chuang C, Sahgal A, Lee L, et al. Effects of residual target motion for image-tracked spine radiosurgery. Med Phys 2007;34(11):4484–90.

40. Gerszten PC, Burton SA, Ozhasoglu C. CyberKnife radiosurgery for spinal neoplasms. Prog Neurol Surg 2007;20:340–58.

41. Guckenberger M, Meyer J, Wilbert J, et al. Precision required for dose-escalated treatment of spinal metastases and implications for image-guided radiation therapy (IGRT). Radiother Oncol 2007;84(1):56–63.

42. Sahgal A, Larson DA, Chang EL. Stereotactic body radiosurgery for spinal metastases: a critical review. Int J Radiat Oncol Biol Phys 2008;71(3):652–65.

43. Wang H, Shiu A, Wang C, et al. Dosimetric effect of translational and rotational errors for patients undergoing image-guided stereotactic body radiotherapy for spinal metastases. Int J Radiat Oncol Biol Phys 2008;71(4):1261–71.

44. Yin FF, Ryu S, Ajlouni M, et al. Image-guided procedures for intensity-modulated spinal radiosurgery. technical note. J Neurosurg 2004;101(Suppl 3):419–24.

45. Schultheiss TE. The radiation dose-response of the human spinal cord. Int J Radiat Oncol Biol Phys 2008;71(5):1455–9.

46. Ryu S, Jin JY, Jin R, et al. Partial volume tolerance of the spinal cord and complications of single-dose radiosurgery. Cancer 2007;109(3):628–36.

47. Gagnon GJ, Henderson FC, Gehan EA, et al. CyberKnife radiosurgery for breast cancer spine metastases: a matched-pair analysis. Cancer 2007;110(8):1796–802.

48. Kavanagh BD, McGarry RC, Timmerman RD. Extracranial radiosurgery (stereotactic body radiation therapy) for oligometastases. Semin Radiat Oncol 2006;16(2):77–84.

49. Teh BS, Paulino AC, Lu HH, et al. Versatility of the Novalis system to deliver image-guided stereotactic body radiation therapy (SBRT) for various anatomical sites. Technol Cancer Res Treat 2007;6(4):347–54.

50. Cheshier SH, Hanft SJ, Adler JR, et al. CyberKnife radiosurgery for lesions of the foramen magnum. Technol Cancer Res Treat 2007;6(4):329–36.

51. Gerszten PC, Germanwala A, Burton SA, et al. Combination kyphoplasty and spinal radiosurgery: a new treatment paradigm for pathological fractures. J Neurosurg Spine 2005;3(4):296–301.

52. Gerszten PC, Ozhasoglu C, Burton SA, et al. CyberKnife frameless stereotactic radiosurgery for spinal lesions: clinical experience in 125 cases. Neurosurgery 2004;55(1):89–98 [discussion: 98–9].

53. Gerszten PC, Welch WC. CyberKnife radiosurgery for metastatic spine tumors. Neurosurg Clin N Am 2004;15(4):491–501.

54. Ho AK, Fu D, Cotrutz C, et al. A study of the accuracy of cyberKnife spinal radiosurgery using skeletal structure tracking. Neurosurgery 2007;60(2 Suppl 1):ONS147–56 [discussion: ONS156].

55. Mahan SL, Ramsey CR, Scaperoth DD, et al. Evaluation of image-guided helical tomotherapy for the retreatment of spinal metastasis. Int J Radiat Oncol Biol Phys 2005;63(5):1576–83.

56. Gerszten PC, Burton SA, Ozhasoglu C, et al. Stereotactic radiosurgery for spinal metastases from renal cell carcinoma. J Neurosurg Spine 2005;3(4):288–95.

57. Gerszten PC, Burton SA, Quinn AE, et al. Radiosurgery for the treatment of spinal melanoma metastases. Stereotact Funct Neurosurg 2005;83(5-6):213–21.

58. Gerszten PC, Burton SA, Welch WC, et al. Single-fraction radiosurgery for the treatment of spinal breast metastases. Cancer 2005;104(10):2244–54.

Solitary Vertebral Metastasis

Daniel M. Sciubba, MD*, Trang Nguyen, BS, Ziya L. Gokaslan, MD

KEYWORDS
- Spine • Tumor • Metastasis • Treatment • Solitary

There are more than 1.4 million newly diagnosed cases of cancer per year in the United States and more than 500,000 deaths are expected annually from the disease.[1] Osseous metastasis is common; the spine is the most frequent site with about 20,000 cases per year.[2,3] Although 10% to 30% of patients who have cancer develop symptomatic spinal metastases,[3,4] in postmortem studies up to 90% of patients who had terminal cancer had evidence of metastatic spinal disease.[5–9] Some 12% to 20% of malignancies initially present because of symptomatic spinal metastasis.[4,10] As survival time increases for many cancers, it is likely that the incidence and prevalence of spinal metastases will increase also. Given that most patients first present with solitary lesions in the spine, proper initial diagnosis and management are of paramount importance in minimizing pain, improving neurologic function, and potentially lengthening survival.

EPIDEMIOLOGY

The most common primary cancers to have metastatic disease of the spine are cancers of the lung, breast, and prostate.[11–13] The greatest incidence of spinal metastatic lesions occurs during midlife (40–65 years of age), correlating to the age group with a higher cancer risk.[3] Slightly more males are affected than females, reflecting the slightly higher incidence of prostate cancer compared with breast cancer.[3] The location of spinal metastasis correlates to volume, with thoracic spinal metastasis being the most common at 60%, followed by 30% lumbosacral and 10% cervical.[14,15] Most spinal lesions are solitary and multiple spinal lesions reportedly occur in up to 35% of patients.[13–15] In one prospective study, recurrent spinal metastases occurred in 20% of patients.[16] Over the past 20 years, improvements in neuroradiologic imaging, especially MRI, have drastically improved the early diagnosis of metastatic spinal disease. As a result, single lesions are more commonly being identified. Such solitary metastases are then defined if no additional radiographic studies reveal any other site of disease.[17]

PATHWAYS OF SPREAD

Malignant cells can disseminate to the spine by various mechanisms—through the arterial system, through venous drainage, by cerebrospinal fluid, or by direct extension. With the vertebrae's rich blood supply, the hematogenous route is the most common out of these pathways. Arterial seeding initially occurs in the vertebral bone marrow, following which metastatic cells can invade the medullary cavity and subsequently spread to the spinal canal.[18] Venous spread occurs by way of the Batson plexus of valveless veins that allow retrograde travel paravertebrally and communicate with the drainage of multiple organs.[19–21] This route may explain the method in which breast, prostate, kidney, thyroid, and lung cancers metastasize to the spine.[2]

Tumor spread by direct extension from the paraspinal region to the epidural space is less frequent and is usually due to hemopoietic malignancies, such as lymphoma.[14,22] Locally aggressive tumors may also invade the spine, such as lung cancer in the thoracic region, and prostate, bladder, and colon cancer in the lumbosacral region.[20] Recently, focus has shifted away from anatomic pathways of spread toward molecular and cellular determinants, such as the interaction between surface

Department of Neurosurgery, Johns Hopkins University, Baltimore, MD, USA
* Corresponding author. 600 North Wolfe Street, Meyer 8-161, Baltimore, Maryland 1287, USA.
E-mail address: dsciubb1@jhmi.edu (D.M. Sciubba).

Orthop Clin N Am 40 (2009) 145–154
doi:10.1016/j.ocl.2008.09.003

proteins and adhesion molecules on tumor and host cells.[23,24]

PRESENTATION

Although many patients who have spinal metastases may present with significant neurologic deficits, patients who have solitary spinal lesions may have limited epidural extension with minimal neurologic deficits.[17] Despite this, however, solitary spinal lesions can have substantial debilitating effects on quality of life. Across multiple metastatic cancer types, skeletal-related complications occur on average every 3 to 6 months clustered around periods of progression.[25] Pain is the most common and earliest symptom, occurring in up to 95% of patients and before other neurologic deficits.[26–28] Cancer-related pain may be differentiated from other causes by its nocturnal nature.[29,30] Most commonly, the pain is in the form of local neck or back pain from tumor invasion out of the pain receptor–deficient bone marrow to the periosteum or beyond. Mechanically induced pain from spinal cord compression, vertebral body collapse, and pathologic fractures may also occur. The pain can also be of a radicular nature caused by compression of nerve roots yielding sharp, shooting pain in a dermatomal fashion. The presentation of pain occurs on average about 7 months before any other neurologic compromise.[14]

Motor dysfunction is the second most common symptomatic manifestation of vertebral metastases. Those who have a solitary spine lesion may have varying degrees of epidural extension, however, and therefore minimal neurologic dysfunction until a significant amount of spinal compression has occurred.[17] At the time of diagnosis, weakness can be found in 60% to 85% of patients who have metastatic epidural spinal cord compression.[27,28,31] Muscle weakness is usually asymmetric with the iliopsoas most often affected. The most severe weakness is present with thoracic spinal epidural metastases because of the relatively narrow spinal canal and spinal cord vascular supply in this region.[27,28,31] Prompt work-up of neurologic dysfunction is important because neurologic status at time of diagnosis is correlated with ambulatory outcome.[18,32,33]

Many patients also have sensory dysfunction when weakness occurs or shortly after. This dysfunction may occur in a dermatomal distribution with radicular pain or weakness. With cord compression, sensory deficits may occur one to five segments below the myelopathy.[21] Lhermitte sign can occur with cervical or thoracic metastases.[34] Late neurologic deficits include bowel, bladder, and sexual dysfunction, of which bladder dysfunction is the most common autonomic dysfunction and parallels the severity of motor dysfunction.[35]

MANAGEMENT

Management of solitary metastatic bone disease has traditionally been focused on palliation of the debilitating symptoms, such as the pain and motor deficits. Factors such as life expectancy, age, tumor burden, and functional status must be considered when deciding among treatment options. Many clinicians consider external irradiation to be the initial treatment of choice in all patients who have spinal metastases instead of surgery because functional outcomes after both methods have been shown to be comparable in previous studies.[36,37] Such studies, generalized to the patients who had solitary lesions not causing instability or neurologic decline, seem to be especially relevant.

Several studies have suggested, however, that prior irradiation increases the complication rates of spinal surgery and the functional outcome.[38–40] In addition, in rare circumstances in which the primary site of cancer has been removed and systemic disease is well controlled, some authors have postulated that radical resection may lead to long-term control of tumor or even cure.[38,41–44] For instance, following nephrectomy for renal cell carcinoma, some authors have conducted en bloc vertebral body resections for solitary renal cell carcinoma spinal metastasis.[45]

BIOPSY

Accurate diagnosis is especially important when there is no prior history of cancer and patients present initially with a solitary spinal lesion. An increasing number of studies suggest that the primary histology of the spine lesion has an extremely large effect, if not the most important effect, on patient survival, regardless of treatments offered for the spine lesion.[46–48] Dramatic differences in survival are seen not only between different sites of origin of the tumor (breast versus lung) but also between specific subtypes of site of origin. For instance, Sciubba and colleagues[46] showed that patients who had estrogen receptor–positive breast cancer survived significantly longer following spine surgery for metastatic lesions than patients who did not have estrogen receptors. Similarly, early data from M.D. Anderson Cancer Center suggest that in patients who have prostate cancer metastatic to the spine, Gleason grade of tissue obtained from the original prostate gland biopsy is independently associated with survival following spine surgery for metastatic lesions.[49]

Percutaneous image-guided biopsy is a safe and accurate method that can be used when surgery is not indicated and when there are no other systemic lesions that could be biopsied.[21,30] The success rates range from up to 76% for sclerotic lesions to 93% for lytic lesions.[50,51] Because 5% of patients who have spinal cord compression may have extradural plasmacytoma (solitary form of multiple myeloma), immunoelectrophoresis of urine or serum for monoclonal proteins should also be considered.[52] There have been some data from the M.D. Anderson Cancer Center that suggest patients who have solitary spine lesions and no sites of primary disease have worse prognosis following spine surgery when the origin of disease cannot be conclusively determined (ZL Gokaslan, unpublished, 2001). It has been postulated that such patients suffer from more poorly differentiated, aggressive pathologies.

STANDARD RADIATION TREATMENT

The mainstay of treatment of painful lesions without mechanical instability that do not involve neural elements is conventional external beam radiotherapy (XRT). XRT, usually in total doses of 25 to 40 Gy over 8 to 20 daily fractions,[30,53] can help provide pain relief, prevent pathologic fractures or vertebral collapse, and delay or reverse neurologic dysfunction.[21] The outcome of XRT depends on the radiation sensitivity of the tumor. Those who have a solitary spinal metastasis tend to do better, whereas those who have multiple vertebral lesions, visceral or brain lesions, or lung cancer have been shown to have shorter survival.[34,54,55] In addition, slow onset of neurologic deficit often predicts a better radiotherapy response compared with those who have a rapid decline.[56] XRT should be the primary modality for highly sensitive tumors, such as multiple myeloma, lymphoma, plasmacytoma, small cell lung cancer, testicular seminoma, neuroblastoma, and Ewing sarcoma. Moderately sensitive cancers include breast, lung, prostate, and colon metastases. Although poorly sensitive tumors, such as melanoma, renal cell, and thyroid metastases, may need a more aggressive surgical approach, radiation can provide substantial pain relief.[30]

Although radiation therapy can reduce pain, it is not effective against bone destruction and instability for which surgery should be considered.[57] Radiation alone thus does not suffice in patients who have solitary metastases and obvious mechanical instability. The spine usually also cannot be re-irradiated for recurrence because of risk for

neurologic toxicity, particularly myelopathy.[58] The limited precision of conventional XRT and the low tolerance of the spinal cord to radiation commonly restrict the amount of radiation that can be given below the optimal therapeutic dose.[36,59,60] Some studies have looked into whether radiation could be given at a high dose in one fraction compared with traditional multifraction therapy with smaller individual doses. Several phase III prospective randomized trials and a meta-analysis showed that multifraction radiation therapy and single fraction therapy at 8 to 10 Gy were equivalent in providing pain relief and survival.[61–65] More patients in the single fraction groups needed to be retreated, however.[63]

STEREOTACTIC RADIOSURGERY

More modern unconventional radiotherapies, such as stereotactic radiosurgery (SRS) and intensity-modulated radiotherapy (IMRT), which have step dose fall-off outside the targeted area, may allow higher radiation doses to reach the lesion with less risk for injury to the spinal cord and surrounding normal tissue.[21,30] Such techniques are especially attractive for patients who have solitary spine metastasis who present with pain but without spinal instability or cord compression. Doses are typically 8 to 18 Gy over one to two sessions.[21] Because a theoretic 3-mm positioning error could reportedly double the dose delivered to the spinal cord, the high accuracy (1.36 mm from target center) and precision (±0.11 mm) of these new techniques is particularly attractive.[66,67] Radiosurgery requires well-defined targets and immobilization or accurate tracking of the target. The radiation is delivered by the convergence of multiple beam orientations with intensity modulation of each beam (**Fig. 1**).

SRS and IMRT are especially attractive options for solitary lesions without epidural spinal cord compression or mechanical instability in which pain is the primary complaint. The largest report to date of the use of SRS is a prospective, nonrandomized cohort study of 500 spinal metastatic lesions from 393 patients.[68] The maximum dose ranged from 12.5 to 25 Gy. The study showed that 86% had long-term pain improvement, 90% had long-term tumor control when SRS was the primary treatment modality, and 88% had tumor control when SRS was used for radiographic tumor progression after previous irradiation. At a median follow-up of 21 months there was no acute radiation toxicity or new neurologic deficits.

Another large SRS study included almost 200 patients who had metastatic spinal lesions treated

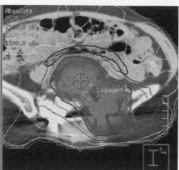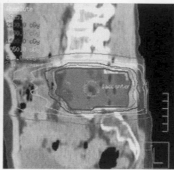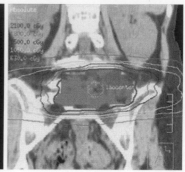

Fig. 1. Computed tomography images of a solitary spinal metastasis in the axial, sagittal, and coronal planes showing superimposed spinal stereotactic radiosurgery (SRS) dosing plans.

with doses from 8 to 18 Gy, with the lower dosage given for lesions near the spinal cord so that only 10 Gy was exposed to 10% of the adjacent spinal cord volume.[69,70] Eighty-five percent of patients had pain relief within 4 weeks. Overall the treatment was well tolerated with one case of radiation-induced myelopathy after 13 months in a patient who had previous radiotherapy.[70] A phase I/II study also supports that SRS can be safe and effective with an 84% 1-year tumor progression–free incidence in 63 patients. Failure tended to occur in two patterns: in the bone adjacent to the treatment site and in the epidural space adjacent to the spinal cord.[71,72]

Although SRS is still experimental, there are many advantages that may encourage its widespread practice for solitary or oligometastatic spinal lesions.[73] Irradiation of large proportions of the bone marrow may be avoided, thus reducing the effect on the hematopoietic and immunologic reserve.[73–75] The ability to treat patients in one day versus several for conventional radiation therapy may be a significant deciding factor for a patient who has a short life expectancy. SRS can also be given in cases wherein there is local recurrence following surgical or conventional radiation therapy or as salvage therapy for those who cannot undergo those alternative options.[74] It may also be more helpful for more radio-resistant tumors, such as melanoma, sarcoma, and renal cell carcinoma, because higher doses of radiation are given.

PERCUTANEOUS VERTEBROPLASTY AND KYPHOPLASTY

For patients who have solitary lesions who present with painful pathologic vertebral compression fractures without neurologic compromise, percutaneous vertebroplasty or kyphoplasty is an effective minimally invasive treatment option that can

be done in an outpatient or short-stay basis It is effective in treating pain and preventing further deformity, theoretically by providing structural support and minimizing mechanical pain. Additionally, the cement itself may have analgesic properties and antitumor properties. Although this procedure can provide immediate results, there is a 10% risk for symptomatic complications and estimated 73% risk for asymptomatic cement leakage.[76–82] Kyphoplasty differs from vertebroplasty in that initial placement and inflation of a balloon in the vertebral body creates a cavity into which polymethylmethacrylate is then injected under low pressure, thus theoretically decreasing the risk for cement leakage. Vertebroplasty and kyphoplasty, although effective, are relatively contraindicated for patients who have epidural spinal cord compression. The exception is for patients who are poor surgical candidates, in which case vertebroplasty or kyphoplasty can be done in combination with single fraction radiosurgery with favorable pain relief.[83,84]

SURGERY

Traditionally, irradiation has been considered the primary treatment of spinal metastases. Surgery is generally indicated, however, in cases of spinal instability, progressive neurologic deficit from neural compression, enlarging radio-resistant tumor, need for open biopsy, and intractable pain unrelieved by nonsurgical treatment.[57] The potential benefits of surgery must be considered along with the patient's expected length of survival because treatment is mainly palliative. It is typically regarded that surgery should only be recommended for patients who have a life expectancy of more than 3 to 6 months (Fig. 2).[21,85]

Historically, solitary spinal masses with cord compression were treated with decompressive laminectomy. This procedure created posterior

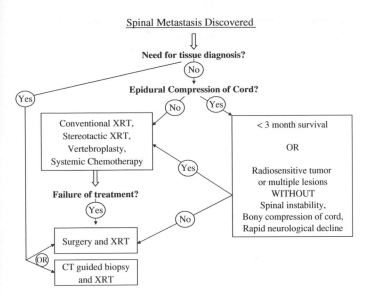

Spinal Metastasis Discovered

Need for tissue diagnosis?

No

Epidural Compression of Cord?

Yes

No   Yes

Conventional XRT,
Stereotactic XRT,
Vertebroplasty,
Systemic Chemotherapy

Yes

Failure of treatment?

Yes   No

Surgery and XRT

OR

CT guided biopsy
and XRT

< 3 month survival

OR

Radiosensitive tumor
or multiple lesions
WITHOUT
Spinal instability,
Bony compression of cord,
Rapid neurological decline

Fig. 2. Algorithm for management of spinal metastatic lesions.

spinal instability, however, and combined with the most commonly located anterior instability by the tumor, this resulted in worse symptomatic outcomes.[57] As surgical techniques, especially anterior approaches, and instrumentation systems have improved, surgery is being reconsidered as another initial treatment option.[86–90] In a randomized, prospective clinical trial, direct circumferential spinal cord decompression with spinal stabilization and radiotherapy was compared with radiotherapy alone.[91] The study showed a statistically significant increase in the percentage of patients who were ambulatory following treatment in the surgery plus XRT group versus the XRT-alone group. Those treated with surgery were also more likely to retain continence, muscle strength, functional ability, and had increased

survival times. Having surgery in addition to radiotherapy has also been calculated to be cost effective in cost per additional day of ambulation and cost per life-year gained.[92]

Radiation should be given after surgery if possible; higher complication rates, in particular wound healing, occur because radiation changes affect the surgical field.[93] Patient selection is also important. Although there are no strict criteria, patient-related factors (paraparesis severity, pain) and tumor-related factors (histologic type, prognosis, and extent of disease) should be considered on a case-by-case basis. Preoperative scoring systems include one by Tomita and another by Tokuhashi.[47,48] Both scoring paradigms take into account the number of metastatic lesions, with a worse prognosis for survival in patients who

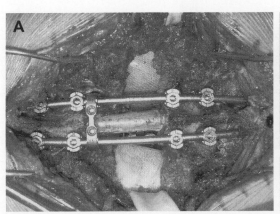
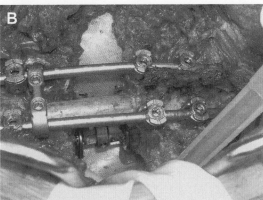

Fig. 3. Intraoperative photographs following spondylectomy for a solitary breast cancer metastasis at T4. Posterior view of surgical exposure following vertebrectomy and reconstruction with pedicle screws and rods (*A*) and oblique view showing anterior column reconstruction with expandable cages (*B*).

have an increased number of lesions. As a result, these authors generally suggest that a more aggressive approach (eg, surgical excision) should be initially considered for patients who have fewer lesions, compared with more conservative or palliative, nonsurgical approaches for multiple lesions. Others, including Sundaresan and colleagues,[17] have reported that surgery for solitary metastases specifically can have favorable outcomes, including long-term survival.

Aggressive surgery, consisting of wide or marginal resection, has gained increasing support in the management of solitary metastases, because it has the potential to minimize local recurrence. Oncologically, total tumor resection is the optimum treatment to improve local control. Most studies have limited their surgical approaches to intralesional curettage using posterolateral or extracavitary approaches to minimize morbidity. As a result, the incidence of local recurrences has ranged from 20% to 50%, with few long-term survivors. To minimize local recurrences, en bloc techniques have been proposed for solitary metastases.[44,45,94] In the case of renal cell carcinoma it may even lead to curative therapy.[45]

CASES

At our own institution, patients have undergone spondylectomy procedures for solitary metastatic lesions of the mobile spine. Specifically, one patient underwent a T4 spondylectomy for treatment of a solitary breast cancer metastasis following bilateral mastectomy, chemotherapy, and radiation (**Fig. 3**). Since surgery, the patient has been doing well in remission of her disease. In another patient who had a solitary metastatic parathyroid carcinoma lesion, spondylectomy was done for metabolic control of hyperparathyroidism to treat malignant osteoporosis (**Fig. 4**). In this case, the

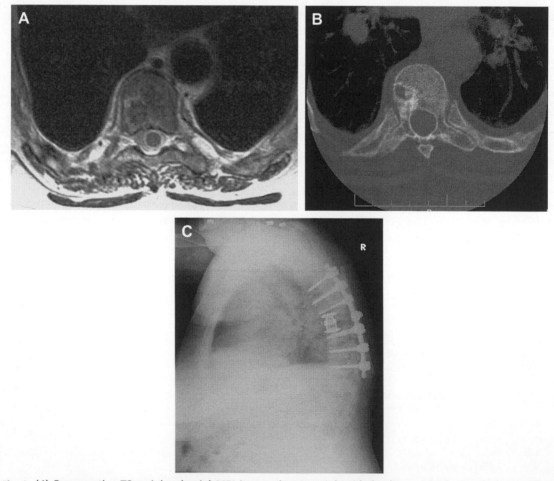

Fig. 4. (*A*) Preoperative T2-weighted axial MRI image showing right-sided solitary spinal metastasis consistent with parathyroid carcinoma. (*B*) Preoperative CT scan showing same lesion. (*C*) Lateral radiograph following complete spondylectomy and reconstruction with cage and pedicle screws.

patient's endocrine abnormalities subsided, and she no longer suffers from frequent skeletal fractures. As systemic therapies improve for various cancers, it is likely that such radical surgery will be more commonly used for local control of solitary spine metastases in selected patients who have good potential for systemic control.

SUMMARY

Most metastatic lesions of the spine present first as solitary growths. It is imperative for the primary care provider and the surgeon to appreciate the classic presenting signs and symptoms, which usually involve pain with or without neurologic dysfunction. Rapid diagnosis of the histology in concert with oncologic work-up aids in determining the appropriate management options. Although historically treated by only palliative measures (eg, pain control, decompressive surgery, and standard radiation), patients who have solitary spinal metastatic lesions can be expected to have substantial improvements in pain, neurologic recovery, and in some cases potential for local control and improved survival with current treatment options. Although pain control and standard radiation are still used, spinal stereotactic radiosurgery, vertebroplasty and kyphoplasty, and spinal cord decompression and fusion are now consistently used in aggressive management and offer exciting preliminary results. As advancements in the treatment of systemic malignancies continue to occur, allowing increases in survival time for patients who have metastatic disease, more and more patients will present with symptomatic spinal metastases. For such patients, multispecialty and multimodality treatment with surgery, radiation, or percutaneous procedures will undoubtedly become the standard of care.

REFERENCES

1. American Cancer Society. Cancer facts & figures 2008. Atlanta: American Cancer Society; 2008.
2. Coleman RE. Clinical features of metastatic bone disease and risk of skeletal morbidity. Clin Cancer Res 2006;12(20 Pt 2):6243s–9s.
3. Perrin RG, Laxton AW. Metastatic spine disease: epidemiology, pathophysiology, and evaluation of patients. Neurosurg Clin N Am 2004;15(4):365–73.
4. Wu AS, Fourney DR. Evolution of treatment for metastatic spine disease. Neurosurg Clin N Am 2004; 15(4):401–11.
5. Cobb CA 3rd, Leavens ME, Eckles N. Indications for nonoperative treatment of spinal cord compression due to breast cancer. J Neurosurg 1977;47(5): 653–8.
6. Jaffe W. Tumors and tumorous conditions of the bones and joints. Philadelphia: Lea & Febiger; 1958.
7. Lenz M, Freid J. Metastases to the skeleton, brain and spinal cord from cancer of the breast and effect of radiotherapy. Ann Surg 1931;93:278–93.
8. Sundaresan N, Krol G, DiGiacinto G. Metastatic tumors of the spine. In: Sundaresan N, Schmidek H, Schiller A, editors. Tumors of the spine: diagnosis and clinical management. Philadelphia: WB Saunders; 1990.
9. Wong DA, Fornasier VL, MacNab I. Spinal metastases: the obvious, the occult, and the impostors. Spine 1990;15(1):1–4.
10. Schiff D, O'Neill BP, Suman VJ. Spinal epidural metastasis as the initial manifestation of malignancy: clinical features and diagnostic approach. Neurology 1997;49(2):452–6.
11. Constans JP, de Divitiis E, Donzelli R, et al. Spinal metastases with neurological manifestations. Review of 600 cases. J Neurosurg 1983;59(1):111–8.
12. Feiz-Erfan I, Rhines LD, Weinberg JS. The role of surgery in the management of metastatic spinal tumors. Semin Oncol 2008;35(2):108–17.
13. Helweg-Larsen S, Hansen SW, Sorensen PS. Second occurrence of symptomatic metastatic spinal cord compression and findings of multiple spinal epidural metastases. Int J Radiat Oncol Biol Phys 1995;33(3):595–8.
14. Gabriel K, Schiff D. Metastatic spinal cord compression by solid tumors. Semin Neurol 2004;24(4): 375–83.
15. Schiff D. Spinal cord compression. Neurol Clin 2003; 21(1):67–86.
16. van der Sande JJ, Boogerd W, Kroger R, et al. Recurrent spinal epidural metastases: a prospective study with a complete follow up. J Neurol Neurosurg Psychiatr 1999;66(5):623–7.
17. Sundaresan N, Rothman A, Manhart K, et al. Surgery for solitary metastases of the spine: rationale and results of treatment. Spine 2002;27(16):1802–6.
18. Arguello F, Baggs RB, Duerst RE, et al. Pathogenesis of vertebral metastasis and epidural spinal cord compression. Cancer 1990;65(1):98–106.
19. Batson OV. The function of the vertebral veins and their role in the spread of metastases. Ann Surg 1940;112(1):138–49.
20. Ross J, Brant-Zawadzki M, Moore KR, et al. Neoplasms, cysts, and other masses. In: Ross J, editor. Diagnostic imaging: spine. Altona, Manitoba, Canada: Amirsys; 2005. p. IV1–126.
21. Sciubba DM, Gokaslan ZL. Diagnosis and management of metastatic spine disease. Surg Oncol 2006; 15(3):141–51.
22. Jacobs WB, Perrin RG. Evaluation and treatment of spinal metastases: an overview. Neurosurg Focus 2001;11(6):e10.

23. Choong PF. The molecular basis of skeletal metasta-ses. Clin Orthop Relat Res 2003;(Suppl 415): S19–31.

24. Yuh WT, Quets JP, Lee HJ, et al. Anatomic distribu-tion of metastases in the vertebral body and modes of hematogenous spread. Spine 1996;21(19): 2243–50.

25. Coleman RE. Bisphosphonates: clinical experience. Oncologist 2004;9(Suppl 4):14–27.

26. Bach F, Larsen BH, Rohde K, et al. Metastatic spinal cord compression. Occurrence, symptoms, clinical presentations and prognosis in 398 patients with spinal cord compression. Acta Neurochir (Wien) 1990;107(1–2):37–43.

27. Helweg-Larsen S, Sorensen PS. Symptoms and signs in metastatic spinal cord compression: a study of progression from first symptom until diagnosis in 153 patients. Eur J Cancer 1994;30A(3):396–8.

28. Posner J. Neurological Complications of Cancer. Philadephia: FA Davis; 1995.

29. Aydinli U, Ozturk C, Bayram S, et al. Evaluation of lung cancer metastases to the spine. Acta Orthop Belg 2006;72(5):592–7.

30. White AP, Kwon BK, Lindskog DM, et al. Metastatic disease of the spine. J Am Acad Orthop Surg 2006;14(11):587–98.

31. Greenberg HS, Kim JH, Posner JB. Epidural spinal cord compression from metastatic tumor: results with a new treatment protocol. Ann Neurol 1980; 8(4):361–6.

32. Henson R, Urich H. Cancer of the Nervous System. Oxford: Blackwell Scientific Publications; 1982.

33. Levack P, Graham J, Collie D, et al. Don't wait for a sensory level—listen to the symptoms: a prospec-tive audit of the delays in diagnosis of malignant cord compression. Clin Oncol (R Coll Radiol) 2002; 14(6):472–80.

34. Mut M, Schiff D, Shaffrey ME. Metastasis to nervous system: spinal epidural and intramedullary metasta-ses. J Neurooncol 2005;75(1):43–56.

35. Botterell EH, Fitzgerald GW. Spinal cord compres-sion produced by extradural malignant tumours; early recognition, treatment and results. Can Med Assoc J 1959;80(10):791–6.

36. Loblaw DA, Laperriere NJ. Emergency treatment of malignant extradural spinal cord compression: an evidence-based guideline. J Clin Oncol 1998; 16(4):1613–24.

37. Maranzano E, Latini P. Effectiveness of radiation therapy without surgery in metastatic spinal cord compression: final results from a prospective trial. Int J Radiat Oncol Biol Phys 1995;32(4):959–67.

38. Fourney DR, Abi-Said D, Rhines LD, et al. Simulta-neous anterior-posterior approach to the thoracic and lumbar spine for the radical resection of tumors followed by reconstruction and stabilization. J Neu-rosurg 2001;94(2 Suppl):232–44.

39. Pascal-Moussellard H, Broc G, Pointillart V, et al. Complications of vertebral metastasis surgery. Eur Spine J 1998;7(6):438–44.

40. Wise JJ, Fischgrund JS, Herkowitz HN, et al. Com-plication, survival rates, and risk factors of surgery for metastatic disease of the spine. Spine 1999; 24(18):1943–51.

41. Abe E, Sato K, Tazawa H, et al. Total spondylectomy for primary tumor of the thoracolumbar spine. Spinal Cord 2000;38(3):146–52.

42. Heary RF, Vaccaro AR, Benevenia J, et al. "En-bloc" vertebrectomy in the mobile lumbar spine. Surg Neurol 1998;50(6):548–56.

43. Sundaresan N, DiGiacinto GV, Krol G, et al. Spondy-lectomy for malignant tumors of the spine. J Clin Oncol 1989;7(10):1485–91.

44. Tomita K, Kawahara N, Baba H, et al. Total en bloc spondylectomy for solitary spinal metastases. Int Or-thop 1994;18(5):291–8.

45. Boriani S, Biagini R, De Iure F, et al. En bloc resec-tions of bone tumors of the thoracolumbar spine. A preliminary report on 29 patients. Spine 1996; 21(16):1927–31.

46. Sciubba DM, Gokaslan ZL, Suk I, et al. Positive and negative prognostic variables for patients undergo-ing spine surgery for metastatic breast disease. Eur Spine J 2007;16(10):1659–67.

47. Tokuhashi Y, Matsuzaki H, Oda H, et al. A revised scor-ing system for preoperative evaluation of metastatic spine tumor prognosis. Spine 2005;30(19):2186–91.

48. Tomita K, Kawahara N, Kobayashi T, et al. Surgical strategy for spinal metastases. Spine 2001;26(3): 298–306.

49. Williams B, Fox B, Sciubba DM, et al. Surgical man-agement of metastatic prostate cancer to the spine. J Neurosurg Spine, in press.

50. Lis E, Bilsky MH, Pisinski L, et al. Percutaneous CT-guided biopsy of osseous lesion of the spine in pa-tients with known or suspected malignancy. AJNR Am J Neuroradiol 2004;25(9):1583–8.

51. Rimondi E, Staals EL, Errani C, et al. Percutaneous CT-guided biopsy of the spine: results of 430 biop-sies. Eur Spine J 2008;17(7):975–81.

52. McLain RF, Markman M, Bukowski RM, et al. Cancer in the Spine: Comprehensive Care. Totowa (NJ): Humana Press; 2006.

53. Klimo P Jr, PSchmidt MH. Surgical management of spinal metastases. Oncologist 2004;9(2):188–96.

54. Sioutos PJ, Arbit E, Meshulam CF, et al. Spinal me-tastases from solid tumors. Analysis of factors af-fecting survival. Cancer 1995;76(8):1453–9.

55. Tatsui H, Onomura T, Morishita S, et al. Survival rates of patients with metastatic spinal cancer after scinti-graphic detection of abnormal radioactive accumu-lation. Spine 1996;21(18):2143–8.

56. Rades D, Blach M, Nerreter V, et al. Metastatic spinal cord compression. Influence of time between onset of

motoric deficits and start of irradiation on therapeutic effect. Strahlenther Onkol 1999;175(8):378–81.

57. Simmons ED, Zheng Y. Vertebral tumors: surgical versus nonsurgical treatment. Clin Orthop Relat Res 2006;443:233–47.

58. Raizer JJ. The evolving role of radiosurgery for metastatic spine tumors. Nat Clin Pract Neurol 2007; 3(9):492–3.

59. Faul CM, Flickinger JC. The use of radiation in the management of spinal metastases. J Neurooncol 1995;23(2):149–61.

60. Ryu SI, Chang SD, Kim DH, et al. Image-guided hypo-fractionated stereotactic radiosurgery to spinal lesions. Neurosurgery 2001;49(4):838–46.

61. 8 Gy single fraction radiotherapy for the treatment of metastatic skeletal pain: randomised comparison with a multifraction schedule over 12 months of patient follow-up. Bone Pain Trial Working Party. Radiother Oncol 1999;52(2):111–21.

62. Gaze MN, Kelly CG, Kerr GR, et al. Pain relief and quality of life following radiotherapy for bone metastases: a randomised trial of two fractionation schedules. Radiother Oncol 1997;45(2):109–16.

63. Kaasa S, Brenne E, Lund JA, et al. Prospective randomised multicenter trial on single fraction radiotherapy (8 Gy × 1) versus multiple fractions (3 Gy × 10) in the treatment of painful bone metastases. Radiother Oncol 2006;79(3):278–84.

64. Nielsen OS, Bentzen SM, Sandberg E, et al. Randomized trial of single dose versus fractionated palliative radiotherapy of bone metastases. Radiother Oncol 1998;47(3):233–40.

65. Steenland E, Leer JW, van Houwelingen H, et al. The effect of a single fraction compared to multiple fractions on painful bone metastases: a global analysis of the Dutch bone metastasis study. Radiother Oncol 1999;52(2):101–9.

66. Chang EL, Shiu AS, Lii MF, et al. Phase I clinical evaluation of near-simultaneous computed tomographic image-guided stereotactic body radiotherapy for spinal metastases. Int J Radiat Oncol Biol Phys 2004;59(5):1288–94.

67. Ryu S, Fang Yin F, Rock J, et al. Image-guided and intensity-modulated radiosurgery for patients with spinal metastasis. Cancer 2003;97(8):2013–8.

68. Gerszten PC, Burton SA, Ozhasoglu C, et al. Radiosurgery for spinal metastases: clinical experience in 500 cases from a single institution. Spine 2007; 32(2):193–9.

69. Jin JY, Chen Q, Jin R, et al. Technical and clinical experience with spine radiosurgery: a new technology for management of localized spine metastases. Technol Cancer Res Treat 2007;6(2):127–33.

70. Ryu S, Jin JY, Jin R, et al. Partial volume tolerance of the spinal cord and complications of single-dose radiosurgery. Cancer 2007;109(3): 628–36.

71. Chang EL, Shiu AS, Mendel E, et al. Phase I/II study of stereotactic body radiotherapy for spinal metastasis and its pattern of failure. J Neurosurg Spine 2007;7(2):151–60.

72. Ryu S, Rock J, Rosenblum M, et al. Patterns of failure after single-dose radiosurgery for spinal metastasis. J Neurosurg 2004;(Suppl 3):402–5.

73. Romanelli P, Adler JR Jr. Technology insight: image-guided robotic radiosurgery–a new approach for noninvasive ablation of spinal lesions. Nat Clin Pract Oncol 2008;5(7):405–14.

74. Gerszten PC, Burton SA. Clinical assessment of stereotactic IGRT: spinal radiosurgery. Med Dosim 2008;33(2):107–16.

75. Burton AW, Hamid B. Kyphoplasty and vertebroplasty. Curr Pain Headache Rep 2008;12(1):22–7.

76. Aebli N, Goss BG, Thorpe P, et al. In vivo temperature profile of intervertebral discs and vertebral endplates during vertebroplasty: an experimental study in sheep. Spine 2006;31(15):1674–8 [Discussion: 9].

77. Pilitsis JG, Rengachary SS. The role of vertebroplasty in metastatic spinal disease. Neurosurg Focus 2001;11(6):e9.

78. Wu JC, Tang CT, Wu DL, et al. Treatment of adjacent vertebral fractures following multiple-level spinal fusion. Acta Neurochir Suppl 2008;101:153–5.

79. Cotten A, Dewatre F, Cortet B, et al. Percutaneous vertebroplasty for osteolytic metastases and myeloma: effects of the percentage of lesion filling and the leakage of methyl methacrylate at clinical follow-up. Radiology 1996;200(2):525–30.

80. Burton AW, Rhines LD, Mendel E. Vertebroplasty and kyphoplasty: a comprehensive review. Neurosurg Focus 2005;18(3):e1.

81. Choe DH, Marom EM, Ahrar K, et al. Pulmonary embolism of polymethyl methacrylate during percutaneous vertebroplasty and kyphoplasty. AJR Am J Roentgenol 2004;183(4):1097–102.

82. Chen YJ, Chang GC, Chen WH, et al. Local metastases along the tract of needle: a rare complication of vertebroplasty in treating spinal metastases. Spine 2007;32(21):E615–8.

83. Gerszten PC, Germanwala A, Burton SA, et al. Combination kyphoplasty and spinal radiosurgery: a new treatment paradigm for pathological fractures. J Neurosurg Spine 2005;3(4):296–301.

84. Gerszten PC, Germanwala A, Burton SA, et al. Combination kyphoplasty and spinal radiosurgery: a new treatment paradigm for pathological fractures. Neurosurg Focus 2005;18(3):e8.

85. Heary RF, Bono CM. Metastatic spinal tumors. Neurosurg Focus 2001;11(6):e1.

86. Byrne TN. Metastatic epidural cord compression. Curr Neurol Neurosci Rep 2004;4(3):191–5.

87. Mannion RJ, Wilby M, Godward S, et al. The surgical management of metastatic spinal disease: prospective

assessment and long-term follow-up. Br J Neurosurg 2007;21(6):593–8.

88. Wai EK, Finkelstein JA, Tangente RP, et al. Quality of life in surgical treatment of metastatic spine disease. Spine 2003;28(5):508–12.

89. Weigel B, Maghsudi M, Neumann C, et al. Surgical management of symptomatic spinal metastases. Postoperative outcome and quality of life. Spine 1999;24(21):2240–6.

90. Witham TF, Khavkin YA, Gallia GL, et al. Surgery insight: current management of epidural spinal cord compression from metastatic spine disease. Nat Clin Pract Neurol 2006;2(2):87–94 quiz 116.

91. Patchell RA, Tibbs PA, Regine WF, et al. Direct decompressive surgical resection in the treatment of spinal cord compression caused by metastatic cancer: a randomised trial. Lancet 2005;366(9486): 643–8.

92. Thomas KC, Nosyk B, Fisher CG, et al. Cost-effectiveness of surgery plus radiotherapy versus radiotherapy alone for metastatic epidural spinal cord compression. Int J Radiat Oncol Biol Phys 2006; 66(4):1212–8.

93. Ghogawala Z, Mansfield FL, Borges LF. Spinal radiation before surgical decompression adversely affects outcomes of surgery for symptomatic metastatic spinal cord compression. Spine 2001; 26(7):818–24.

94. Sakaura H, Hosono N, Mukai Y, et al. Outcome of total en bloc spondylectomy for solitary metastasis of the thoracolumbar spine. J Spinal Disord Tech 2004; 17(4):297–300.

Minimally Invasive Management of Spinal Metastases

Onder Ofluoglu, MD[a,b],*

KEYWORDS

- Spine • Metastasis • Minimally invasive treatment
- Vertebroplasty • Kyphoplasty • Thoracoscopy

The surgical treatments of spinal metastases remain controversial. Many local and systemic factors have to be considered in the treatment of metastatic lesions of the spine, including tumor type, extent of metastatic disease in the spine and the body, stability of the spine, neurologic status, comorbid conditions, and life expectancy of the patient. The standard open operations are suitable for patients in healthier conditions and with a longer life expectancy. The en bloc resections of solitary metastases of certain cancer types (kidney, breast, and thyroid) require conventional approaches. In most patients, the treatment is largely palliative and aims to achieve relief of pain and to regain function, thus improving the quality of the life of the patient as quickly as possible. Because of their immunocompromised status from ongoing chemotherapy, poor nutrition, and comorbid medical conditions, these patients cannot tolerate the conventional surgical methods.

Minimally invasive spinal interventions are reasonable alternatives to treat spinal metastatic disease. These procedures can result in less soft tissue trauma, lower blood loss, and shorter hospitalization time. These methods rarely interfere with the adjuvant treatments. The overall morbidity is considerably lower in comparison to conventional spine surgery.

PERCUTANEOUS VERTEBRAL AUGMENTATION: VERTEBROPLASTY AND KYPHOPLASTY

Vertebroplasty (VP) is a minimally invasive procedure that consists of image-guided percutaneous injection of bone cement into the vertebral body. Galibert and colleagues[1] first used the procedure for structural augmentation of a C2 vertebral body destroyed by an aggressive hemangioma. With a successful outcome, six more patients were treated with the same method, and these researchers reported their results. Because the short-term results were promising for pain relief and strengthening of mechanically compromised vertebra and the complication rates were low, the indications for the procedure were expanded widely to treat benign and malignant osteolytic lesions and osteoporotic fragility fractures.

Kyphoplasty (KP), also called balloon-assisted VP, was developed more recently. It involves an inflatable bone tamp to restore the original shape of the compressed vertebra before cement injection. Unlike VP, it offers more controlled and low-pressure cement injection into a previously created cavity to reduce the risk for extraosseous cement leak and subsequent complications.[2] Currently, both procedures are used widely.[3–7]

Indications and Patient Selection

Percutaneous vertebral augmentation (PVA) is regarded as a palliative procedure for the treatment of patients who have spinal metastasis and are not ideal candidates for conventional open surgery because of a limited life span (less than 3 months) or high risk for morbidity. Painful vertebral fractures and severe osteolysis with impending fracture related to benign (eg, hemangioma, eosinophilic granuloma) or malignant (eg,

ᵃ Department of Orthopedics, Lutfi Kirdar Research Hospital, Şemsi Denizer Cd. E-5 Karayolu Cevizli Mevkii 34890, Kartal, Istanbul, Turkey
ᵇ Cakmak m. Soyak Yenisehir Palmiye, C2 D27 Umraniye, Istanbul 34770, Turkey
* Cakmak m. Soyak Yenisehir Palmiye, C2 D27 Umraniye, Istanbul 34770, Turkey.
E-mail address: oofluoglu@gmail.com

Orthop Clin N Am 40 (2009) 155–168
doi:10.1016/j.ocl.2008.09.006

myeloma, metastasis) tumors constitute primary indications. PVA provides immediate stabilization and pain relief and dramatically improves the quality of the life in these patients. It is not indicated in patients with asymptomatic lesions or in patients who respond to medical therapy. Absolute contraindications are infection of the target vertebra(e), uncorrectable coagulopathy or hemorrhagic diathesis, and allergy to any component required for the procedure. Patients with progressive neurologic deficit from spinal cord compression should undergo surgical decompression.[8,9] Diffuse spinal pain attributable to disseminated metastases responds poorly to PVA.[10] Relative contraindications are radicular pain that is more severe than axial pain, lytic involvement of posterior cortex, and severe collapse of a vertebral body (more than two thirds of vertebral height).[9,10] Although involvement of the epidural space is also regarded as a relative contraindication by some investigators, successful results with low complication rates were reported.[5]

Preprocedural Evaluation

A detailed clinical history and examination with specific emphasis on neurologic signs and symptoms to rule out other causes, such as degenerative spondylosis or radiculopathy, are necessary. It is also important to differentiate between malignant vertebral compression fractures and osteoporotic or metastatic fractures. Imaging studies in patients who have spinal tumors include plain radiographs; MRI, particularly T1, T2, and short tau inversion recovery sequences; CT; and bone scans.[4,11,12] Whole-spine MRI is indicated in patients with suspected cord compression, because the additional information may alter the management plan, such as multilevel metastatic fractures.[13] Not all affected levels may require treatment, and it is crucial to distinguish the symptomatic level(s). Contrast-enhanced MRI should be acquired when the unenhanced appearances do not correlate with the clinical findings or when they suggest intradural or intramedullary disease.[14]

Technique of the Procedure

An anesthesiologist must monitor the patient during the procedure, and surgical and resuscitative backup must be available. In most cases, the procedure can be done under local anesthesia with conscious sedation. This provides feedback from the patient from cement leakage, because there may be a change in the quality or severity of pain or change in the neurologic status.[5] Prophylactic antibiotics are administered before the procedure.

In immunocompromised patients, the use of antibiotic-impregnated cement may be considered.

The cervical spine can be approached by an anterolateral route. A right-sided approach is preferred to avoid the esophagus. The carotid-jugular complex is pushed laterally and downward and separated from the trachea and esophagus. The upper cervical vertebrae (C1–C4) can be accessed by a direct lateral approach, anterior to the vertebral artery and posterior to the carotid artery.[15] A posterior approach to C1 after occlusion of the involved vertebral artery to prevent vertebrobasilar embolism has been described.[16] The second cervical vertebra can be accessed by a transoral approach. This procedure carries a high risk for infection and requires disinfection of the pharyngeal mucosa and pre- and postoperative antibiotic coverage.[17]

In the upper and midthoracic regions, a parapedicular approach can be used because the pedicles are too small. Here, the needle is positioned between the posterior surface of the neck of the rib and the anterior surface of the transverse process. The parapedicular approach carries a higher risk for pneumothorax and paraspinous hematoma than a transpedicular approach.[10,18,19] In the lumbar vertebra, a transpedicular or posterolateral approach (if the pedicles are involved by tumor or cannot be visualized during fluoroscopy) is used (**Fig. 1**).

Cement can be applied by means of unilateral or bilateral needles. Bilateral application is recommended in thoracic and lumbar vertebrae. It is not advisable to fill the whole tumoral cavity because of the risk for displacing the neoplastic tissue into the canal.[3] In the cervical vertebrae, a single needle centered on a lytic lesion permits good filling. Sacroplasty requires multiple injections depending on the topographic features of the lesions.

In neoplastic conditions, PVA is best done under dual guidance with a combination of fluoroscopy and CT (**Fig. 2**).[20] CT can demonstrate the small cement leaks much better than fluoroscopy. Especially in patients with epidural tumoral involvement, small cement leaks may be symptomatic. CT is also helpful to visualize upper thoracic vertebrae commonly obscured by the shoulders on fluoroscopy. Similarly, for applications of cervical or sacral tumors, CT imaging is preferred.[16]

Effect on Pain Relief

The retrospective and prospective studies have shown that VP and KP resulted in marked reduction of spinal pain in approximately 90% of the

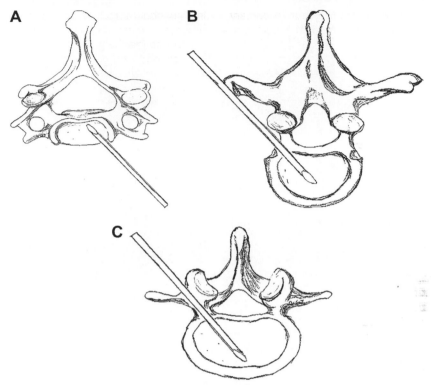

Fig. 1. Percutaneous VP: anterolateral (*A*), transcostovertebral (*B*), and transpedicular (*C*) approaches to cervical, lumbar, and thoracic vertebrae.

patients.[2,6,21–23] Analgesic efficacy remained stable up to 1 year in most cases (**Table 1**).

Fourney and colleagues[24] retrospectively reviewed 97 (65 VP and 32 KP) procedures in a group of patients who had cancer (21 who had myeloma and 35 who had other malignancies). All patients had intractable spinal pain. Patients noted marked or complete pain relief after 49 procedures (84%) and no change in the rest. Reductions in visual analog scale pain scores remained significant for up to 1 year.

The mechanism of pain relief after PVA is not clearly understood. The analgesic effect of VP may derive from immobilization of trabecular microfractures by cement injection, thus regaining vertebral strength and stiffness.[3,6] The chemical and thermal cytotoxicity of bone cement may also cause necroses of tumor tissue and nerve endings in the surrounding bone.[25,26] The strength and stiffness of involved vertebrae are weakly correlated with the percentage fill-volume of cement injected during VP. It was demonstrated that to restore strength, 16.2% cement fill of the affected vertebral body was sufficient and that to restore stiffness, 29.8% cement fill of the affected vertebral body was sufficient.[27] Cement injection in the amount of 2 mL could restore strength,

whereas larger volumes (4 mL in thoracic and thoracolumbar areas and 6–8 mL in the lumbar spine) were necessary to restore stiffness.[27,28]

Complications

The frequency of complications of PVA procedures is higher in patients who have tumors (5%–10%) than in patients who have osteoporotic fractures (1%–3%) or hemangiomas (2%–5%).[29,30] This is correlated with the frequency of cortical breakdown in metastatic lesions.[5,6,26] The most common minor complications are infection; fracture of the ribs, posterior vertebral elements, and pedicles; allergic reaction; bleeding; and hematoma formation at the puncture site.

Cement Leak

The common pattern of cement extravasation in osteoporotic fractures is intradiscal. In metastatic lesions, however, cement may leak into various locations because of cortical breakdown. In most cases, cement extravasation does not cause symptoms or clinical problems. Cotten and colleagues[26] performed VP in 40 patients who had metastases or multiple myeloma. Tumoral

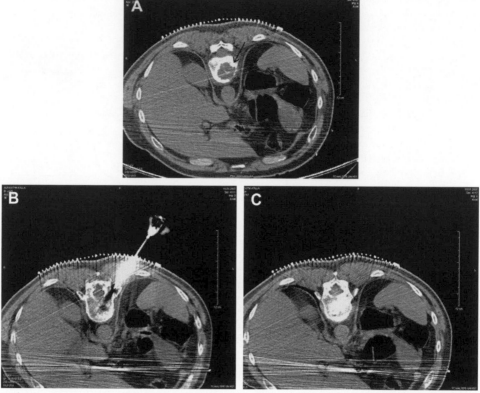

Fig. 2. CT-guided VP for painful spinal metastasis in a patient who has lung cancer. (*A*) Osteolytic compression fracture of T7. (*B*) Percutaneous VP by a transcostovertebral approach. (*C*) Cement filling into the tumoral cavity without leakage.

involvement of the epidural space and neural foramina was noted in 17 patients at presentation. These researchers evaluated the patients with CT after the procedure and detected cement leaks in 29 of 40 patients. Most of the leaks were located in paravertebral tissue (21 leaks), followed by leaks in the spinal canal, neural foramina, adjacent disks, and lumbar venous plexus. Despite the high rate of cement leaks, only 2 patients with a foraminal leak underwent decompressive surgery.[26]

Barragán-Campos and colleagues[31] performed VP in 117 patients who had metastatic lesions

Table 1				
Pain response after percutaneous vertebral augmentation in spinal metastases				
Study	Procedure	No. Patients	No. Procedures	Patients with Excellent / Good Pain Relief (%)
Weil and colleagues[6]	VP	37	52	94
Cotten and colleagues[25]	VP	37	40	97
Fourney and colleagues[23]	VP-KP	56	97	84
Alvarez and colleagues[20]	VP	21	27	81
Dudeney and colleagues[2]	KP	18	55	100
Pflugmacher and colleagues[40]	KP	31	64	100
Appel and Gilula[21]	VP	23	27	87
Calmels and colleagues[22]	VP	52	103	92
Total		275	465	91.8

and identified a total of 423 instances of leakage of cement from the 304 treated vertebrae. Three hundred thirty-two (78.5%) leakages were located in the venous network, which were classified as vascular leakages. More than half of the vascular leakages were located in epidural veins or paravertebral plexus. The remaining 91 leakages (21.5%) were nonvascular. Among the 423 cement leaks in 117 patients, only 8 resulted in (6.8%) complications: 6 (5.1%) local and 2 (1.7%) systemic. Four patients developed radicular pain that responded to medical therapy. Two pulmonary emboli associated with cement migration through the vena cava were observed, one of which resulted in death.[31]

The incidence of pulmonary cement embolism was reported to be relatively higher (4.6%) when patients were routinely screened by chest radiography.[32] Although the cement embolism is asymptomatic in most cases, reports of potentially life-threatening cases have been getting attention.[33,34] The frequency of this complication may increase secondary to the widespread use of these percutaneous procedures. Because there is no existent therapy for cement embolism, prophylactic measures (eg, using a smaller volume of cement injection, avoiding multiple injections in the same session, low-pressure cement injection, use of high-viscose bone cement) is the only way to avoid this complication.

Neurologic complications associated with epidural, intradural, foraminal, and perivertebral cement extravasation can be seen. Of those, foraminal leaks are most likely to be symptomatic and may require surgical decompression. Although small asymptomatic cement leaks into the epidural space are common in PVA, cord compression resulting in neurologic impairment is rare (0.1%). The cement leak is seen especially in cases with tumoral destruction of the posterior wall.[35]

Intraosseous venography was used for predicting polymethylmethacrylate (PMMA) flow characteristics within the vertebral body and potential undesirable sites of cement deposition, such as through cortical defects and within venous structures.[36] The results regarding the utility of the antecedent venography in determining improved clinical outcomes or decreased complications during VP are conflicting, however.

The subsequent fractures of adjacent level vertebrae after PVA are a potential complication, probably related to an increase in stiffness of treated vertebrae. The risk for adjacent level fracture is greater in patients undergoing KP than in patients undergoing VP.[37] The risk for subsequent fractures in patients who have myeloma and

undergo KP was 23% at 18 months of follow-up and was higher than that of osteoporosis (12.5% per year).[9]

Because PVA is not an ablative procedure, the use of adjuvant radiotherapy to prevent tumoral progress and related complications is recommended in radiosensitive tumors.[38]

Vertebroplasty Versus Kyphoplasty

Currently, there are no prospective randomized or nonrandomized controlled trials to compare the efficacy of the methods. Both procedures were shown to be safe and effective to achieve pain control and spinal stabilization. Laboratory and clinical studies showed that the KP generated better height compensation than VP in osteoporotic vertebrae.[39] Similar results were reported in patients who had myeloma and metastatic lesions.[2,40,41] It was also suggested that KP is associated with a lower risk for cement extravasation than VP (7% versus 19.7%) because of low-pressure fill of higher viscosity cement into the created cavity.[7,42] KP is a more expensive, complex, and time-consuming procedure than VP. As previously stated, there is a lack of strong scientific evidence to support one technique over the other in metastatic conditions. VP can be preferred in patients with minimal collapse of the vertebra or vertebra plana that is unlikely to gain height. VP is also the safer procedure if the posterior wall of the vertebra is destroyed by the tumor so as to avoid further displacement of the fragments or tumor by inflation of the balloon. In patients with multiple wedge fractures of the vertebrae, KP is a reasonable option.[2,3]

PERCUTANEOUS RADIOFREQUENCY ABLATION

Image-guided radiofrequency ablation (RFA) is used to treat the benign (osteoid osteoma) and metastatic spinal neoplasms. The procedures are performed using partially insulated electrodes placed under CT guidance. When attached to an appropriate radiofrequency (RF) generator, RF current is emitted from the noninsulated portion (ie, exposed tip) of the active electrode and the current attempts to find the path to the ground. The current passing through the tissue from the active electrode leads to ion agitation, which is converted to heat as a result of the friction. The process of cellular heating induces immediate and irreparable cellular damage, which leads to coagulation necrosis. Because ion agitation, and thus tissue heating, is greatest in areas of highest current density (ie, closest to the active electrode tip), necrosis is limited to a relatively small volume of tissue surrounding the RF electrode.[43]

For spinal metastasis, RFA is a useful tool to reduce pain and related disability in patients with end-stage disease for whom there are no other options. The procedure is performed under a combination of conscious sedation and local anesthesia and is fairly well tolerated (**Fig. 3**). Pain reduction occurs within the first 24 hours for some and in the first week in most patients. The proposed mechanisms by which RFA decreases pain may involve pain transmission inhibition by destroying sensory nerve fibers in the periosteum and bone cortex; reduction of lesion volume with decreased stimulation of sensory nerve fibers; destruction of tumor cells that are producing nerve-stimulating cytokines (eg, tumor necrosis factor-α [TNFα], interleukins) and inhibition of osteoclast activity.[44]

In spite of a large number of skeletal lesions treated with RFA, only a limited number of reports have been published concerning the treatment of spinal neoplasms. The lesions within 1 cm of the spinal cord were considered ineligible because of the risk for thermal injury to the spinal cord.[45] Ex vivo studies demonstrated the decreased heat transmission in cancellous bone and an insulative effect of the cortical bone.[46]

Nakatsuka and colleagues[47] reported the largest series: 17 patients who had spinal metastases treated with RFA, with a high technical and clinical success rate of up to 96%. Four patients (24%) experienced neurologic complications because of the proximity of the lesions to the posterior cortex or pedicles. A later study was published by the same group on the safety and clinical utility of bone RFA with real-time monitoring of the spinal canal temperature for the treatment of spinal tumors located 1 cm or less from the spinal cord. The thermocouple was placed in the spinal canal under CT fluoroscopic guidance, and RFA application was stopped when the spinal canal temperature reached 45°C. In 9 of the 10 patients, the spinal canal temperature did not exceed 45°C. In the remaining patient, the temperature rose to 48°C, resulting in transient neural damage. Clinical success was achieved within 1 week in all patients.[48]

Buy and colleagues[45] described saline-infused bipolar RFA. In this technique, one electrode was thermally shielded by the opposing second electrode, which also actively heats nearby tissue. The heat is trapped between the two electrodes,

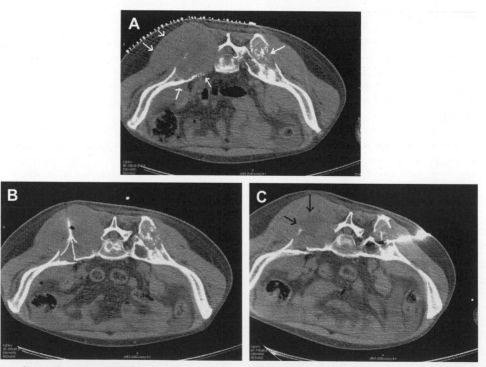

Fig. 3. RFA of sacroiliac metastasis in a patient who has end-stage pancreatic cancer. (*A*) Large soft tissue mass of the left posterior iliac spine extends into the sacroiliac joint and spinal canal. Metastatic involvement of the opposite side and ascites are noted (*arrows*). (*B*) RFA with a starburst electrode (RITA Medical Systems, Mountain View, California) was placed on bone-tumor interfaces and on the soft tissue part of the tumor. (*C*) Procedure was repeated for the other side. Note the central necrosis of the tumor mass immediately after ablation (*arrows*). There was considerable pain relief after the procedure.

obviating diversion of current from the ablation site to any other direction. High-concentration saline infusion was used to increase energy conductivity, limiting tissue carbonization around the electrodes, and thus reducing tissue impedance. No major complications were observed even in cases with involvement of the posterior wall and soft tissue around the vertebral body with destruction of the cortex.

In patients with spinal instability, the combination of RFA and PVA results in stable and painless vertebrae. RFA before PVA may reduce the risk for cement extravasation by destroying the tumoral tissue and thrombosing the paravertebral and intravertebral venous plexus.[49–51]

MINIMALLY INVASIVE SPINAL SURGERY

The surgical treatment of spinal metastases was restricted to decompressive laminectomy until 1980s; however, significant failures were reported because of progressive instability. In more recent years, circumferential decompression and stabilization are being used by means of posterior and anterior or posterolateral approaches. Although the results are more favorable than laminectomy, the surgical morbidity of the procedure is high, especially in patients who have immunocompromised and comorbid conditions. Preoperative radiotherapy is also a risk factor for wound healing. Therefore, the minimally invasive surgery (MIS) of spine tumors was introduced to minimize surgical trauma to soft tissue and to accelerate postoperative recovery without losing the surgical effectiveness.

Essentially, endoscopic approaches, including thoracoscopic and laparoscopic techniques and mini-open surgeries for the treatment of spinal pathologic conditions, have been described. Patients with single or adjacent level involvement with neurologic symptoms from tumor compression or vertebral collapse who have a life expectancy of at least 3 months are considered as candidates for MIS. Because the resection is all intralesional in MIS, the procedure is not appropriate for the treatment of primary tumors or a solitary metastasis, which may benefit from en bloc resection.

Endoscopic Surgery

Video-assisted thoracoscopic surgery
The video-assisted thoracoscopic surgery (VATS) procedure provides visualization and magnification of the entire ventral spine from T1 to T12 without the need for open thoracotomy. In comparison to open thoracotomy, pulmonary morbidity is lower and the mechanics of chest wall motion are better in thoracoscopy because of reduced

surgical trauma and resultant pain.[52] Thoracoscopy avoids scapular dysfunction and may decrease the incidence of intercostal neuralgia. The spine can be decompressed, reconstructed, and stabilized by means of a thoracoscopic approach.

Mack and colleagues[53] first reported the use of VATS for the treatment of spinal disorders in 1993. These researchers performed VATS on various conditions that included the drainage of spinal abscesses, biopsy of vertebral bodies, discectomy for a herniated nucleus pulposus, and anterior releases for kyphoscoliosis.[53] More recently, the procedure was modified so that vertebrectomy, vertebral body reconstruction, and stabilization can be performed.[54] In 1996, Rosenthal and colleagues[55] described anterior spinal decompression and stabilization by means of a thoracoscopic approach in four patients with progressive neurologic dysfunction and pain attributable to metastatic spinal involvement. All the patients were ambulatory, and their preoperative neurologic deficits improved after resection of the tumor, decompression of the cord, and reconstruction with autologous bone or bone cement followed by stabilization with an anterior plate.[55]

Surgical technique
The surgery is performed in a large operating room because the procedure requires a large number of personnel and equipment, including C-arm fluoroscopy, endoscopic devices, video monitors, and an instrument table. A double-lumen endotracheal tube is inserted for selective collapse of the lung on the involved side. The patient is positioned in a lateral decubitus position with the tumor mass directed upward. The number, position, and size of the portals depend on the surgeon's preference and location of the tumor. First, a blunt trocar is inserted, passing through the intercostal muscles over the superior surface of the rib. This is the only portal inserted without visual control, and it has to be done with caution. It is usually positioned at the fifth or sixth intercostal space between the middle and posterior axillary lines. The thoracic cavity is entered and inspected, followed by release of any pleural adhesions. The affected segment is identified visually if obvious or is confirmed radiographically (fluoroscopy or plain radiographs). At this stage, the operating table is tilted approximately 30° toward the surgeon to facilitate displacement of the lung and mediastinal structures. The next portal is placed, based on the location of the tumor, at the midaxillary line above or below the first portal. The third portal is usually placed slightly ventral to the others at the ninth or tenth intercostal space. These working channels are introduced under visual control to

minimize injuries to the mediastinal structures. The parietal pleura are sectioned, starting at the medial aspect of the affected vertebra and extending cranially and caudally to reach uninvolved segments. The diaphragm can be opened if extension of exposure lower than the insertion of the diaphragm is necessary. The corpectomy is performed starting with discectomy one level below and above the involved vertebra, followed by removal of the tumor from the periphery to the center of the vertebral body until the posterior longitudinal ligament is reached. The ligament is opened, and decompression of the dural sac and spinal cord is completed. Reconstruction and stabilization are performed depending on the size of the defect and surgeon's preference.[56,57]

In the upper thoracic region, working portals are placed in the third or fourth intercostal space. The first two intercostal spaces are avoided because of the risks to axillary neurovascular structures. The endoscope is introduced more posteriorly in the fourth intercostal space anterior to the latissimus dorsi muscle. Le Huec and colleagues[58] described an alternative endoscopic approach for levels T1 to T3. These investigators added an endoscope to a Smith-Robinson incision to provide visualization of the T1 to T3 levels, therefore being less invasive than previously described techniques. Two patients who had spine metastasis underwent the resection and strut graft fixation. A satisfactory neurologic decompression, confirmed by improvement of the postoperative Frankel's score, was achieved in both patients.[58]

Huang and colleagues[59] treated 12 patients who had anterior spinal pathologic findings in the thoracolumbar junction using a three-portal or modified two-portal technique. The size of the thoracoscopic portals was greater than usual to perform conventional spinal instrumentation. Eight patients in this series presented with metastatic lesions. The procedure was completed successfully in all but two patients. In one patient, the procedure was converted to open surgery because of pleural adhesions from a previous operation. Massive bleeding was reported in the other patient who had renal cell carcinoma, resulting in an incomplete corpectomy.

Laparoscopic retroperitoneal approach to the thoracolumbar spine

The endoscopic approach to the lumbar spine can be performed by a combination of thoracoscopic and laparoscopic approaches. In this technique, an initial portal is introduced into right seventh intercostal space after the right lung is deflated. The junction of right twelfth costal cartilage is exposed under direct vision until retroperitoneal fat

can be seen. The origin balloon is used to dissect retroperitoneal space by introducing saline (1 L) into a distensible balloon. The balloon is subsequently deflated, and insufflation of carbon dioxide (CO_2) is performed in the retroperitoneum. The diaphragm can be visualized from its superior and inferior aspects and is transected. Once the diaphragm is cut, the air seal is lost and thoracoscopic instruments can be introduced into the lumbar spine. Optimal exposure is obtained by retracting the lung, diaphragm, and retroperitoneal contents. The corpectomy, reconstruction, and anterior stabilization can then be performed (Fig. 4).[56]

Limitations and contraindications of the thoracoscopic approach

The surgical team and the anesthesia team must be familiar with the procedure. Patients with severe pulmonary dysfunction cannot tolerate the procedure because it requires a prolonged period of single-lung ventilation. Extensive pleural adhesions attributable to radiotherapy, previous surgery, or trauma may also complicate the procedure, and other approaches may be chosen (eg, conventional thoracotomy, posterolateral decompression). The procedure is contraindicated in the presence of pachypleuritis and contralateral pneumonectomy.[57,60]

Complications

Although the number of thoracoscopic procedures has increased, most spine surgeons have limited experience with the procedure. This is because it is not widely accepted as a routine procedure and has a steep learning curve, prolonged surgical time, problems with intraoperative bleeding-control, and lack of specific endoscopic equipment.[61] The simpler or moderately complex pathologic conditions (ie, sympathectomy, moderate-sized disk herniation, paraspinal tumors) can be treated with an acceptable complication rate; however, thoracoscopic decompression of metastatic tumors and subsequent spinal reconstruction may be associated with higher rates of complications.[52]

Huang and colleagues[61] evaluated 90 patients treated with thoracoscopy. Of those, 41 patients had spine metastases and experienced a higher rate and more severe complications than the others. Intraoperative bleeding (>2 L) occurred in 5 of 41 patients and was the most common complication. It was noted that the sources of bleeding were epidural veins, tumor feeding vessels, and intercostal vessels. Two of the patients who had metastasis died (the first patient from complications of coagulopathy and respiratory failure and the

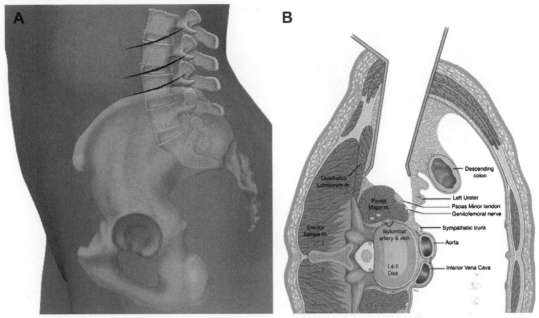

Fig. 4. Endoscopic retroperitoneal approach to the lumbar spine. (*A*) Localization of skin incisions as determined with fluoroscopy. (*B*) Axial schematic representation demonstrates anatomic considerations. (*From* Kim DH, Jaikumar S, Kam AC. Minimally invasive spine instrumentation. Neurosurgery 2002;51(Suppl):S21; with permission.)

other from postoperative pneumonia and sepsis) from the complications. Intercostal neuralgia (3 patients), superficial wound infection (3 patients), pharyngeal pain (3 patients), atelectasis (2 patients), inadvertent pericardial penetration (1 patient), and graft dislodgement and implant failure (1 patient) were the other complications noted in patients who had metastatic lesions.

Endoscopy-assisted posterolateral decompression

This technique is recommended in patients who need combined posterior and anterior stabilization because of poor bone quality.[62] Additionally, the patients who have upper and lower thoracic lesions or extensive pleural adhesions in which thoracoscopic access is difficult can be treated.

In this technique, endoscopy is used to achieve better neural decompression than is achieved by the standard posterolateral approach in the thoracic spine. The procedure begins with a midline posterior incision and incorporates a costotransversectomy approach combined with a standard transpedicular approach. Anterior tumor is removed under direct vision until a cavity is formed in the vertebral body. A 4-mm 30° scope is then introduced to visualize the posterior vertebral cortex, floor of the spinal canal, and any tissues just anterior to the cord. Decompression of the cord is followed by corpectomy. The procedure is

completed by anterior spinal reconstruction and posterior stabilization (**Fig. 5**).

McLain[62] successfully treated nine tumor cases with endoscopy-assisted posterolateral decompression, including four with upper thoracic involvement. Six patients with preoperative neurologic deficit recovered completely.[62]

Minimal Access Spine Surgery

Despite its advantages, endoscopic surgeries have not been used in common surgical practice in the spine. These techniques are noted as having a steep learning curve and require adequate training before performance. Prolonged operative times and substantial bleeding may be encountered frequently because of complexity of the procedure. Expensive equipment is necessary for endoscopic setup. Therefore, the initial enthusiasm for endoscopic anterior spinal procedures has drifted to minimally access posterior and anterior approaches.[63–65] Compared with endoscopic surgery, mini-open anterior lumbar surgery is easier to learn and less expensive, and it offers safer mobilization of neurovascular structures, faster decompression of the spinal canal, and easier reconstruction of the anterior column under three-dimensional direct vision.[66]

Minimal access surgery (MAS) was initially developed for the treatment of spinal trauma,

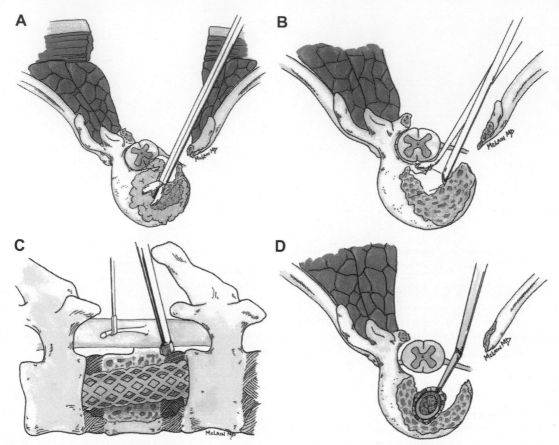

Fig. 5. (*A*) Endoscopy-assisted posterolateral approach. (*B*) Removal of the tumor and cancellous bone after resection of the pedicle and medial rib under direct vision. (*C*) Removal of the whole tumor tissue and posterior cortex under endoscopic visualization. (*D*) Reconstruction of the cavity with a cage. (*From* McLain RF. Spinal cord decompression: an endoscopically assisted approach for metastatic tumors. Spinal Cord 2001;39:483,485; with permission.)

deformity, or degeneration. In 1997, Mayer[67] described the microsurgical approach to cover all lumbar levels from L2 to S1. Twenty-five patients were treated with mini-open retroperitoneal (20 patients) or transperitoneal (5 patients) anterior lumbar fusion. No systemic or technique-related complications were reported. The morbidity of the procedure was low, and all the patients showed solid bone fusion.[67] Similar results have been reported subsequently.[66,68]

Surgical techniques

Mini-open thoracotomy The patient is placed in the right or left lateral decubitus position depending on the location and extent of the tumor. Generally, the right-sided approach is used for the upper thoracic region, and the left-sided approach is used for the thoracolumbar junction. The procedure begins with radiologic identification of the affected vertebral body. A 5- to 10-cm skin incision is

made over the rib. After subperiosteal exposure, 5 to 10 cm of the rib is resected and the lung is deflated. The parietal pleura are opened, and the lung is pushed medially with surgical sponges.[64,65] An alternative approach performed without resection of the rib and lung deflation was described by Kossmann and colleagues[64] A specially designed table-mounted retractor system is required to facilitate exposure and surgery. After the thoracic cavity is exposed, the corpectomy and reconstruction are performed (**Fig. 6**). In the thoracolumbar junction, a combined transthoracic-transdiaphragmatic approach is used from T12 to L2. The lesser invasive approach, the "extracoelomic miniapproach," avoiding the peritoneal and pleural cavities, was also described.[69]

Retroperitoneal miniapproach This approach is used for access to L3 and L4. The level of the affected vertebra was identified by fluoroscopy and marked laterally on the flank. A left-sided

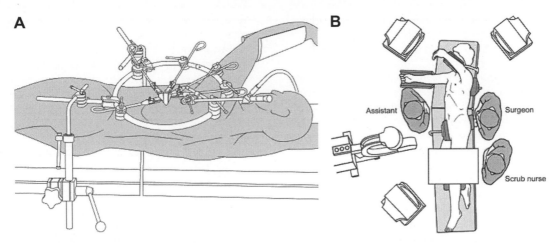

Fig. 6. (*A*) Access to upper thoracic vertebra by a special table-mounted anterior retractor in a mini-open thoracotomy. (*B*) Surgical setup for the procedure. (*From* Kossmann T, Jacobi D, Trentz O. The use of a retractor system (SynFrame) for open, minimal invasive reconstruction of the anterior column of the thoracic and lumbar spine. Euro Spine J 2001;10:398; with permission.)

approach is preferred. The surgery starts with a 4- to 6-cm incision. The external and internal oblique muscles with their fascia are opened. After dividing the transversus abdominis muscle and pushing the underlying peritoneum, the retroperitoneal space is entered. Further medial retraction of the peritoneum exposes the quadratus lumborum and psoas muscles. The retractor is inserted as medial blades retract the peritoneal sac medially: one blade retracts the rib cage cranially, and one blade retracts the abdominal muscle medially. The ureter is retracted medially with the visceral peritoneum. The ilioinguinal and iliohypogastric nerves may cross the surgical field and should be preserved. The psoas muscle is mobilized and pushed laterally. The table is tilted toward the surgeon to ease access. The retractor is readjusted to aid in the exposure during the corpectomy and to protect the vessels and visceral organs. The spinal reconstruction and stabilization are then performed similar to the open procedure.[64,65]

Although the experience of MAS in patients who have a tumor is limited, encouraging results have been reported. Kossmann and colleagues[64] treated 65 patients who had various spinal pathologic conditions by minithoracotomy or the retroperitoneal approach. Six patients had metastatic lesions. After corpectomy, reconstruction of the anterior column was performed with expandable cages or plates filled with bone cement. The operation time was short (112 minutes on average), and blood loss was minimal in most of the patients. No intra- or postoperative complications related to the procedure were observed. One patient who had multiple metastases died during surgery as the result of an acute thromboembolic event.

Huang and colleagues[63] compared the results of open thoracotomy versus minithoracotomy in patients who had thoracic spinal metastasis involving T3 to T12 vertebrae. Twenty-nine patients had a minithoracotomy, and 17 had a standard thoracotomy. The mean operative time, blood loss, and time required for postoperative chest tube retention were found to be similar for both groups. Postoperative intensive care unit stays were significantly shorter for the minithoracotomy group, however. Neurologic improvement and overall survival rates were also similar for both groups.

Payer and Sottas[65] recently reported the results of mini-open anterior corpectomy in 37 patients (26 who had fractures and 11 who had tumors). Posterior fixation was performed as a first step in all the patients, followed by anterior surgery during the same anesthesia session for tumor cases and postponed 7 to 10 days for trauma patients. Average blood loss was 711 mL in patients who had a tumor. Six perioperative complications were encountered from the anterior approach, including dural tear, pneumothorax, paralytic ileus, inguinal hypoesthesia, and superficial infection. Neurologic status improved in 20 of 22 patients.

SUMMARY

The minimally invasive treatment of spinal metastases is increasingly preferred in patients who are not able to tolerate open surgery or who have a limited life expectancy Image-guided percutaneous interventions, VP, and KP afford effective pain palliation and regaining of the strength and stiffness of involved vertebrae. The main concern is cement leakage and related complications. KP provides low-pressure injection and may reduce the complications related to cement leak.

RFA is another effective method to reduce pain and related disability in patients who have end-stage disease for whom there are no other options. Its combination with VP can reduce the risk for cement leak while providing immediate stability.

Minimally invasive surgical techniques are attractive options in patients with neurologic symptoms from tumor compression or vertebral collapse. The functional and oncologic results are comparable to those of conventional open procedures, whereas surgical morbidity from the procedure is lower. The mini-open approaches have gained more popularity recently because the endoscopic approaches have a steep learning curve and require special and costly equipment.

REFERENCES

1. Galibert P, Deramond H, Rosat P, et al. Preliminary note on the treatment of vertebral angioma by percutaneous acrylic vertebroplasty. Neurochirurgie 1987; 33(2):166–8.
2. Dudeney S, Lieberman IH, Reinhardt MK, et al. Kyphoplasty in the treatment of osteolytic vertebral compression fractures as a result of multiple myeloma. J Clin Oncol 2002;20(9):2382–7.
3. Carrino JA, Chan R, Vaccaro AR. Vertebral augmentation: vertebroplasty and kyphoplasty. Semin Roentgenol 2004;39(1):68–84.
4. Jakobs TF, Trumm C, Reiser M, et al. Percutaneous vertebroplasty in tumoral osteolysis. Eur Radiol 2007;17(8):2166–75.
5. Shimony JS, Gilula LA, Zeller AJ, et al. Percutaneous vertebroplasty for malignant compression fractures with epidural involvement. Radiology 2004;232(3): 846–53.
6. Weill A, Chiras J, Simon JM, et al. Spinal metastases: indications for and results of percutaneous injection of acrylic surgical cement. Radiology 1996;199(1): 241–7.
7. Binning MJ, Gottfried ON, Klimo P Jr, et al. Minimally invasive treatments for metastatic tumors of the spine. Neurosurg Clin N Am 2004;15(4):459–65.
8. Wise JJ, Fischgrund JS, Herkowitz HN, et al. Complication, survival rates, and risk factors of surgery for metastatic disease of the spine. Spine 1999;24(18): 1943–51.
9. Lieberman I, Reinhardt MK. Vertebroplasty and kyphoplasty for osteolytic vertebral collapse. Clin Orthop Relat Res 2003;(415 Suppl):S176–86.
10. Mathis JM. Percutaneous vertebroplasty: procedure technique. In: Mathis JM, Deramond H, Belkoff SM, editors. Percutaneous vertebroplasty and kyphoplasty. 2nd edition. New York: Springer; 2006. p. 112–33.
11. Yu SW, Chen WJ, Lin WC, et al. Serious pyogenic spondylitis following vertebroplasty. Spine 2004; 29(10):209–11.
12. Halpin RJ, Bendok BR, Liu JC. Minimally invasive treatments for spinal metastases: vertebroplasty, kyphoplasty, and radiofrequency ablation. J Support Oncol 2004;2(4):339–51.
13. Husband DJ, Grant KA, Romaniuk CS. MRI in the diagnosis and treatment of suspected malignant spinal cord compression. Br J Radiol 2001;74(877): 15–23.
14. Loughrey GJ, Collins CD, Todd SM, et al. Magnetic resonance imaging in management of suspected spinal canal disease in patients with known malignancy. Clin Radiol 2000;55(11):849–55.
15. Huegli RW, Schaeren S, Jacob AL, et al. Percutaneous cervical vertebroplasty in a multifunctional image-guided therapy suite: hybrid lateral approach to C1 and C4 under CT and fluoroscopic guidance. Cardiovasc Intervent Radiol 2005;28(5):649–52.
16. Wetzel SG, Martin JB, Somon T, et al. Painful osteolytic metastasis of the atlas: treatment with percutaneous vertebroplasty. Spine 2002;27(22):E493–5.
17. Monterumici DA, Narne S, Nena U, et al. Transoral kyphoplasty for tumors in C2. Spine J 2007;7(6): 666–70.
18. Boszczyk BM, Bierschneider M, Hauck S, et al. Transcostovertebral kyphoplasty of mid and high thoracic spine. Eur Spine J 2005;14(10):992–9.
19. Beall DP, Braswell JJ, Martin HD, et al. Technical strategies and anatomic considerations for parapedicular access to thoracic and lumbar vertebral bodies. Skeletal Radiol 2007;36(1):47–52.
20. Gangi A, Guth S, Imbert JP, et al. Percutaneous vertebroplasty: indications, technique and results. Radiographics 1998;18(3):621–33.
21. Alvarez L, Pérez-Higueras A, Quiñones D, et al. Vertebroplasty in the treatment of vertebral tumors: post procedural outcome and quality of life. Eur Spine J 2003;12(4):356–60.
22. Appel NB, Gilula LA. Percutaneous vertebroplasty in patients with spinal canal compromise. AJR Am J Roentgenol 2004;182(4):947–51.
23. Calmels V, Vallée JN, Rose M, et al. Osteoblastic and mixed spinal metastases: evaluation of the analgesic efficacy of percutaneous vertebroplasty. AJNR Am J Neuroradiol 2007;28(3):570–4.
24. Fourney DR, Schomer DF, Nader R, et al. Percutaneous vertebroplasty and kyphoplasty for painful vertebral body fractures in cancer patients. J Neurosurg 2003;98(1 Suppl):21–30.
25. Belkoff SM, Molloy S. Temperature measurements during polymerization of polymethylmethacrylate cement used for vertebroplasty. Spine 2003;28(14): 1555–9.

26. Cotten A, Dewatre F, Cortet B, et al. Percutaneous vertebroplasty for osteolytic metastases and myeloma: effects of the percentage of lesion filling and the leakage of methyl methacrylate at clinical follow-up. Radiology 1996;200(2):525–30.

27. Molloy S, Mathis JM, Belkoff SM. The effect of vertebral body percentage fill on mechanical behavior during percutaneous vertebroplasty. Spine 2003; 28(14):1549–54.

28. Belkoff SM, Mathis JM, Jasper LE, et al. The biomechanics of vertebroplasty: the effect of cement volume on mechanical behavior. Spine 2001;26(14): 1537–41.

29. Singh K, Samartzis D, Vaccaro AR, et al. Current concepts in the management of metastatic spinal disease. The role of minimally-invasive approaches. J Bone Joint Surg Br 2006;88(4):434–42.

30. Deramond H, Depriester C, Galibert P, et al. Percutaneous vertebroplasty with polymethylmethacrylate. Technique, indications and results. Radiol Clin North Am 1998;36(3):533–46.

31. Barragán-Campos HM, Vallée JN, Lo D, et al. Percutaneous vertebroplasty for spinal metastases: complications. Radiology 2006;238(1):354–62.

32. Choe DH, Marom EM, Ahrar K, et al. Pulmonary embolism of polymethyl methacrylate during percutaneous vertebroplasty and kyphoplasty. AJR Am J Roentgenol 2004;183(4):1097–102.

33. Abdul-Jalil Y, Bartels J, Alberti O, et al. Delayed presentation of pulmonary polymethylmethacrylate emboli after percutaneous vertebroplasty. Spine 2007; 32(20):589–93.

34. Zaccheo MV, Rowane JE, Costello EM. Acute respiratory failure associated with polymethylmethacrylate pulmonary emboli after percutaneous vertebroplasty. Am J Emerg Med 2008;26(5):636, e5–7.

35. Mathis JM, Deramond H. Complications associated with vertebroplasty and kyphoplasty. In: Mathis JM, Deramond H, Belkoff SM, editors. Percutaneous vertebroplasty and kyphoplasty. 2nd edition. New York: Springer; 2006. p. 210–22.

36. McGraw JK, Heatwole EV, Strnad BT, et al. Predictive value of intraosseous venography before percutaneous vertebroplasty. J Vasc Interv Radiol 2002; 13(2 Pt 1):149–53.

37. Frankel BM, Monroe T, Wang C. Percutaneous vertebral augmentation: an elevation in adjacent-level fracture risk in kyphoplasty as compared with vertebroplasty. Spine J 2007;7(5):575–82.

38. Jang JS, Lee SH. Efficacy of percutaneous vertebroplasty combined with radiotherapy in osteolytic metastatic spinal tumors. J Neurosurg Spine 2005;2(3): 243–8.

39. Hiwatashi A, Sidhu R, Lee RK, et al. Kyphoplasty versus vertebroplasty to increase vertebral body height: a cadaveric study. Radiology 2005;237(3): 1115–9.

40. Gaitanis IN, Hadjipavlou AG, Katonis PG, et al. Balloon kyphoplasty for the treatment of pathological vertebral compressive fractures. Eur Spine J 2005; 14(3):250–60.

41. Pflugmacher R, Beth P, Schroeder RJ. Balloon kyphoplasty for the treatment of pathological fractures in the thoracic and lumbar spine caused by metastasis: one-year follow-up. Acta Radiol 2007; 48(1):89–95.

42. Eck JC, Nachtigall D, Humphreys SC, et al. Comparison of vertebroplasty and balloon kyphoplasty for treatment of vertebral compression fractures: a meta-analysis of the literature. Spine J 2008;8(3): 488–97.

43. Gazelle GS, Goldberg SN, Solbiati L, et al. Tumor ablation with radio-frequency energy. Radiology 2000;217(3):633–46.

44. Thanos L, Mylona S, Galani P, et al. Radiofrequency ablation of osseous metastases for the palliation of pain. Skeletal Radiol 2008;37(3):189–94.

45. Buy X, Basile A, Bierry G, et al. Saline-infused bipolar radiofrequency ablation of high-risk spinal and paraspinal neoplasms. AJR Am J Roentgenol 2006;186(5 Suppl):S322–6.

46. Dupuy DE, Hong R, Oliver B, et al. Radiofrequency ablation of spinal tumors: temperature distribution in the spinal canal. AJR Am J Roentgenol 2000; 175(5):1263–6.

47. Nakatsuka A, Yamakado K, Maeda M, et al. Radiofrequency ablation combined with bone cement injection for the treatment of bone malignancies. J Vasc Interv Radiol 2004;15(7): 707–12.

48. Nakatsuka A, Yamakado K, Takaki H, et al. Percutaneous radiofrequency ablation of painful spinal tumors adjacent to the spinal cord with real-time monitoring of spinal canal temperature. Cardiovasc Intervent Radiol I: 26 Epub ahead of print.

49. Grönemeyer DH, Schirp S, Gevargez A. Image-guided radiofrequency ablation of spinal tumors: preliminary experience with an expandable array electrode. Cancer J 2002;8(1):33–9.

50. Schaefer O, Lohrmann C, Markmiller M, et al. Technical innovation. Combined treatment of a spinal metastasis with radiofrequency heat ablation and vertebroplasty. AJR Am J Roentgenol 2003;180(4): 1075–7.

51. Halpin RJ, Bendok BR, Sato KT, et al. Combination treatment of vertebral metastases using image-guided percutaneous radiofrequency ablation and vertebroplasty: a case report. Surg Neurol 2005; 63(5):469–74.

52. Han PP, Kenny K, Dickman CA. Thoracoscopic approaches to the thoracic spine: experience with 241 surgical procedures. Neurosurgery 2002;51(5 Suppl):S88–95.

53. Mack MJ, Regan JJ, Bobechko WP, et al. Application of thoracoscopy for diseases of the spine. Ann Thorac Surg 1993;56:736–8.

54. McAfee PC, Regan JR, Fedder IL. Anterior thoracic corpectomy for spinal cord compression performed endoscopically. Surg Laparosc Endosc 1995;5(5): 339–44.

55. Rosenthal D, Marquardt G, Lorenz R, et al. Anterior decompression using a microsurgical endoscopic technique for metastatic tumors of the thoracic spine. J Neurosurg 1996;84(4):556–72.

56. Kim DH, Jaikumar S, Kam AC. Minimally invasive spine instrumentation. Neurosurgery 2002;51(5 Suppl):S15–25.

57. Rosenthal D. Endoscopic approaches to the thoracic spine. Eur Spine J 2000;9(Suppl 1):8–16.

58. Le Huec JC, Lesprit E, Guibaud JP, et al. Minimally invasive endoscopic approach to the cervicothoracic junction for vertebral metastases: report of two cases. Eur Spine J 2001;10(5):421–6.

59. Huang TJ, Hsu RW, Liu HP, et al. Video-assisted thoracoscopic treatment of spinal lesions in the thoracolumbar junction. Surg Endosc 1997;11(12): 1189–93.

60. Amini A, Beisse R, Schmidt MH. Thoracoscopic spine surgery for decompression and stabilization of the anterolateral thoracolumbar spine. Neurosurg Focus 2005;6:1–9.

61. Huang TJ, Hsu RW, Sum CW, et al. Complications in thoracoscopic spinal surgery: a study of 90 consecutive patients. Surg Endosc 1999;13(4):346–50.

62. McLain RF. Spinal cord decompression: an endoscopically assisted approach for metastatic tumors. Spinal Cord 2001;39(9):482–7.

63. Huang TJ, Hsu RW, Li YY, et al. Minimal access spinal surgery (MASS) in treating thoracic spine metastasis. Spine 2006;31(16):1860–3.

64. Kossmann T, Jacobi D, Trentz O. The use of a retractor system (SynFrame) for open, minimal invasive reconstruction of the anterior column of the thoracic and lumbar spine. Eur Spine J 2001;10(5):396–402.

65. Payer M, Sottas C. Mini-open anterior approach for corpectomy in the thoracolumbar spine. Surg Neurol 2008;69(1):25–31.

66. Lin RM, Huang KY, Lai KA. Mini-open anterior spine surgery for anterior lumbar diseases. Eur Spine J 2008;17(5):691–7.

67. Mayer HM. A new microsurgical technique for minimally invasive anterior lumbar interbody fusion. Spine 1997;22(6):691–9.

68. Dewald CJ, Millikan KW, Hammerberg KW, et al. An open minimally invasive approach to the lumbar spine. Am Surg 1999;65(1):61–8.

69. El Saghir H. Extracoelomic mini approach for anterior reconstructive surgery of the thoracolumbar area. Neurosurgery 2002;51(5 Suppl):S118–22.

Spine Oncology: Daedalus, Theseus, and the Minotaur

Rakesh Donthineni, MD, MBA[a,b,*], Onder Ofluoglu, MD[c]

KEYWORDS
• Spine • Tumor • Surgery • Outcome

Over the past 3 decades, the management of spine tumors has progressed dramatically. With emerging diagnostic technologies, novel adjuvant agents, and improved surgical techniques, the survival and quality of life of patients has considerably improved. With Stener's early report on vertebrectomy; improved techniques introduced by Tomita; the design, use, and validation of staging methodologies developed by Tomita and by Weinstein, Boriani, and Biagini; and the progress of algorithmic approaches to metastatic disease to the spine, the overall approach to these disease-afflicted axial areas of the body has made tremendous advancements.[1–9]

In comparison to surgical management of the appendicular skeleton, surgical management of spine lesions is more challenging because of the complex anatomy, the need to preserve vital adjacent structures, the lack of adequate reconstruction options, and the high risks of acute and late complications of surgical and adjuvant treatments. Also, because of the considerable delay in detecting spinal tumors, most tumors at presentation tend to be larger and have more extensive infiltration and lower chances of a good outcome than tumors in other areas of the body.

Advancement in imaging technologies and the widespread availability of such technologies at costs within reach have lowered the threshold for scanning to investigate persistent common symptoms originating in the axial locations or in patients with a history of malignancy. These concepts have contributed to both earlier detection and earlier intervention.

CT and MRI have greatly enhanced the ability of the surgeon to accurately delineate the extension of the lesion within the bone, the soft tissue, and the spinal canal. Such enhancements have led to great leaps forward in preoperative planning and postoperative evaluation, resulting in improved outcomes.

The introduction of positron emission tomography (PET) imaging as an increasingly useful, noninvasive method for staging tumors, assessing response, and detecting disease recurrence has further altered treatment strategies for malignant tumors. Future prospective studies will investigate the correlation between PET response to chemotherapy and patient outcomes.

While imaging technology brought about great advancements in techniques for defining spinal lesions, histologic diagnosis is still essential. Needle biopsies are now obtainable throughout most of the spine, either under fluoroscopy or CT guidance. Biopsies under MRI guidance will increase the rate of obtaining viable tumor tissue. Increasingly aware of risks of contamination along the needle track, interventionists have altered their methods, turning to smaller needles and approaches less likely to raise contamination. Interventionists have also found that it is normally a safe practice to discuss needle placement with the surgeon, as the needle track may need to be excised in future tumor management.

Computer-assisted orthopedic surgery and navigation applications combine preoperative imaging with real-time views of anatomic landmarks during surgery. The usefulness and accuracy of

[a] Spine and Orthopaedic Oncology, 5700 Telegraph Avenue, Suite 100, Oakland, CA 94609, USA
[b] Department of Orthopaedics, University of California Davis, Suite 3800, Y Street, Sacramento, CA 95817, USA
[c] Department of Orthopedics, Lutfi Kirdar Research Hospital, Istanbul, Turkey
* Corresponding author.
E-mail address: rdmd.inc@gmail.com (R. Donthineni).

Orthop Clin N Am 40 (2009) 169–171
doi:10.1016/j.ocl.2008.09.007

these applications are still evolving in the clinical and research setting in orthopedic operations, such as knee ligament reconstruction, total joint arthroplasty, and pedicle screw placement. The few but promising reports show a potential role for computer-assisted orthopedic surgery and navigation applications in the treatment of spine tumors.[10–12]

Multimodal intraoperative neurologic monitoring of the functional integrity of the spinal motor descending pathways has provided valid and reliable contributions to improved surgical results. Such monitoring aids in reducing or preventing neurologic damage during gross tumor resections.[13]

Modern multiagent chemotherapy has boosted survival rates for chemo-sensitive sarcomas from 20% to 70%. However, the prognosis of those with metastatic or recurrent disease has changed little over the past 3 decades. Encouraging results have recently been reported with new biological and molecular agents in this era of targeted therapy for patients with poor prognosis. The new agents have also been tested on tumors for which chemotherapy has long been known to be ineffective. In metastatic patients, bisphosphonates have emerged in recent years as a highly effective therapeutic option for the prevention of skeletal complications. These agents have inhibitory effects on osteoclast generation, maturation, and activity, thereby reducing osteoclast-mediated bone resorption. Also, considerable preclinical evidence suggests that bisphosphonates have antitumor effects. The role of bisphosphonates will continue to evolve as further clinical trial data become available.[14,15]

Radiotherapy is often the first-line treatment for spinal metastasis. Recently developed options, including intensity-modulated radiation therapy, stereotactic radiosurgery, or stereotactic radiotherapy, allow very large doses of radiation, provide satisfactory dose coverage of tumor, and avoid excessive radiation to the surrounding normal tissue.

With the gradual transition from the use of hooks to pedicle and facet screws, a widening array of reconstructive options for the vertebral body, and improved preoperative planning assisted by modern imaging modalities, surgeons have gained greater confidence to tackle more challenging cases. Biocompatible devices (eg, polyetheretherketone and carbon fiber cages) have facilitated easier follow-up for any local recurrences. The use of such devices and capabilities are publicized in the scientific literature, although the high costs have somewhat limited their use. Similarly, minimally invasive approaches have garnered a new following, encouraging the industry to develop further tools to assist in these surgical approaches. The conventional surgical techniques are poorly tolerated by patients with disseminated metastasis. The image-guided percutaneous vertebral augmentations—vertebroplasty and kyphoplasty—offer effective pain palliation and vertebral stabilization in such patients. Tumoral ablation procedures, including radiofrequency, cryotherapy or laser applications, can lower the risk of cement leak and subsequent complications. Additional prospective randomized studies in large cohorts of patients are needed to establish the indication, safety profile, and cost of such procedures.

Daedalean efforts are needed to not only contain tumors, but also to extinguish them (ergo the Minotaur and its demise by Theseus). Efforts of experts in spine oncology are slowly gathering momentum and, with the formation of interstudy groups (eg, Global Spinal Tumor Study Group and others),[16] validation of staging, algorithms, and management methods can be conducted both as a retrospective, but more importantly, as prospective randomized controlled trials. Such accumulation of knowledge and expertise will precipitate studies leading to improved outcomes through evidence-based medicine. It also behooves us to educate our physician colleagues (both spine and nonspine specialists) about the importance of early recognition, appropriate staging, and proper management to give the best results. If such knowledge is lacking, the physician should refer the distraught patient to a center of excellence for better outcomes.

ACKNOWLEDGMENTS

We acknowledge our esteemed colleagues for contributing the wonderful articles in this issue focused on spine oncology and helping not only bring forward the latest ideas and expertise, but in the process allowing the vast others to be able to extract the relevant information pertaining to the management of their patients.

REFERENCES

1. Stener B. Total spondylectomy in chondrosarcoma arising from the seventh thoracic vertebra. J Bone Joint Surg Br 1971;53:288–95.
2. Stener B. Complete removal of vertebrae for extirpation of tumors. A 20-year experience. Clin Orthop 1989;245:72–82.

3. Enneking WF, Spainer SS, Goodman MA. A system for the surgical staging of musculoskeletal sarcomas. Clin Orthop 1980;153:106–20.

4. Boriani S, Weinstein JN, Biagini R. Spine update. Primary bone tumors of the spine. Spine 1997;22:1036–44.

5. Hart RA, Boriani S, Biagini R, et al. A system for surgical and management of spine tumors. Spine 1997;22:1773–83.

6. Tomita K, Toribatake Y, Kawahara N, et al. Total en bloc spondylectomy and circumspinal decompression for solitary spinal metastasis. Paraplegia 1994;32:36–46.

7. Tomita K, Kawahara N, Baba H, et al. Total en bloc spondylectomy: a new surgical technique for primary malignant vertebral tumors. Spine 1997;22:324–33.

8. Tokuhashi Y, Matsuzaki H, Oda H, et al. A revised scoring system for preoperative evaluation of metastatic spine tumor prognosis. Spine 2005;30:2186–91.

9. Gasbarrini A, Cappuccio M, Mirabile L, et al. Spinal metastases: treatment evaluation algorithm. Eur Rev Med Pharmacol Sci 2004;8:265–74.

10. Arand M, Hartwig E, Kinzl L, et al. Spinal navigation in tumor surgery of the thoracic spine: first clinical results. Clin Orthop 2002;399:211–8.

11. Hufner T, Kfuri M, Galanski M, et al. New indications for computer-assisted surgery. Clin Orthop 2004;426:219–25.

12. Cho HS, Kang HG, Kim HS, et al. Computer-assisted sacral tumor resection. J Bone Joint Surg Am 2008;90A:1561–6.

13. Sutter M, Eggspuehler A, Grob D, et al. The validity of multimodal intraoperative monitoring (MIOM) in surgery of 109 spine and spinal cord tumors. Eur Spine J 2007;16(Suppl 2):S197–208.

14. Coleman RE. Bisphosphonates: clinical experience. Oncologist 2004;9(Suppl 4):14–27.

15. Corey E, Brown LG, Quinn JE, et al. Zoledronic acid exhibits inhibitory effects on osteoblastic and osteolytic metastases of prostate cancer. Clin Cancer Res 2003;9:295–306.

16. Ibrahim A, Crockard A, Antonietti P, et al. Does spinal surgery improve the quality of life for those with extradural (spinal) osseous metastases? An international multicenter prospective observational study of 223 patients. J Neurosurg Spine 2008;8:271–8.

Index

Orthop Clin N Am 40 (2009) 173–177
doi:10.1016/S0030-5898(08)00096-5
0030-5898/08/$ – see front matter © 2008 Elsevier Inc. All rights reserved.

orthopedic.theclinics.com

Moving?

Make sure your subscription moves with you!

To notify us of your new address, find your **Clinics Account Number** (located on your mailing label above your name), and contact customer service at:

E-mail: elspcs@elsevier.com

800-654-2452 (subscribers in the U.S. & Canada)
314-453-7041 (subscribers outside of the U.S. & Canada)

Fax number: 314-523-5170

Elsevier Periodicals Customer Service
11830 Westline Industrial Drive
St. Louis, MO 63146

*To ensure uninterrupted delivery of your subscription, please notify us at least 4 weeks in advance of move.

Printed and bound by CPI Group (UK) Ltd, Croydon, CR0 4YY

15/10/2024

01774723-0001